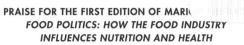

PRAISE FOR THE FIRST EDITION OF MARION NESTLE'S
FOOD POLITICS: HOW THE FOOD INDUSTRY
INFLUENCES NUTRITION AND HEALTH

"Anyone who cares about what they put in their body ought to read *[Food Politics]* carefully and think long and hard about the choices. Your life just might depend on it." —*Newsday*

"'Voting with [our] forks' for a healthier society, Nestle shows us, is within our power." —*Los Angeles Times*

"Educating the public is a start, and *Food Politics* is an excellent introduction to how decisions are made in Washington—and their effects on consumers. Let's hope people take more notice of it than they do of the dietary guidelines." —*The Nation*

"Nestle has written a provocative and highly readable book arguing that America's agribusiness lobby has stifled the government's regulatory power, helped create a seasonless and regionless diet, and hampered the government's ability to offer sound, scientific nutritional advice." —*The Economist*

"What a book this is! Of course we have always suspected and known some of the truth, but never in such bold detail! In this fascinating book we learn how powerful, intrusive, influential, and invasive big industry is and how alert we must constantly be to prevent it from influencing not only our personal choices, but those of our government agencies. Marion Nestle has presented us with a courageous and masterful exposé." —Julia Child

"Food politics underlie all politics in the United States. There is no industry more important to Americans, more fundamentally linked to our well-being and the future well-being of our children. Nestle reveals how corporate control of the nation's food system limits our choices and threatens our health. If you eat, you should read this book." —Eric Schlosser, author of *Fast Food Nation*

"Nestle is in a unique position to have seen firsthand how food purveyors, government and academicians end up as bedfellows when it comes to suggesting to people what and how much to eat." —*Eating Well*

"*Food Politics* . . . has nudged [Nestle's] argument into the mainstream of consideration—not quite fodder for an installment of *Oprah,* but no longer the heady stuff of National Public Radio, either. And that has some restaurant-industry officials more than a little upset." —*Restaurant Business*

"Nestle tells us a series of engaging and surprising stories and gives us a lively presentation of the politics, as she perceives them, of advice on diet and health during the past century . . . This book is thought-provoking, and I recommend it." —*The New England Journal of Medicine*

"Some of Nestle's shocking revelations about the behavior of Big Food will shock only those who are easily shocked; others will be welcomed less as news than as occasions for those so inclined to make public displays of moral outrage." —*London Review of Books*

"*Food Politics* is written to interest and be accessible to a wide range of readers, whether they have training in nutrition or not. The book has achieved this objective by keeping jargon to a minimum, explaining terms as needed, and being written in a lively, engaging style." —*Journal of Nutrition Education*

"A real page turner, this book will give you metaphoric indigestion—unless, of course, you believe that McDonald's offers 'a nutritious addition to a balanced diet' (as one U.S. Senator declared in 1977)." —*Natural Health*

"Regardless of who is to blame for the obesity epidemic, Nestle has laid down a challenge that won't easily go away. It will be interesting to see how the food industry responds." —*Food Chemical News*

"The case examples are remarkable and the value here is in Nestle's clear, thorough documentation, which provides missing pieces in the puzzle of poor nutrition in a country where food is all too abundant." —*The Lancet*

"This superbly documented book encourages readers to think about what they eat and to ask, who profits?" —Gambero Rosso

"*Food Politics* is an academically scrupulous account of how the food industry in the United States controls government nutrition policies. It's important and eye-opening reading for anyone looking to make intelligent and informed food choices." —*EarthSave Magazine*

"*Food Politics* is a carefully considered, calmly stated, devastating criticism of the nation's food industry and its efforts to get people to eat excessive amounts of unhealthy food." —*Social Policy*

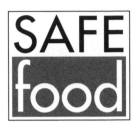

CALIFORNIA STUDIES IN FOOD AND CULTURE

Darra Goldstein, Editor

MARION NESTLE

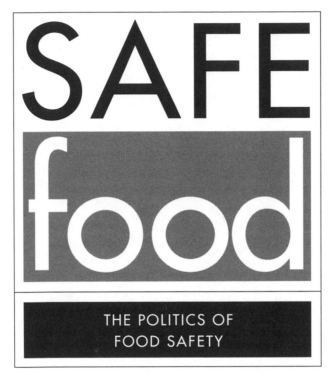

SAFE
food

THE POLITICS OF
FOOD SAFETY

Updated and Expanded

UNIVERSITY OF CALIFORNIA PRESS
Berkeley Los Angeles London

University of California Press, one of the most distinguished university presses in the United States,
enriches lives around the world by advancing scholarship in the humanities, social sciences, and natural
sciences. Its activities are supported by the UC Press
Foundation and by philanthropic contributions from
individuals and institutions. For more information,
visit www.ucpress.edu.

University of California Press
Berkeley and Los Angeles, California

University of California Press, Ltd.
London, England

ISBN 978-0-520-26606-3 (pbk. : alk. paper)

The Library of Congress has cataloged an earlier
edition of this book as follows:

Library of Congress Cataloging-in-Publication Data

Nestle, Marion.
   Safe food : bacteria, biotechnology, and bioterrorism /
Marion Nestle.
      p.   cm.— (California studies in food and culture ; 5)
   Includes bibliographical references and index.
   ISBN 978-0-520-23292-1 (cloth : alk. paper)
   1. Food—Safety measures.   2. Food—Biotechnology.
3. Bioterrorism.   I. Title.   2. Series.

RA601.N465   2003
363.19'26—dc21   2002027172

Manufactured in the United States of America

18   17   16   15   14   13   12   11   10   09
10   9   8   7   6   5   4   3   2   1

This book is printed on Natures Book, which contains
50% post-consumer waste and meets the minimum
requirements of ANSI/NISO Z39.48–1992 (R1997)
(*Permanence of Paper*).

CONTENTS

PREFACE TO THE 2010 EDITION

WHEN *SAFE FOOD* FIRST APPEARED IN 2003, FOOD SAFETY HARDLY appeared on the public agenda. American food safety advocates struggled to be heard but generated little public interest or congressional action. I wrote *Safe Food* to explain the political history of our fragmented and ineffective food safety system and how politics gets in the way of efforts to improve the system. Having no illusions that the book would do what Upton Sinclair's *The Jungle* accomplished in 1906, I hoped that it would at least generate some creative thinking about food safety problems and their solutions.

I spent the next few years dealing with invitations to speak about the health implications of food marketing discussed in my earlier book, *Food Politics*. I also wrote *What to Eat,* a book that uses supermarket aisles as an organizing device for thinking about food issues, safety among them. By the time that book came out in 2006, I thought I was done with food safety. I had nothing more to say about it.

Then came September 14, 2006. On that day, one that California vegetable growers still refer to as 9/14, the Food and Drug Administration (FDA) announced the recall of spinach contaminated with *E. coli* O157:H7, the pathogen introduced in chapter 1 and discussed throughout this book. This incident brought the inadequacies of our food safety system to public attention as never before and renewed calls for mandatory regulation. As always, these calls were ignored. The result was an astonishing series of national outbreaks and food recalls, one right after another.

To my surprise, I began to receive invitations to write and speak about food safety issues. These came with further invitations to visit farms, packing plants, and food manufacturing and processing operations. I was appointed to the Pew Commission on Industrial Farm Animal Production, which visited both large and small cattle, pig, and chicken farms. I also visited a free-range bison ranch. Following the pet food recalls of 2007, as part of the research for my account of those events, *Pet Food Politics* (2008), I visited factories that produce pet foods, raw and cooked. I had plenty of opportunity to see how food is produced under safe and unsafe conditions, and plenty to talk about.

In question sessions following my talks, I could hear how abstract the regulation of microbes in food feels to most people. Americans assume that the government keeps food free of contaminants and give food safety little thought. Instead, questions are about dread-and-outrage factors, topics covered in this book such as food biotechnology and irradiation, but also the right to consume raw milk, raw oysters, and other foods the government considers unsafe. Films such as *The Future of Food* and *Our Daily Bread* and, later, *Food, Inc.* and *Fresh,* dealt with such matters and generated more questions along the same lines.

It soon became clear that *Safe Food* still had plenty to say about current events and, perhaps, could be made more useful to a wider audience. In rereading it, I was relieved to find that it holds up well in establishing the historical basis of our current food safety predicaments. For this new edition, I corrected typos, clarified a few fuzzy points, changed some tenses from present to past, and wrote an epilogue to bring the events up to date. Otherwise, the original text remains. But I did think one additional change was needed. The book's subtitle, *Bacteria, Biotechnology, and Bioterrorism,* did not reflect its overarching theme: that food safety is political. The new subtitle, *The Politics of Food Safety,* is really what this book is about.

Here, I argue that whether we view microbes or genetic modifications as the greater hazard depends on whether we look at foods through the lens of scientific or other value systems. Microbial contamination is responsible for an estimated 76 million illnesses, 325,000 hospitalizations, and 5,000 deaths in the United States each year. Food biotechnology is responsible for no measurable human illness to date. Yet public dread and outrage about food safety problems continues to be much more about genetic modification than about the unlucky victims of severe food poisonings.

In part, the disconnect between science and values explains why it is so difficult to get Congress to act on matters of food safety. Congress also views microbes as so familiar and so much under personal control that no governmental action is needed. Food industry pressures encourage this view. I have long said that nothing short of the death of a close relative of a senior senator by food poisoning will induce Congress to fix the food safety system. Otherwise, Congress will continue to respond to pressures from food corporations willing to cut safety corners and place their customers at risk to protect profit margins.

At the time of this writing, Congress is about to pass a new food safety bill, but one designed to fix only the FDA, not the system as a whole. Absent from the current debate is public dread and outrage about microbial contaminants and the politics of food safety. Without stronger public support for coordinated mandatory regulation of the entire food safety system, we can expect outbreaks and massive food recalls to continue, and even more people to suffer from illnesses that easily could have been prevented.

A NOTE ON THE NOTES

Serious researcher that I am, I must mention the alarming challenge posed by updating the endnotes to this book. Seven years after publication of the first edition, I could not find more than a handful of the eighty or so Internet references at their original addresses (URLs). Using titles, I was able to find most at new locations, but some seem to have vanished into cyberspace. I was dismayed to discover that the Internet is not the permanently tamperproof file cabinet I had imagined it to be. Fortunately, the titles are permanent. At the time of this writing they could be found at the listed URLs, but these must be considered ephemeral.

New York
February 2010

PREFACE TO THE FIRST EDITION

FOOD SAFETY IS A MATTER OF HUGE PUBLIC INTEREST. HARDLY a day goes by without a front-page account of some new and increasingly alarming hazard in our food supply. As an academic nutritionist with a long-standing interest in how food affects health, I cannot help but deal with issues of food safety, daily. Students, colleagues, and friends often ask me whether it is safe to eat one or another food or ingredient. My department at New York University offers degree programs in the new field of food studies as well as in nutrition, and many instructors and colleagues associated with these programs work in restaurants or specialty food businesses. They also ask safety questions, as their livelihoods depend on serving safe food.

Nevertheless, I did not set out to write a book about food safety. My academic training is in science (molecular biology, but long lapsed) as well as in public health nutrition, and for many years my research has focused on the ways in which science and politics interact to influence government policies that affect nutrition and health. In that context, I have been speaking and writing about food biotechnology since the early 1990s. I immediately saw that genetically engineered foods raise questions about politics as much as about safety. Indeed, the safety questions seemed overshadowed by issues related to the implications of such foods for society and democratic values.

I originally intended to include several chapters on such issues in a book about the ways in which food companies use the political system to achieve commercial goals. That book, *Food Politics: How the Food Industry Influences Nutrition and Health*, came out in 2002 from the

University of California Press. In the course of events, however, it became clear that the subject of food safety deserved a book in its own right.
To begin with, during the years I worked on *Food Politics* (1999 to 2001),
food safety crises popped up one after another, especially in Europe. Mys-
teriously contaminated soft drinks, cows sick with mad cow and foot-
and-mouth disease, and outbreaks of what my friend and colleague
Claude Fischler calls "*Listeria* bacteria hysteria" were eliciting headlines
and destroying economies as well as confidence in the food supply. On
the domestic front, one food after another—hamburger and such unlikely suspects as raspberries, apple juice, and bean sprouts—appeared
as sources of bacterial infections. Because some of the contaminating bacteria resisted antibiotics, the illnesses were difficult to treat. Product recalls because of microbial contamination also seemed to be growing both
in size and public attention.

Furthermore, I was receiving increasingly urgent queries from purveyors of small-scale, artisanal cheeses who wanted to know: can cheeses
in general, and raw milk cheeses in particular, transmit bacterial diseases,
mad cow disease, or foot-and-mouth disease? The answers to such questions were not easy to find, and I was soon engaged in reading veterinary reports and badgering experts and federal officials for information.
Eventually, I could provide a scientific answer: cheese has a low probability of transmitting these or any other diseases, but the possibility cannot be excluded. This answer is either satisfactory or not depending on
whether one is an optimist or a pessimist, and it raises its own set of questions. Does a low probability of harm mean that a risk is negligible and
can be ignored? Or is it unreasonable to take the chance? Would pasteurization (heating milk briefly to a temperature high enough to kill most
bacteria) make cheeses safer? Should the federal government require
cheese makers to pasteurize milk or to follow other special safety procedures? Is the benefit of eating prized specialty cheeses worth any risk,
no matter how small? The answers to such questions involve judgments
based in part on science, but also on more personal considerations—how
much one values the taste of cheeses made from raw milk, for example,
or the social contribution of artisanal cheese making. Because such judgments are based on opinion and point of view, and sometimes on commercial considerations, and because they affect the regulation, marketing, and financial viability of food products, they bring food safety into
the realm of politics.

I have been a minor participant in making such judgments. As a member of the Food Advisory Committee to the Food and Drug Adminis-

tration (FDA) in the mid-1990s, I learned about other special safety procedures, particularly a scientific method for reducing the risk of harmful bacteria in food called, obscurely, Hazard Analysis and Critical Control Point, or by its equally obscure acronym, HACCP (pronounced "hassip"). Despite its name, HACCP seemed to me to make a lot of sense, and I wondered why food companies—especially those that produce and process beef and chicken—seemed so reluctant to apply HACCP methods for reducing pathogens, and to test for microbial contaminants to make sure that infected meat stayed out of the food supply. Instead, food companies appeared to be using every political means at their disposal to resist having such rules imposed. Here, too, food safety issues seemed to be mired in politics.

On the morning of September 11, 2001, I was at home working on the index to *Food Politics* when terrorists attacked the World Trade Center, just a mile away from my New York City apartment. Among the many consequences of that event were some otherwise insignificant ones having to do with this book. My cheese purveyor colleagues added anthrax to their list of safety questions (answer: another situation of very low probability), and I realized that a book on this subject would also have to deal with food bioterrorism—an extreme example of food safety politics in action.

In some ways, this book extends the arguments set forth in *Food Politics*. There, I discussed the ways in which the food industry (the collective term for companies that produce, process, market, sell, and serve food and beverages) influences what people eat and, therefore, health. To encourage people to eat more of their products, or to substitute their products for those of competitors, food companies spend extraordinary amounts of money on advertising and marketing. More important, they use politics to influence government officials, scientists, and food and nutrition professionals to make decisions in the interests of business— whether or not such decisions are good for public health. In doing so, food companies operate just like any other businesses devoted to increasing sales and satisfying stockholders. One difference is that the food industry is unique in its universality: everyone eats.

To pick just one example: food companies donate campaign funds where they are most likely to buy influence. According to the Center for Responsive Politics, a group that tracks campaign contributions on its Web site, www.opensecrets.org, several food companies and trade associations discussed in this book ranked among the top 20 agribusiness donors in 2001, with contributions ranging from $100,000 to nearly $1 million. The skewed distribution of these donations to Republican rather than to Democratic members of Congress is especially noteworthy. For example, the giant cigarette company Philip Morris, which owns Kraft Foods, donated 89% of more than $900,000 to Republicans. Other companies involved in food safety disputes of one kind or another also donated heavily to Republicans: Archer Daniels Midland (70%), the National Cattleman's Beef Association (82%), the Food Marketing Institute (90%), the National Food Processors Association (96%), and the United Dairy Farmers (100%). When the Republican administration of George W. Bush was in power, these groups expected to receive especially favorable attention to their views on food safety issues, and they usually did.

Underlying discussions of such matters of influence in *Food Politics* and in this present volume are several recurrent themes:

- The increasing concentration of food producers and distributors into larger and larger units
- The overproduction and overabundance of food in the United States
- The competitiveness among food companies to encourage people to eat more food or to substitute their products for those of competing companies
- The relentless pressures exerted by food companies on government agencies to make favorable regulatory decisions
- The invocation of science by food companies as a means to achieve commercial goals
- The clash in values among stakeholders in the food system: industry, government, and consumers
- The ways in which such themes demonstrate that food is political

Food safety, however, would seem to be the least political of food issues. Who could possibly *not* want food to be safe? Consumers do not want to worry about unsafe food and do not like getting sick. Unsafe food is bad for business (recalls are expensive, and negative publicity hurts sales) as well as for government (through loss of trust). As this book explains, food safety is political for many of the same reasons discussed in *Food Politics*: economic self-interest, stakeholder differences, and collision of values. At stake are issues of risk, benefit, and control. Who bears the risk of food safety problems? Who benefits from ignoring them? Who makes the policy decisions? Who controls the food supply? For the most part, these are political—not scientific—questions, and they demand political responses. Because billions of dollars are involved, food safety issues are "hot topics" demanding attention from everyone involved in the food system: producers, distributors, regulators, and the public.

I wrote this book for everyone—from general readers to scientists—who would like to know more about the issues underlying disputes about food safety issues. How concerned should we be about the safety of the food we eat? What aspects of food safety issues should concern us? What issues really are involved? The purpose of the book is to establish a basis for a better understanding of the issues, the positions of the various stakeholders, and the ways in which the political system operates in matters as fundamental as the safety of the food we eat. I hope this book will help everyone interested in food, whether trained in science or not, to develop more considered opinions about food safety issues.

In part because I want the book to reach a wide audience, I have worked hard to make it accessible, readable, and free of jargon, and have defined terms that might be unfamiliar whenever they appear. Although nontechnical discussions of science necessarily omit crucial details, I have tried to provide enough sense of the complexity to make the political arguments understandable. Because any discussion of government policy inevitably requires abbreviations, I define them in the text and in a list (page xv). For readers who might like a quick reminder of the science underlying genetic engineering, an appendix provides a brief summary.

Although I do not try to disguise my own views on the issues discussed in this book, I attempt to present a reasonably balanced account of them. Because any book expressing a political point of view is likely to be controversial, I extensively document my sources. I refer to articles in traditional academic journals and books, of course, but also to newspaper accounts, press releases, and advertisements. These days, many previously inaccessible documents are available on the Internet, and I cite numerous Web addresses in the notes that conclude this book. The notes begin with an explanation of the citation method and the definitions of whatever abbreviations seemed most convenient to use. Because I have been a member of federal committees dealing with some of the issues considered here, and because I frequently attend conferences on these subjects, I sometimes refer to events that I witnessed personally, but I have tried to keep such undocumented observations to a minimum.

I hope that *Safe Food* will interest consumer advocates, students, college and university instructors, people who work for food companies, those employed in government agencies, and everyone else who is concerned about matters of food, nutrition, health, international trade, and, in these difficult times, "homeland security." If, as I argue, food safety is as much a matter of politics as it is of science, then food safety problems require political solutions. My deepest hope for the book is that it will encourage readers to become more active in the political process.

ACKNOWLEDGMENTS

THE GENESIS OF THIS BOOK LIES WITH WARREN BELASCO, JOAN Gussow, and Sheldon Margen, who read the manuscript of *Food Politics* and argued that the food safety material would work better as a separate entity. My dear sponsor at the University of California Press, Stan Holwitz, agreed to take on this second project. The formidable editor John Bergez guided the manuscript reconstruction; I could not have a better writing teacher. Extraordinarily generous friends, colleagues, and relatives read and commented on specific chapters or sections of the manuscript at various stages of preparation: Philip Benfey, Jennifer Berg, Elinor Blake, Lee Compton, Laramie Dennis, Beth Dixon, Carol Tucker Foreman, Jeffrey Fox, Mark Furstenberg, Janna Howley, Kristie Lancaster, Trish Lobenfeld, Mimi Martin, Margaret Mellon, Richard Novick, Domingo Piñero, Robert Moss, and Fred Tripp. I am greatly indebted to Joanne Csete, Ellen Fried, and Rebecca Nestle, who read the *entire* draft of the book—acts of courage that extended well beyond the demands of friendship, collegiality, and filial affection.

Many people provided information or documents to which I might not otherwise have had access: James Behnke, Jennifer Cohen, Dennis Dalton, Caroline Smith DeWaal, Carol Tucker Foreman, Rebecca Goldburg, Karen Heisler, Michael Jacobson, James Liebman, Charles Margulies, Robert Marshak, George Pillsbury, Sarah Pillsbury, Krishnendu Ray, Michael Taylor, Catherine Woteki, Annette Yonke, and Lisa Young. For several years, Christine McCullum has been forwarding information on biotechnology gleaned from the Internet, carefully filtered to include just what I most needed to know. Kristie Lancaster, Domingo Piñero, and

Sheldon Watts graciously dropped whatever they were doing to help me deal with computer emergencies. Rob Kaufelt (Murray's Cheese) and Peter Kindel (Artisanal) asked questions about cheese, and Sara Firebaugh helped answer them. I also thank all the other contributors of information and materials who preferred to remain anonymous. Finally, I "borrowed" the title of this book from *Safe Food: Eating Wisely in a Risky World* (Living Planet Press, 1991, but now sadly out of print), for which I thank Michael Jacobson and his colleagues at the Center for Science in the Public Interest.

At a particularly difficult moment during the manuscript revision, Margaret Mellon provided inspiration. For encouragement throughout I am grateful to my agent, Lydia Wills; to Wendel Brunner, Loma Flowers, Ruth Rosen, JoAnn Silverstein, and Sam Silverstein; to my Moss cousins, and to my children and their partners: Rebecca Nestle and Michael Suenkel, and Charles Nestle and Lidia Lustig. I owe special thanks to my extraordinary colleagues in the Department of Nutrition and Food Studies at NYU for their forbearance and assistance and review of the manuscript at every stage of preparation, particularly to Alyce Conrad for designing several of the more complicated illustrations, Fred Tripp for his daily clipping service to the *Wall Street Journal*, Ellen Fried for expert research assistance and review of the manuscript at every stage of preparation, and Jessica Fischetti and Kelli Ranieri for office life support. Dean Ann Marcus granted sabbatical leave, and Deans LaRue Allen, Gabriel Carras, and Thomas James granted much else in the way of encouragement. I recognize and very much appreciate the unusual level of care and attention given to *Safe Food* by the production and design teams at the University of California Press and BookMatters. Preparation of this book was supported in part by research development grants from New York University and its Steinhardt School.

LIST OF ABBREVIATIONS

APHA	American Public Health Association
APHIS	Animal and Plant Health Inspection Service (of USDA)
BGH	Bovine growth hormone (see bST)
BIO	Biotechnology Industry Organization
BSE	Bovine spongiform encephalopathy (mad cow disease)
bST	Bovine somatotropin (see BGH)
Bt	*Bacillus thuringiensis*
CDC	Centers for Disease Control and Prevention (of DHHS)
CFSAN	Center for Food Safety and Applied Nutrition (of FDA)
CJD	Creutzfeldt-Jakob Disease
CNI	Community Nutrition Institute
CSPI	Center for Science in the Public Interest
DHHS	U.S. Department of Health and Human Services
DNA	Deoxyribonucleic acid
EC	European Commission (of the EU)
EMS	Eosinophilia-Myalgia Syndrome
EPA	Environmental Protection Agency
ERS	Economic Research Service (of USDA)
EU	European Union
FDA	Food and Drug Administration (of DHHS)
FIFRA	Federal Insecticide, Fungicide and Rodenticide Act of 1988
FSIS	Food Safety and Inspection Service (of USDA)

Additional abbreviations are defined in the Notes.

GAO	General Accounting Office (of Congress) (since 2004, the Goverment Accountability Office)
GM	Genetically modified
GMO	Genetically modified organism
HACCP	Hazard Analysis and Critical Control Point
IGF-I	Insulin-like growth factor-I
IOM	Institute of Medicine (of the National Academies)
NAS	National Academy of Sciences (now National Academies)
NFPA	National Food Processors Association (since 2005, the Food Products Association)
NIH	National Institutes of Health (of DHHS)
OMB	Office of Management and Budget (of the White House)
OSTP	Office of Science and Technology Policy (of the White House)
OTA	Office of Technology Assessment (formerly of Congress, now defunct)
rBGH	Recombinant bovine growth hormone (see rBST)
rbST	Recombinant bovine somatotropin (see rBGH)
USDA	U.S. Department of Agriculture
vCJD	Variant Creutzfeldt-Jakob Disease
WHO	World Health Organization
WTO	World Trade Organization

FOOD SAFETY IS POLITICAL

FOOD SAFETY IS A MATTER OF INTENSE PUBLIC CONCERN, AND for good reason. Food "poisonings," some causing death, raise alarm not only about the food served in restaurants and fast-food outlets but also about the food bought in supermarkets. The introduction in the 1990s of genetically modified foods—immediately dubbed "Franken-foods"—only added to the general sense of unease. Finally, the September 11, 2001, terrorist attacks on the World Trade Center and Pentagon further heightened such concerns by exposing the vulnerability of food and water supplies to food bioterrorism.

Discussions of food safety in the media and elsewhere tend to focus on scientific aspects: the number of illnesses or deaths, the level of risk, or the probability that a food might cause harm. Such discussions overlook a central fact: food safety is a highly political issue. Preventing foodborne illness involves much more than washing hands or cooking foods to higher temperatures. It involves the interests of huge and powerful industries that use every means at their disposal to maximize income and reduce expenses, whether or not these means are in the interest of public health. Like other businesses, food businesses put the interests of stockholders first. Because food is produced, processed, distributed, sold, and cooked before it is eaten, its safety is a shared responsibility, meaning that blame also can be shared. Any one company in the food chain can deny responsibility and pass accountability along to another. Furthermore, food companies can and do use their considerable financial power to influence government regulations that might affect balance sheets, again whether or not such influence is in the public interest. Although consumer groups concerned about food safety also participate in these political processes, they rarely have equivalent resources or the ability to gain similar levels of attention. In this book, we will see how conflicts between business and consumer interests involve politics in three areas of food safety: foodborne illness, food biotechnology, and food bioterrorism.

To illustrate the many ways in which food safety is as much a matter of politics as it is of science, I begin this book with a familiar example: the front-page disclosure late in 2000 that a prohibited variety of genetically engineered corn—StarLink—had turned up in supermarket taco shells. The StarLink example reveals many of the themes that recur throughout this book and sets the stage for the rest of our discussion.

THE STARLINK CORN AFFAIR

Our story opens on September 18, 2000, with a report from the *Washington Post:* a group called Genetically Engineered Food Alert discovered genetic traces of StarLink corn in taco shells made by Taco Bell. StarLink was not supposed to be in the human food supply. Two years earlier, the Environmental Protection Agency (EPA) allowed Aventis Crop-Science, the owner of the genetic engineering technology for this corn, to grow StarLink—but only for animal feed. The EPA wanted Aventis to prove that StarLink corn would not cause allergic reactions before allowing it in the human food supply. If supermarket foods contained Star-Link, something had gone wrong with the regulatory system.

As events unfolded, the StarLink affair displayed all the hallmarks of classic political scandals: new information dribbling out one fragment at a time, lies, cover-ups, and finger-pointing. During the next year or so, international trading partners refused to buy U.S. corn, farmers hesitated to plant genetically modified corn varieties, and Canada spent nearly a million dollars to keep StarLink out of its food supply. Aventis took StarLink off the market, sold off its agricultural division, and owed millions of dollars in lawsuit settlements. Anyone following these events could see that genetically modified corn not only pervaded the U.S. food supply but also grew in places where it was not supposed to be—in fields of conventional corn, organically grown corn, and native corn grown in remote regions of Mexico. The StarLink affair had political consequences.

The StarLink affair also had political causes. For reasons of politics, federal regulatory agencies operate under policies designed to promote the food biotechnology industry, not to obstruct it with demands for extensive safety testing before products get into the food supply or for labeling of these products. In a different regulatory environment, the fact that the key protein in StarLink corn appeared similar to other proteins known to cause allergic reactions (allergenic proteins, or allergens) might have forced Aventis to find out whether this corn caused allergic reactions before allowing it anywhere near the food supply. Instead, the EPA authorized StarLink corn to be grown as food for animals. EPA officials reasoned that animals would be likely to digest the protein and destroy its function; they did not think the intact protein would get into meat. In splitting its decision, however, the EPA assumed that corn grown for animal feed could be segregated—kept separate—from corn intended for human consumption. As later chapters explain, the EPA should have known better, and its decision to permit StarLink to be grown at all suggested that the agency was partial to the interests of Aventis. Because this history is complicated, table 1 provides a chronological outline of the more important events.[1]

To understand why the safety of a genetically engineered corn might be political, we must look back to the early 1990s, when federal agencies ruled that such crops did not raise any special safety considerations and permitted them to be widely grown (chapter 7 discusses these decisions in some detail). Among the more successful of such crops is corn engineered to contain a gene from a species of common soil bacteria, *Bacillus thuringiensis* (*Bt*). The *Bt* gene provides the information needed to make a crystalline protein that is toxic to insect pests. Organic farmers have used the *Bt* protein toxin for decades in the form of a spray that washes off in the rain and decomposes rapidly. Agricultural biotechnologists thought the *Bt* toxin might work even better if it could be genetically engineered into the tissues of the plant. In the mid-1990s, a Belgian firm, Plant Genetic Systems, developed the trademarked StarLink variety of corn. StarLink contains the gene for a novel form of the *Bt* toxin—called Cry9C (for crystalline protein #9C)—that is especially effective against moths, corn borers, bollworms, cutworms, and other destructive insects in their larval stages.[2]

As a reporter from *Fortune* explained, corporate life at that time must have been difficult for the scientists who were developing StarLink. International joint ventures, mergers, and acquisitions put control of the technology successively in the hands of Belgian, German, and French companies, as illustrated in figure 1 (page 7). As StarLink corn was wending its way into the human food supply, the German company AgrEvo, itself formed by a joint venture of Hoechst and Schering, acquired Plant Genetic Systems. By September 2001, when the StarLink gene turned up

TABLE 1. Key events in the political history of StarLink corn,* 1995 to 2002

Year	Month	Selected Events
1995		Plant Genetic Systems (Belgium) develops StarLink (Cry9C) variety of *Bt* corn. EPA grants registrations to other *Bt* varieties for 5 years.
1996		Companies plant non-StarLink *Bt* corn varieties.
1997		Plant Genetic Systems applies for EPA registration of StarLink. EPA grants permit for experimental plantings on 3,000 acres in 28 states.
1998		EPA limits registration for StarLink as a plant pesticide, permits use only for animal feed. Farmers plant StarLink on 10,000 acres in United States; registration transferred to AgrEvo.
1999		StarLink planted on 250,000 acres in United States. AgrEvo petitions for extension of registration to human food. EPA seeks comment on StarLink allergenicity.
2000	January to August	EPA panel reviews AgrEvo petition. StarLink is available from 15 seed companies in 33 varieties and is planted by 2,500 farmers on 300,000 acres; registration transferred to Aventis CropScience. Consumer group, Genetically Engineered Food Alert, announces campaign to require testing and labeling of genetically modified ingredients in food products. FDA receives reports of allergic reactions to StarLink corn products.
	September	Genetically Engineered Food Alert reports evidence of StarLink gene (not protein) in Taco Bell taco shells, owned by Kraft Foods. Kraft confirms tests, recalls 2.5 million boxes. Aventis blocks further sales of seeds, announces agreement with government to buy remaining seeds to use for animal feed. Consumers file lawsuit claiming allergic reactions.
	October	FDA confirms presence of StarLink in taco shells and announces plans to test food samples. Consumer groups identify StarLink in Safeway taco shells; Safeway issues recall. Aventis "voluntarily" withdraws EPA registration of StarLink. Mission Foods recalls 298 products distributed in the United States, Canada, and Korea; other companies also issue recalls. Kellogg closes U.S. factory because its supplier mills have no corn. Aventis petitions EPA to permit StarLink in existing foods on basis that amounts are too low to cause allergies; EPA asks for comments. USDA says it has traced all but 1.2 million bushels (1.5%) of StarLink produced in 2000. Japan finds StarLink in imported U.S. corn.
	November	Aventis says it will sell its CropScience division, reports "traces" of StarLink protein in conventional corn produced in 1998. American Seed Trade Association says it cannot guarantee that corn is free of genetic modification, asks USDA to approve a tolerance level of 1%. USDA tells EPA advisory committee that it cannot locate 7 million bushels (11%) of StarLink corn. More than 40 people report allergic reactions to StarLink corn products. EPA committee says StarLink protein has "medium likelihood" of being allergenic but "low probability" of causing problems from food.

TABLE 1. *(continued)*

Year	Month	Selected Events
2000	December	EPA is reported to know since 1997 that StarLink is in the human food supply. Farmers file class action suit against Aventis for not warning them that StarLink was restricted to animal feed. Japan finds 28,000 tons of StarLink corn in food supply.
2001	February	Aventis fires president, vice-president, and chief counsel of CropScience division; company says the StarLink recall cost nearly $100 million.
	March	Aventis reports that 430 million bushels of stored corn from 1999 contain traces of StarLink. USDA reports traces of StarLink in non-StarLink seeds intended for planting in 2001. EPA says it will never issue another split registration. Greenpeace finds StarLink in Kellogg products, demands recall; Kellogg complies.
	April	Aventis asks EPA to set tolerance limit on the amount of StarLink permitted in the human food supply.
	June	CDC and FDA find no evidence of antibodies to StarLink protein in stored blood samples from people who reported allergic reactions. FDA finds no evidence of StarLink gene in yellow corn products but does find the gene in one sample of white corn tortilla chips.
	July	EPA advisory panel confirms December 2000 judgment that StarLink could be allergenic. Corn growers reduce acres planted in genetically modified seeds.
	September	Bayer said to be buying Aventis CropScience for $5 billion and to assume $1.7 billion in debt. U.S. consumer group, Center for Food Safety, obtains Freedom of Information Act information that Aventis knew in 1999—and told EPA in January 2000—that farmers were selling StarLink for use in human food.
	December	Canada reports that keeping StarLink out of its food supply cost its government nearly $1 million.
2002	March	Federal judge approves $9 million settlement of farmers' class-action suit against companies involved in StarLink production and distribution.
	June	Bayer completes purchase of Aventis CropScience; forms Bayer CropScience; divests interests in Starlink.
	October	GeneScan Australia reports traces of StarLink in one-third of test food samples.

SOURCES: *Food Traceability Report. StarLink: Lessons Learned.* Washington, DC: FCN Publishing, 2001. Taylor MR, Tick JS. *The StarLink Case: Issues for the Future.* Washington, DC: Pew Initiative on Food and Biotechnology, October 2001. Online: www.pewagbiotech.org. Also: various reports from the *New York Times,* the *Washington Post, Food Chemical News,* and the Environmental Protection Agency (www.epa.gov/scipoly/sap).

*StarLink™ is corn genetically engineered to contain a protein called Cry9C from a species of bacteria, *Bacillus thuringiensis* (*Bt*), toxic to corn borers and other insect pests.

in taco shells, that company had merged into Aventis CropScience, an agricultural division of the French drug company Aventis, which in turn had been formed by the merger of Hoechst with Rhône-Poulenc.[3] This dizzyingly complex ownership history was typical of corporate dynamics at the turn of the twenty-first century.

To return to our story: in 1997, Plant Genetic Systems (soon to be AgrEvo) applied to the EPA for a "registration"—a planting license— for StarLink corn. Because company data indicated that the StarLink Cry9C *Bt* protein toxin appeared similar in structure to proteins known to cause human allergies, the EPA did something unprecedented: it issued a limited registration. The agency licensed AgrEvo to grow Star-Link corn, but *only* for animal feed or industrial purposes.

Following approval, plantings of StarLink increased rapidly. Farmers grew the corn on about 10,000 acres in 1998, 250,000 acres in 1999, and 300,000 acres in 2000—still just a small fraction of the 80 million U.S. acres planted with corn in any given year.[4]

Once harvested, StarLink corn soon worked its way into the food production and distribution system. Figure 2, which illustrates the principal components of the StarLink food chain, immediately reveals why the question, "how did StarLink get into the human food supply?" is not the one to ask. The real question is how it could possibly have been kept out.

The chain of production begins with Aventis CropScience, the owner of the StarLink technology at the time the gene appeared in taco shells. Aventis does not sell seeds; it licenses the technology to seed companies to grow the plants. In this case, Garst Seeds was the principal (but not the only) licensed company. Garst, in turn, sold StarLink seeds to about 2,500 farmers who grew the corn throughout the Midwest, mainly (40%) in Iowa. The farmers harvested the corn and transported it to about 350 grain elevators. From the elevators, corn seeds traveled to Azteca Milling in Plainview, Texas, to be converted into corn flour. In turn, the flour traveled to Mexico (and other places) to be made into taco shells and corn products distributed throughout the world. Corn plants look alike, and corn seeds are either yellow or white. StarLink is yellow corn and looks no different from any other yellow corn. Unless StarLink is carefully segregated from other varieties, it can easily become mixed with conventional corn at any stage of production—in the fields or in trucks, grain elevators, or processing plants.

During the summer of 2000, Larry Bohlen of Friends of the Earth, one of the groups participating in Genetically Engineered Food Alert, learned

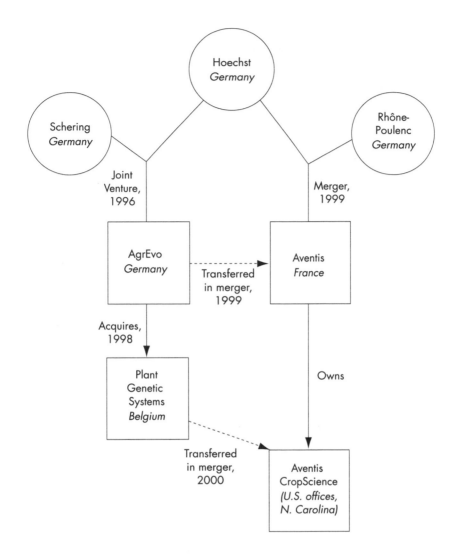

FIGURE 1. The multinational origins of Aventis CropScience, owner of the genetic engineering technology for StarLink corn in 2000, when its gene "illegally" appeared in supermarket taco shells. Bayer (*Germany*) bought Aventis CropScience in 2002.

that neither the growers of StarLink nor the owners of grain elevators were making any special effort to segregate the genetically modified corn from conventional varieties. He knew of a test developed by GeneticID, a company in Iowa, that could identify "foreign" genes in genetically modified foods. Using that test, Friends of the Earth examined corn

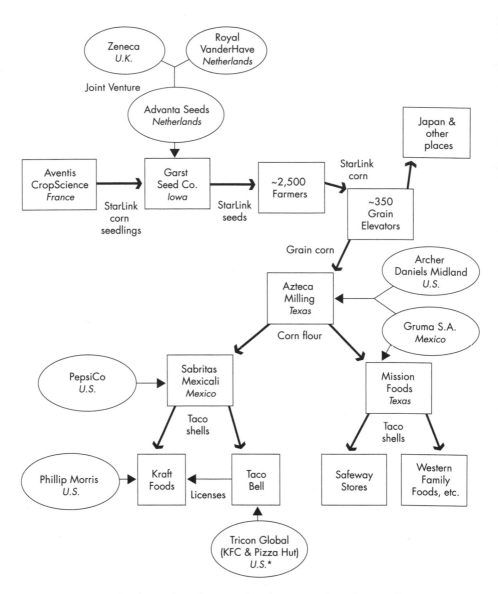

FIGURE 2. The chain of production, distribution, and marketing of StarLink corn through the food system in 2000. Square boxes contain the principal elements in this chain. Ovals indicate corporate ownership. The diagram reveals the difficulties of keeping StarLink corn separated from conventional corn during growth, harvest, storage, and processing.

*Tricon Global changed its name to Yum! Brands, Inc. in 2002.

products on supermarket shelves and hit the jackpot with the shells made by Taco Bell (owned by Kraft Foods, then a division of Philip Morris). Further testing revealed signs of the StarLink gene in other foods: vegetarian corn dogs, seed corn from conventionally grown plants, seeds from other types of genetically modified corn, corn shipped to Japan, and white as well as yellow corn. Because StarLink was not permitted in these products, it would have to be removed—a challenging and costly process involving product recalls, purchases of stored corn, closures of manufacturing plants, testing of samples, legal fees, bail-out funds, loss of sales, lost jobs, lost exports, and, eventually, judgments in class-action lawsuits. Not least, the StarLink affair contributed to further loss of confidence in the food biotechnology industry and in the ability of government agencies to protect the public by regulating genetically modified foods.

The Safety Issue: Allergenicity

The driving force behind these events was the idea that some people might be allergic to the StarLink protein. Food allergies, although rare, can be extremely dangerous and sometimes fatal to susceptible individuals. In the months following the taco shell disclosure, the Food and Drug Administration (FDA) collected accounts from people who said they experienced allergic reactions to products made with StarLink corn, and the EPA asked its Scientific Advisory Panel to advise the agency about scientific issues related to the allergenicity of the StarLink protein.

The panel's responses to the EPA surely constitute the most thorough evaluation of a food allergen ever conducted and provide a vivid example of how difficult it is to make policy decisions based on science that is incomplete and uncertain (which so often is the case). Panel members said they were "uncomfortable with the available data" and did not have enough information to decide whether the StarLink protein could cause allergic reactions. They knew that proteins are strings of amino acids arranged in a particular sequence, and that whether a protein provokes an allergic response depends on how that sequence folds—its structure and shape. Only some proteins are allergenic, but it is not yet possible to predict the structural features that induce allergic reactions. The panel members had to make educated guesses about the size, digestibility, and stability to heat of the Cry9C protein, and about the prevalence of this protein in the food supply.

One reason the Cry9C protein is toxic to insects is that they cannot easily digest it—break it down—to its constituent amino acids; the structure of the protein survives the digestive processes more or less intact. The Cry9C protein also is relatively stable to heat, so cooking might not destroy its ability to cause allergic reactions. Furthermore, preliminary feeding studies showed that the Cry9C protein appeared intact in the blood of rats and provoked immune responses, meaning that rats could not digest it and destroy its allergenicity. No such studies had been conducted in humans, however. Thus, panel members could not dismiss the possibility that the StarLink protein *might* be allergenic to humans. They judged the StarLink protein to have a "medium" likelihood of being allergenic, mainly because its potential to induce allergic reactions could not be disproved. Because processing and cooking were likely to destroy some of the Cry9C proteins, and the amounts were quite small to begin with, they judged Cry9C to have a "low" probability of actually causing allergic reactions in the population. These judgments supported the EPA's precautionary decision not to allow StarLink to enter the human food supply.[5]

A further complication is the question of whether people actually experience allergic reactions when they eat StarLink products. As it turns out, this connection is not easy to prove. Just because people feel sick after eating a food does not necessarily mean that the food—and not something else—caused the illness. Finding the StarLink *gene* in a food does not necessarily mean that the protein it specifies will cause allergic reactions. Like other genes, the StarLink gene is made of DNA (deoxyribonucleic acid), and its constituent components are common to all living species (see appendix). DNA and genes do not induce allergic reactions, but they specify the structure of proteins. Proteins (but not all of them) cause allergies. To prove that the StarLink protein is allergenic, scientists have to show that people reporting allergic reactions ate foods containing the StarLink corn protein and displayed immune responses to the StarLink protein in their blood. To investigate these matters, the FDA had to develop new testing materials and methods, and quickly. By June 2001, 63 people complained to the FDA about allergic reactions to StarLink and agency scientists collected food and blood samples from about 10 of them.

Using the new methods, FDA scientists tested the food samples but could not detect the StarLink *gene* in any of them. They also failed to find the StarLink protein in the foods, although the test was inconclusive in one sample. In the meantime, scientists from the Centers for Disease Control and Prevention (CDC) tested the blood samples for evidence of immune responses to the StarLink protein; they found none. These results led the agencies to conclude that the reported illnesses must have been caused by something other than an allergic reaction to the StarLink protein.[6]

With these results in hand, the EPA Scientific Advisory Panel met again in July 2001 to continue debating issues related to StarLink allergenicity. By this time, the EPA had canceled the StarLink registration, thereby prohibiting further plantings. The U.S. Department of Agriculture (USDA) joined with Aventis to buy the remaining mixtures of conventional and StarLink corn to use for animal feed or industrial uses. Corn handlers, millers, and food processors began testing to see whether their stocks contained the StarLink Cry9C protein, and began selling off the commingled corn.

In the meantime, EPA panel members continued to raise questions about the reliability of the FDA and CDC testing methods and said that they still could not exclude the possibility that StarLink might be allergenic. They saw no reason to change their previous conclusion that the Cry9C protein had a medium chance of being allergenic but a low chance of actually causing allergic reactions in the population. Instead, they said it was time to ask *political* questions: "What went right? What went wrong? What have we learned? How did Cry9C penetrate the human food supply? Why was the adulteration detected by a public interest group rather than through a more formal surveillance program (e.g., Federal agencies or regulated industry)?"[7]

Implications for Stakeholders

The answers to such political questions depend on the point of view—and, therefore, the interests—of the various stakeholders in food safety: the food industry, the government, consumer advocacy groups, and the general public. The StarLink affair revealed how these interests affect opinions and actions related to safety matters.

We can begin by looking at the reactions of the food industry—in this instance, the companies that produce, process, and sell StarLink corn or its products. As indicated in figures 1 and 2, large national and international corporations own many of the companies involved in the StarLink chain of production and distribution. These companies are businesses that must respond to the demands of directors and stockholders, and it seems likely that their managers had more immediate matters to worry about than whether corn intended for animal feed was commingling with conventional corn.

Aventis officials behaved as if they had no doubt that the EPA would approve StarLink for human consumption and would allow it to remain in the food supply. They began with denials and finger-pointing, starting with an attempt to discredit the accuracy of the GeneticID test. When subsequent testing confirmed the presence of the Cry9C gene in supermarket foods, Aventis "volunteered" to give up its right to plant StarLink, reportedly because the EPA threatened to revoke its registration.[8] The company also tried another tack; it petitioned the EPA to allow StarLink to remain in supermarket foods for four more years until virtually all commingled products would be sold. Aventis officials argued that the amounts in food were too small to harm consumers and that having to remove foods containing StarLink from corn supplies and supermarket shelves would greatly disrupt the food system. Indeed, disruptions were likely to be considerable, since the commingled corn for the 2000 crop amounted to 124 million bushels, and Japan and South Korea had rules forbidding any genetically modified corn from entering their countries. For all of these reasons, the Grocery Manufacturers of America and other food industry trade associations strongly supported the Aventis petitions.

Using yet another tactic, Aventis asked the EPA to set a "tolerance" limit for StarLink—a level below which regulatory agencies would ignore traces of the Cry9C gene or protein in food. Aventis warned corn processors that StarLink was so thoroughly commingled in the corn supply that the only way to deal with that situation was to *accept* it: "Will there ever be an end to this? Unfortunately, as of right now, the answer is 'no'—there will never be an 'end' as long as there is zero tolerance for Cry9C in food."[9]

These events led critics to ask the questions raised in any political scandal: What did Aventis and the EPA know, and when did they know it? Reports soon trickled out that both company and government officials knew—perhaps as early as 1997 and certainly by 1998—that StarLink was commingled with conventional corn. At a meeting late in 2000, I heard an official of the EPA say—unfortunately not for direct quotation—that Aventis had worked hard to lobby the White House Office of Science and Technology Policy, the State Department, and the FDA, USDA, and EPA during the months prior to the taco shell disclosure in an effort to convince federal officials that StarLink was not going to cause safety problems. Because Aventis officials acted as if StarLink were demonstrably safe, they were vulnerable to criticism from consumer groups like Friends of the Earth: "Aventis can't possibly have enough information to conclude that StarLink is safe at any level in our food."[10]

Other companies in the StarLink chain joined Aventis in further denial and blame. Officials of Garst Seed said that farmers knew they were supposed to separate StarLink from other corn, and "it's unfortunate some customers say they weren't informed about the program. . . . But we worked hard to get that message out."[11] Farmers, however, denied they had been told to segregate StarLink and filed lawsuits for damages. Operators of grain elevators also denied hearing anything about the need for crop segregation, and at least half of them had forwarded commingled corn for unapproved uses. Overall, the various companies in the chain of production and distribution assumed that their customers would not much care about this issue. As an analyst for J. P. Morgan explained, "If you're eating at Taco Bell, health consciousness is not high on your list of concerns."[12]

The government also is a major stakeholder in food safety, and its responses reflected the peculiar way in which regulatory authority is distributed among no less than three major agencies—the EPA, FDA, and USDA (see chapter 1). EPA officials criticized Aventis for claiming innocence about how StarLink might have gotten into the human food supply, for insufficiently informing growers about the need for crop segregation, and for flagrantly ignoring the terms of the restricted registration. The FDA at first seemed unconcerned; StarLink corn was the EPA's problem, and the taco shells, which do fall under FDA jurisdiction, seemed unlikely to be harmful. One FDA official reassured the *New York Times,* "This is not a case where we have illnesses or health problems."[13] When the FDA had to ask Friends of the Earth for a sample of the taco shells in order to conduct its own after-the-fact testing, however, it seemed clear that the agency was giving "inadequate oversight and attention to a serious matter of public health."[14] The secretary of the USDA blamed Aventis: "Some might argue that the StarLink episode will lead to greater government involvement. . . . It's important to remember that this problem may not have occurred had industry complied with the terms of its license."[15] Nevertheless, the USDA agreed to spend $20 million to buy back commingled seed in an effort to prevent disruption of the corn market.

Consumer advocacy groups used the potential allergenicity of StarLink to bolster their demands that genetically modified foods be tested before entering the food supply and labeled so people can protect themselves against foods to which they might be allergic. They viewed the events as evidence that neither government nor industry were looking out for the public interest. Representatives from Friends of the Earth and Consumers Union argued, "There is no way the taxpayer should bail out

Aventis for the genetic pollution they created," and "EPA should not re-ward Aventis for their failure to follow the law."[16] Even business com-mentators were dismayed: "Almost everybody involved screwed up. . . . The promises made by StarLink's inventors proved worthless, falling prey to managerial inattention, corporate mergers, blind faith, misplaced hope, woeful ignorance, political activism, and probably greedy farmers too, if you can imagine such a thing."[3] Whether or not StarLink really is al-lergenic (a food safety issue) its unlabeled presence in processed foods did nothing to encourage trust in the food supply, and these events re-vealed the markedly different ways in which the various stakeholders view matters of food safety risk.

Implications for Food Safety Politics: Themes

With StarLink products recalled and class action suits settled, we now turn to the food safety interests of the general public. As consumers, we want food to be safe—or safe enough—and we expect the food indus-try and government to make sure that it is. We also are part of the po-litical equation. As stakeholders in the food system, however, our influ-ence depends on the extent to which we recognize the political forces at work in safety matters. Enhancing that understanding is a principal aim of this book. If the StarLink episode teaches us anything, it is that en-suring food safety is a matter of politics as well as science. In conveying this lesson, the StarLink story illustrates several of the themes that recur throughout the chapters that follow.

The first theme is the fragmented, overlapping, and confusing distri-bution of authority among the federal agencies concerned with food safety: the EPA, FDA, and USDA. All three agencies were in some way responsible for making sure that StarLink did not get into the human food supply, yet the system failed to ensure that food companies followed rules designed to protect public health. We will see how this divided au-thority complicates federal oversight of microbial contaminants in food, genetically engineered foods, and protection of the food supply against potential threats of bioterrorism.

A second theme is the food industry's promotion of economic self-in-terest at the expense of public health and safety. We have just seen how the developers of StarLink assumed that the corn was safe to eat, made little effort to keep it out of the human food supply, and blamed other parts of the food distribution chain for its appearance in taco shells. The StarLink affair is just one example of what *Sierra* magazine calls "Brave

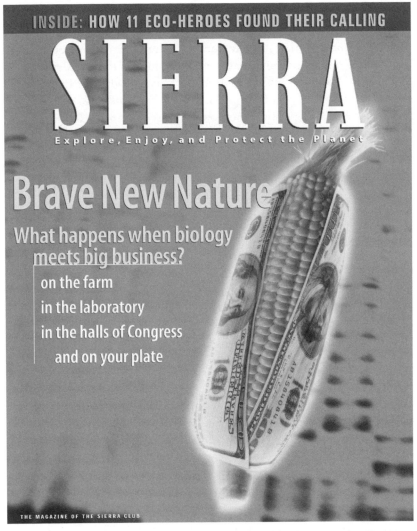

FIGURE 3. Environmental groups recognize political influences on science when they ask what happens when "biology meets big business," as in this cover story from *Sierra*, July/August 2001. (Courtesy of *Sierra* magazine and the photographer, Philip Kaake. Reprinted with permission.)

New Nature—What Happens When Biology Meets Big Business?" (see figure 3). This book provides further examples of situations in which food companies deny responsibility and blame others in matters of food safety, and oppose, resist, and undermine food safety guidelines, following them only when forced to do so by government action or public opinion.

A third theme is the food industry's invocation of science as a rationale for self-interested actions. In the case of StarLink, Aventis used scientific arguments—that the protein was present in amounts too small to cause allergic reactions and that scientists could find no evidence of allergenicity—to divert attention from the ways in which it had ignored the terms of its EPA registration. This book explains how food companies use science as a political tool to oppose requirements to keep harmful microbes out of food, label genetically modified foods, or institute protective measures against bioterrorist threats.

A fourth theme has to do with the use of food safety as a means through which consumer advocacy groups raise issues about the self-interested exercise of corporate power, the imbalance in power between corporate and public interests, and the collusion of government policies with business interests. In the StarLink affair, consumer groups successfully used the EPA's registration rules and uncertainties about allergenicity to challenge the marketing of genetically modified foods and to obtain a large judgment in a class-action lawsuit.[17] This book presents other examples of the ways in which advocacy groups use questions of safety to address much broader social and political concerns.

A fifth theme is the trouble caused by the markedly different ways in which scientists and the public view food safety risks. Because this particular theme is central to understanding why food safety is as much a matter of politics as it is of science, and because this theme emerges as a factor in so many disputes about food safety matters, it comes first in our discussion.

PERCEPTIONS OF FOOD SAFETY RISK: THE "TWO-CULTURE" PROBLEM

Underlying the politics of food safety is a vexing question of definition: What, exactly, is safe? Although it might seem that a food is either safe or not safe, the distinction is rarely unambiguous. Safety is relative; it is not an inherent biological characteristic of a food. A food may be safe for some people but not others, safe at one level of intake but not another, or safe at one point in time but not later. Instead, we can define a safe food as one that does not exceed an *acceptable* level of risk. Decisions about acceptability involve perceptions, opinions, and values, as well as science. When such decisions have implications for commercial or other self-interested motives, food safety enters the realm of politics.[18]

Scientists may be able to settle questions about the allergenicity of Star-

TABLE 2. Comparison of "science-based" and "value-based" approaches to evaluating the acceptability of food safety risks

"Science-Based"	"Value-Based"
Counts and calculates:	Assesses whether risk is:
• Cases	• Voluntary or imposed
• Severity of illnesses	• Visible or hidden
• Hospitalizations	• Understood or uncertain
• Deaths	• Familiar or foreign
• Costs of the risk	• Natural or technological
• Benefits of the risk	• Controllable or uncontrollable
• Costs of reducing the risk	• Mild or severe
• Balance of risk to benefits	• Fairly or unfairly distributed
Balances risk against *benefit and cost*	Balances risk against *dread and outrage*

Link, but science is only one factor among many others that influence opinions about the acceptability of StarLink corn in the food supply. Disputes about food safety often occur as a result of the different ways in which people assess risk. For the sake of discussion, these ways can be divided into two distinct but overlapping approaches to deciding whether a food is safe: from the perspective of "science" and from the perspective of "values." Table 2 summarizes the characteristics of the two approaches. I place them in quotation marks because the two approaches greatly overlap. Science-based approaches are not free of values, and value-based approaches also consider science. With that said, we can use these oversimplified categories to make some further generalizations. From a science-based perspective there is little reason to exclude StarLink from the food supply; the corn has a low probability of causing allergic reactions. From value-based perspectives, however, there may be many reasons to prohibit its use: its lack of labeling or regulatory approval, for example, or simply because it is genetically modified.

These differences in approaching questions of risk were understood long before anyone invented the techniques for genetically modifying foods. In 1959, for example, the scientist and writer C. P. Snow characterized the ways in which people trained in science tend to think about the world—as opposed to those without such training—as representing two distinct cultures separated from one another by a "gulf of mutual incomprehension."[19] Much more recently, the anthropologist Clifford Geertz wrote, "The ways in which we try to understand and deal with the physical world and those in which we try to understand and deal with the social one are not altogether the same. The methods of research, the aims of inquiry, and the standards of judgment all differ, and nothing but confusion, scorn, and accusation—relativism! Platonism! reductionism! verbalism!—results from failing to see this."[20]

The application of the two-culture problem to safety issues also has a long history. In 1979, Philip Handler, then president of the National Academy of Sciences, said, "The *estimation* of risk is a scientific question—and, therefore, a legitimate activity of scientists in federal agencies, in universities and in the National Research Council. The *acceptability* of a given level of risk, however, is a political question to be determined in the political arena."[21] In 1991, Edward Groth, a scientist at Consumers Union, explained that public policy choices lie at the heart of safety debates about food. "Each dispute has two main components, *factual* issues and *value* issues. . . . Factual questions include: What risks are involved? How big are they? Who is at risk? These are scientific questions. The central value question is: Given those facts, what should society *do?*"[22] A more detailed examination of the two approaches to evaluating risks—called, for lack of better terms, science-based and value-based—helps to explain why food safety issues are so political.

Science-Based Approaches: Counting Cases and Costs

Much of what we know about the ways in which people assess safety risks comes from studies by experts in risk communication, a field that deals with questions about how the public is—and should be—informed about matters of potential harm. To explain science-based approaches, risk communication researchers begin by examining how scientists think. Ideally, science begins with an observation. Rather than accepting an observation as a universal truth, scientists question its accuracy, interpretation, and relevance; develop theories to explain its significance; and design and conduct experiments to test those theories. The quality of scientific research depends not only on the question under investigation (some research questions are more interesting and important than others) and the care ("rigor") with which studies are conducted, but also on the ability of the studies to eliminate ("control for") all possible causes of the observation other than the one being tested. Scientific methods also extend beyond observations to suggest probable causes, to exclude irrelevant causes ("confounding variables"), and to estimate the probability that a particular cause is the true reason for the observation of interest.

The point here is that probability is not the same as proof. Biological experiments in humans are complicated by genetic variation and behavioral differences, and study results nearly always depend on probabilities and statistics. This means that they are subject to *interpretation* and, therefore, to perception, opinion, and judgment. Scientists tend to minimize the subjective nature of interpretation and to view knowledge gained through the testing of theories as objective, accurate, evidence-based, hypothesis-driven, and rigorous. As one scientist who consults for the biotechnology industry explains, "The advantage of being a biologist comes not from what I know but from how I think. To me, the greatest value of scientific training is a proclivity for asking questions without being emotionally attached to a specific answer—a willingness to look objectively at data even if the facts contradict our preconceived notions."[23] Scientists who believe that such opinions are objective—and remain unaware of how self-interest might influence them—may well have trouble understanding why the "other culture" questions their impartiality.

In practice, a science-based approach to food safety is one that appears to focus exclusively on the characteristics of the risk itself: annual cases of illness, doctor's visits, hospitalizations, deaths, costs to individuals and to society, the benefits of doing nothing about the risk, and the benefits and costs of risk reduction. From this perspective, risks are measurable and, therefore, "scientific" and "objective." Researchers and federal officials evaluate potential hazards through a formal process of risk assessment that involves identifying the hazard, characterizing it, determining its degree of exposure in the population, and calculating the balance of risk to benefit and cost.[24]

Using this science-based approach, U.S. government agencies identify the primary preventable food safety hazards as microbial infections, antibiotic-resistant *Salmonella*, food allergens, and certain pesticides.[25] For science-based reasons, genetically modified foods do not appear on this list. In this book, we will see how government and industry use science-based approaches to set food safety standards, to regulate genetically modified foods, and to make international decisions about food trade. Because so much self-interest is at stake in such decisions, these areas have political as well as scientific dimensions—whether recognized or not.

The StarLink events, for example, revealed how scientific approaches to risk also are subject to values, opinions, and interpretations. People reported feeling ill after eating products made with StarLink corn, but scientific tests could not confirm that the StarLink protein caused the problem. On that basis, depending on point of view, some experts concluded that StarLink could not possibly cause allergic reactions, whereas others criticized the quality of the testing, the small number of people tested, and other experimental factors that cast doubt on that interpretation. Such differences in opinion among experts should be expected. In 1982, Mary Douglas (an anthropologist) and Aaron Wildavsky (a political scientist) observed that scientific judgments of risk cannot—and, indeed, should not—be separated from value judgments:

> It is a travesty of rational thought to pretend that it is best to take value-free decisions in matters of life and death. One salient difference between experts and the lay public is that the latter, when assessing risks, do not conceal their moral commitments but put them into the argument, explicitly and prominently. . . . The risk expert claims to depoliticize an inherently political problem . . . [But] knowledge of danger is necessarily partial and limited: judgments of risk and safety must be selected as much on the basis of what is valued as on the basis of what is known. . . . Science and risk assessment cannot tell us what we need to know about threats of danger since they explicitly try to exclude moral ideas about the good life.[26]

Value-Based Approaches: Estimating Dread and Outrage

Scientific methods estimate the probability that something in a food might lead to illness, but they do not consider the intangible value or significance of that food to the people eating it. Many people, however, evaluate risks not only for their potential to cause health problems but also from the standpoint of personal beliefs and values that depend on a host of psychological, cultural, and social factors. These personal perspectives about food have also been studied extensively. Anthropologists, for example, tell us that the act of consuming food—taking it into our bodies—is so primal that societies create myths to explain the transformation of food into *us*. Because, in that sense, we truly are what we eat, food raises questions of intimacy and identity and provokes feelings of anxiety. People do not necessarily want food to be perfectly safe (or we would never eat wild mushrooms or raw oysters). We are just more comfortable knowing what we are eating. As the French sociologist Claude Fischler explains, people have an innate tendency to view food as UFOs—unidentified food objects (*objets comestibles non identifiés*). At some deep psychological level, "If we are what we eat, and we don't know what we are eating, then do we still know who we are?"[27]

Specialists in risk communication are well aware of the importance of such anxieties in assessment of safety risks. Paul Slovic and his colleagues, for example, have asked people to rank potential hazards according to the degree of perceived harm. Their findings: people worry most about risks perceived as highly dangerous, particularly to pregnant women and small children (a science-based concept), but they are also concerned about risks perceived as involuntary, unpreventable, unfamiliar, and inequitably distributed—factors based on values. Their studies consistently find people to be less willing to accept risks induced by technology, those poorly understood by science, and those subject to contradictory statements from experts. The more such value-based factors characterize a particular risk, the more the risk generates feelings of anxiety, alarm, dread, and outrage. In fact, risk communication researchers rank such factors on a predictable scale of dread and outrage.[28]

With respect to food, acceptance of risk depends far more on perception of the number and intensity of dread-and-outrage factors than it does on the number of cases of illness. Scientists can identify the probable extent of a foodborne illness in the population, for example, but interpreting what that probability means for the health of any one individual is quite another matter. On a population basis, microbial contaminants unquestionably pose the most prevalent foodborne threat to health. The public, however, also ranks chemical pesticides and additives, irradiation, and genetic engineering high on the list of perceived risks, largely because exposures to them are invisible, involuntary, imposed, and uncontrollable. People make clear, predictable, and understandable distinctions between risks they knowingly accept and those they do not. Many people find the benefits of eating raw fish or raw milk cheeses to greatly exceed the small but finite risk of ingesting harmful microbial contaminants; the choice is voluntary, and the foods are familiar. In contrast, the health risks of genetically modified foods (however remote they may be) are hidden and undemocratically applied—witness StarLink— and as a result are far less acceptable.

Because questions of who imposes risks and who takes risks are crucial in assessing whether a risk is acceptable, decisions about food safety take on political dimensions. During the mid-1990s, when the FDA applied a solely science-based approach to approval of genetically engineered foods, Commissioner David Kessler recognized the political implications of excluding value-based considerations when he told a reporter, "Weighing risks against benefits sounds great, but the truth is there is no magic formula, especially when the risks are taken by one group and the benefits by another."[29]

A comparison of the two approaches to assessing risk explains why whenever someone invokes science in discussions of food safety, we can be reasonably certain that questions of self-interest are at stake but are excluded from debate. Scientists talk about risk as a matter of illness and death. The public wants dread-and-outrage factors to be considered as well. In this book, we will see how the failure of food companies, scientists, and government agencies to recognize the need to address values as well as science in matters of food safety leads to widespread distrust of the food industry and its regulators. When officials and experts dismiss dread-and-outrage concerns as emotional, irrational, unscientific, and indefensible, they raise questions about their own credibility and competence. They fail to recognize their own biases as well as the predictability of public responses to food safety risks. In 1987, Peter Sandman explicitly made this point: "When a risk manager continues to ignore these factors—and continues to be surprised by the public's response of outrage—it is worth asking just whose behavior is irrational."[30]

The Precautionary Principle: Look Before You Leap

The differences in the two approaches to food safety risk have an additional political dimension. They imply different expectations for the ways in which authorities make decisions about the release of new foods and ingredients. The science-based approach works on the proposition "nothing ventured, nothing gained." Regulators determine as well as they can whether a food or ingredient is likely to cause harm and permit those that seem reasonably safe to enter the food supply. The FDA uses this approach for food additives characterized as "generally recognized as safe" (GRAS) and also, with some modifications, for genetically engineered foods. If problems occur, the agency deals with them *after* the foods are marketed. This approach requires neither premarket testing nor labeling; it is based on a standard that requires food manufacturers to demonstrate "reasonable certainty of no harm." This standard, which translates as "safe enough to be acceptable," leaves plenty of room for subjective opinion and judgment.

An alternative approach is one that has come to be known as the principle of precautionary action, or the "precautionary principle." This principle, which emerged in Europe as a guideline for environmental protection, can be summarized as "look before you leap," meaning test the products first, then introduce them into the marketplace. Although this approach may seem so sensible as to be politically neutral, it is nothing of the kind. As the European Commission explains:

Decision-makers are constantly faced with the dilemma of balancing the freedom and rights of individuals, industry and organizations with the need to reduce the risk of adverse effects to the environment or to health. . . . Whether or not to invoke the Precautionary Principle is a decision exercised where scientific information is insufficient, inconclusive, or uncertain and where there are indications that the possible effects on the environment or human, animal or plant health may be potentially dangerous and inconsistent with the chosen level of protection. . . . The appropriate response in a given situation is thus the result of a political decision, a function of the risk level that is "acceptable" to the society on which the risk is imposed.[31]

In practice, invocation of the precautionary principle can be used to require companies to demonstrate that foods are safe *before* they are marketed. As we have seen, the EPA followed this principle to some extent when it ruled that StarLink could not enter the human food supply. On the basis of such precautions, the European Union banned American and Canadian beef from cattle treated with growth hormones and delayed introduction of genetically modified crops. Thus, the precautionary principle has implications for international trade as well as domestic food policy and has become a major rallying point for advocates who favor environmental protection or oppose food biotechnology.[32] In January 1998, for example, a group of such advocates met in Wingspread, Wisconsin, to formulate what is now known as the Wingspread statement on the precautionary principle: "When an activity raises threats of harm to human health or the environment, precautionary measures should be taken even if some cause and effect relationships are not fully established scientifically. In this context, the proponent of the activity, rather than the public, should bear the burden of protection."[33]

As a result of such advocacy, international agreements increasingly incorporate the precautionary principle in policy statements. For example, European and United States experts on food biotechnology issued a joint statement in 2000 saying, "When substantive uncertainties prevent accurate risk assessment, governments should act protectively on the side of safety."[34] Even so mild a statement suggests that companies will have to do more to demonstrate safety in advance. But because testing can *never* prove that a food is perfectly safe, public willingness to accept a new food depends on how well it meets the value concerns summarized in table 2. If a food ranks high in dread and outrage, it will *never* appear safe enough, no matter how much effort goes into attempts to prove it harmless.

In their frustration with dread-and-outrage factors, industry leaders and their supporters argue that no matter what they do, they will never be able to satisfy opponents. Instead, they argue, the true purpose of the precautionary principle is to inhibit business. Elizabeth Whelan, who directs the industry-sponsored American Council on Science and Health, explains why the principle so infuriates her and other science-based assessors of food safety risks: "As a corollary to the Precautionary Principle, consumer activists now insist that if the public *perceives* something as risky, that perception should carry the day regardless of whether there truly is a risk or not. In essence these people argue that science should take a back seat to fear—*whether that fear is justified or not*—when it comes to setting policy."[35]

Such comments reveal that much of the controversy about food safety appears as a conflict between a strictly scientific assessment of risk and an approach that also considers a much broader range of issues that affect society. Underlying the controversy, as this book explains, are industry concerns about economic self-interest as opposed to concerns of consumer advocates about the distribution of risk, benefit, and control in matters of public policy. We will see how scientific decisions about food safety cannot be separated from such political and social matters.

ABOUT THIS BOOK

This book traces the interweaving of science, values, and politics through an examination of three broad areas of food safety: bacteria, biotechnology, and bioterrorism. The first part of the book examines the politics of foodborne microbial illness. These chapters describe government attempts to force food producers, particularly those that slaughter and process meat, to take steps to prevent bacterial contamination of their products, and they explain how those industries consistently resist such safety measures. From a science-based approach to risk assessment, foodborne illness is the single most important food safety problem; it is responsible for millions of cases of stomach upset and thousands of deaths each year. Bacteria rank low on the dread-and-outrage scale, however, because meat is familiar, eating it is voluntary, food "poisonings" are common, and most people survive them. Politics enters this picture at the level of responsibility for preventing foodborne illness. We will see how the meat industry exploits the relatively low level of organized public outrage about microbial safety to oppose federal regulations and, instead, to argue that *consumers* bear the principal burden of ensuring safe food. Part 1 also describes the fragmentation of government oversight as a basis for developing a more coherent approach to dealing with problems of food safety.

Part 2 shifts the discussion to a different issue: genetically modified foods. By the standards of scientific risk assessment—counting cases of illness and death—such foods appear no less safe than foods developed through traditional plant genetics, but, as the StarLink affair indicates, they present many reasons for distrust and alarm. These chapters describe how the food biotechnology industry, in dismissing dread-and-outrage factors as emotional and unscientific, lobbied for—and won—a largely science-based approach to regulation of its products. The chapters explain how the dismissal of consumer concerns about value issues related to food biotechnology forced advocacy groups to use safety as the only "legitimate" basis of discussion. In the StarLink affair, for example, advocates could not use concerns about corporate control of the food supply as an argument against approval of genetically modified foods. They could, however, use the remote risk of allergenicity as a basis for opposition because of the double negative: it is *not* possible to prove that the StarLink protein is *not* allergenic. These chapters describe the origin of disputes about genetically modified foods that arise from conflicting interests and values.

The concluding chapter takes up a third area: food bioterrorism—the deliberate poisoning or contamination of the food supply to achieve some political goal. Questions about food bioterrorism take us into the realm of emerging food safety hazards that might be used as biological weapons: mad cow disease, foot-and-mouth disease, and anthrax. From a science-based perspective, these problems are of uncertain or low overall risk to human health, but they rank high as causes of dread and outrage. The terrorist attacks of September 2001 increased the level of anxiety, particularly about the country's vulnerability to bioterrorism in general, and to food bioterrorism in particular. In concluding this discussion, I offer suggestions for ways in which the government, the food industry, and consumers might engage in political action to deal with this and the other food safety issues raised in this book. Finally, a short appendix briefly summarizes some of the basic scientific concepts that underlie the debates about food safety issues.

With this introduction, we can now begin our discussion by examining the historical and modern reasons why government attempts to keep harmful bacteria out of food have proved so controversial and why they raise issues of politics as well as of science.

PART ONE

RESISTING FOOD SAFETY

FRIENDS AND COLLEAGUES, KNOWING THAT I WAS WRITING about harmful bacteria in food, wondered why anyone would care about things so invisible, tasteless, unpronounceable, and, for the most part, innocuous. Like most people, they view occasional episodes of food "poisoning" as uncomfortable (sometimes *very* uncomfortable), but certainly more a matter of random bad luck than of decades of industry and government indifference, dithering, and outright obstructionism. They accept at face value the endlessly intoned mantra of industry and government: the United States has the safest food supply in the world.

Whether this assertion is true is a matter of some debate. Safety is relative. The most authoritative estimate of the yearly number of cases of foodborne disease in the United States defies belief: 76 million illnesses, 325,000 hospitalizations, 5,000 deaths. As the chapters in part 1 explain, such numbers undoubtedly *underestimate* the extent of the problem. Although the most frequent causes of these illnesses are viruses and species of bacteria—*Campylobacter, Salmonella, Shigella,* and *Escherichia coli* (*E. coli*)—most episodes are never reported to health authorities and their cause is unknown.[1] From a science-based perspective, the risks and costs of foodborne illness are extremely high.

Furthermore, although outbreaks of foodborne illness have become more dangerous over the years, food producers resist the attempts of government agencies to institute control measures, and major food industries oppose pathogen control measures by every means at their disposal. They lobby Congress and federal agencies, challenge regulations in court, and encourage local obstruction of safety enforcement. We will see, for example, that the culture of opposition to food safety measures so permeates the beef industry that it led, in one shocking instance, to the assassination of federal and state meat inspectors.

To explain this culture of resistance, we need to understand that current problems of food safety are not new but are *different*. A century ago, the main sources of foodborne illness were milk from infected cows and spoiled meat from sick animals. Public health measures that we now take for granted—water chlorination and milk pasteurization, for example—eliminated typhoid fever, cholera, and most lethal diarrheal diseases. The food supply depended on local production and was largely decentralized. Fish, for example, were caught wild from the sea. Even though cattle were transported to common areas for slaughter and kept in close quarters—conditions ripe for spreading infections—federal inspection and veterinary care kept most sick animals from entering the food supply.

Today, centralized food production has created even more favorable conditions for dissemination of bacteria, protozoa, and viruses. We call these organisms by collective terms: microbes, microorganisms, or "bugs." If harmful, they are pathogens. Many pathogens infect the animals we use for food without causing any visible signs of illness. Infected animals excrete pathogenic microbes in feces, however, and pass them along to other food animals, to food plants, and to us. If the pathogens survive cooking, stomach acid, and digestive enzymes, they can multiply, produce toxins, upset digestive systems, and do worse. Their effects are especially harmful to people with immature or weakened immune systems—infants, young children, the elderly, and those ill from other causes. Even from this brief description, it should be evident that people involved with every stage of food production, from farm to fork, must take responsibility for food safety to prevent animal infections (producers), avoid fecal contamination (processors), and destroy pathogens (food handlers and consumers).

Sharing of responsibility, however, also permits sharing of blame. As these chapters explain, producers blame processors for foodborne illness, and processors blame producers; government regulators blame both, and everyone blames consumers. The role of government in food safety demands particular notice. Current laws grant regulatory agencies only limited authority to prevent microbial contamination before food gets to consumers. Federal oversight of food safety remains unshakably rooted in policies established almost a century ago, in 1906. Congress designed those policies to ensure the health of *animals,* in an era long before most of the current microbial causes of foodborne illness were even suspected, let alone recognized. Although food safety experts have complained for years about the gap between hazards and oversight practices, attempts to give federal agencies the right to enforce food safety regulations have been blocked repeatedly by food producers and their supporters in Congress, sometimes joined by the agencies themselves, and more recently by the courts. Some progress has occurred, driven by the appearance in common foods of new and more deadly pathogens such as *E. coli* O157:H7, an exceptionally virulent strain of an otherwise normal and relatively harmless bacterial inhabitant of the human digestive tract. The multimillion-dollar costs of product recalls, legal counsel, and liability payments, and the associated costs of damaged reputation and loss of sales, have made the need for more forceful government oversight of food safety apparent to all but the staunchest protectors of food industry self-interest.

For the most part, the events described in this part of the book are *political* and outside the daily experience of most people in our society. Most of us do not worry much about the possibility that foods in our supermarkets might be contaminated and dangerous, and we act on the basis of what Nicols Fox calls the "unspoken contract" among food producers, government regulators, and the public to ensure that food is safe.[2] On a daily basis, most of us think the risks are so small, so familiar, and so voluntary that we can ignore them. Microbial risks generate little dread and virtually no outrage.

I most clearly recognized the extent of our collective denial about the hazards of food pathogens in the summer of 1999 when I served as a member of an American Cancer Society committee developing dietary guidelines for cancer survivors—people diagnosed with cancer and treated for it. Because surgery, radiation, and chemotherapy can cause a temporary decline in immune function, our committee wanted to stress the importance of preventing microbial infections during periods of treatment and recovery. This advice, we realized, firmly precludes even a taste of raw cookie dough, not to mention avoidance of a host of other foods: Caesar salads, homemade ice cream, and anything else made with raw or partially cooked eggs; rare or medium-cooked hamburger and beef tartare; sushi and other raw seafood; raw milk and cheeses made from it; freshly squeezed juices; unpeeled vegetables and unwashed salad greens and berries; and raw sprouts. For people with weakened immune systems, eating uncooked and unpasteurized foods means taking a risk, and not just of minor discomfort but perhaps of hospitalization, long-term disability, or death.[3]

But what about those of us with healthy immune systems? As these chapters explain, *everyone* takes a risk when eating uncooked foods, but the extent of that risk is uncertain. In the absence of better oversight of safety at the production end, federal agencies now advise us to follow safety guidelines that used to be reserved for travelers to developing countries. Such advice converts the act of eating to a matter of risk management rather than of nourishment or pleasure, and must be understood as a political act in itself. Because federal policies cannot ensure that food is safe before people bring it home, government agencies shift the burden of responsibility to consumers. *Of course* all of us should learn to prepare foods properly, but the industry can and should do its share as well.

As these chapters explain, for reasons of history, inertia, turf disputes, and just plain greed, government oversight of food safety has long tended to provide far more protection to food producers than to the public. Only in recent years, when foodborne illness began to raise serious issues of liability, have food companies and federal agencies been forced to consider measures—albeit grudgingly—to prevent microbial pathogens in food.

Like the events related to the StarLink affair, those recounted in these chapters reflect certain recurrent themes. With respect to government, one theme is the fragmented, overlapping, and ultimately obstructive distribution of authority between two federal agencies: the Food and Drug Administration (FDA) and the Department of Agriculture (USDA). Another is the historic closeness of working relationships among congressional agriculture committees, federal regulatory agencies, and food producers. We will see how food producers repeatedly deny responsibility for foodborne illness, invoke science to promote self-interest and divert public attention from harm caused by their products, and express outright hostility to federal oversight. From the standpoint of consumer advocacy, an additional theme bears on the ways in which food safety relates to much broader societal concerns. As Eric Schlosser discussed so compellingly in *Fast Food Nation* (Houghton Mifflin, 2001), much of the actual work in the food industry—in agriculture, slaughterhouses, processing plants, and places where food is served—is carried out by immigrants, teenagers, and other groups paid the minimum wage. People can only produce safe food if they know how to do so, if they follow the rules, and if they are themselves in good health. Thus, the production of safe food also depends on the adequacy of fundamental social support systems such as public education and health care.

In this part of the book, chapter 1 sets the stage by reviewing the origins of the present system of governmental oversight of food safety. Chapters 2 and 3 review some of the landmark incidents leading to the current "crisis" over bacterial pathogens. They also explain how government agencies attempted to deal with such crises in the face of resistance by food producers and processors. In chapter 4, I discuss some political alternatives for improving oversight of our food safety system.

For the most part, these chapters focus on the actions of producers and processors of meat—in this case, beef. Unlike the producers of most other foods, the beef industry makes little attempt to hide its self-interested political activities. Beef industry pressures on Congress and federal regulators are more transparent than those of other food industries, and are better documented. Nevertheless, many of the food safety issues raised by beef production are similar to matters that affect poultry, eggs, seafood (especially the farmed variety), and pork, as well as to those that affect fruits and vegetables inadvertently contaminated as they move from farm to table, sometimes from one country to another.

CHAPTER 1

THE POLITICS
OF FOODBORNE ILLNESS
ISSUES AND ORIGINS

IN THE EARLY 1970S, A TIME WHEN FOOD SAFETY WAS BECOMING a matter of public debate, my young family went to a dinner hosted by a colleague. I don't remember much about the party, but its aftermath remains vivid. Within hours, all but one of us became violently ill. I will spare the details, as nearly everyone has had a similar experience. A flurry of telephone calls the next day made it clear that we were not the only ones who suffered after that dinner. In retrospect, what seems most remarkable about that event was how *ordinary* it was. We survived. We felt better in a day or two. We did not report our illness to health authorities, and neither did anyone else. We did not try to trace the source of the outbreak (although our one son who did not become ill, and who ate nothing green in those days, insisted that the salad must have been at fault).

We assumed that minor food poisonings were a normal part of daily living; they were low on our dread-and-outrage scale. It did not occur to us that microbial illness transmitted by food might be anything more serious than a minor inconvenience and a mess to clean up. If we gave any thought to cholera, typhoid, or botulism (let alone anthrax), we viewed them as diseases of the past, eliminated by basic public health measures such as water chlorination, milk pasteurization, or canning at appropriate temperatures. We were quite unaware of the emerging bacterial pathogens that I discuss in these chapters. At the time, if we worried at all about food safety, it was about agricultural pesticides or food additives—the chemical colors, flavors, and preservatives then increasingly used to make processed foods look and taste better. We were not alone in worrying about food additives: a 1979 report recommended a complete revision of the food safety laws to strengthen our ability to control the use of food chemicals such as saccharin, the artificial sweetener that had just been linked to cancer risk.[1]

Additives and pesticides remained primary public safety concerns through the mid-1980s. Dr. David Kessler, who later became commissioner of the Food and Drug Administration (FDA), said that food safety laws needed an overhaul to control food additives—without even mentioning microbial hazards. Surveys of public attitudes toward food safety often asked about additives and pesticides but rarely probed knowledge or opinions about bacterial pathogens. When the surveys did include such questions, most people continued to rank additives and pesticides first among food safety concerns. At the time, less than 1% of food samples contained chemical additives and pesticides at "unacceptable" levels. Even if such levels were still too high—and any level of pesticides in food continues to raise safety questions—harm from food chemicals paled in comparison to that caused by pathogens. In the late 1980s, health officials found *Salmonella* in one-third of all poultry and estimated that 33 million Americans experienced at least one episode of foodborne microbial illness each year.[2]

A few farsighted advocacy groups such as the Community Nutrition Institute in Washington, DC, pressed for more action to prevent pathogens from entering the food supply. They were aware of the emergence in the early 1980s of an especially nasty variant of *Escherichia coli* (*E. coli*), usually a relatively harmless inhabitant of the human digestive tract. As reports of toxic pathogens in food became more frequent, food safety priorities began to shift. By 1989, both *Time* and *Newsweek* had published cover stories on microbial food hazards. In 1991, the Center for Science in the Public Interest (CSPI), which had led public debate about food additives, published a consumer guide to food safety with exceptionally clear instructions about what needed to be done to prevent foodborne infections.[3]

In the early 1990s, such publicity encouraged Congress to introduce more than 30 bills—a record number—related to food safety, and at least eight states were trying to develop their own rules. Ellen Haas, then president of the consumer advocacy group Public Voice, called food safety "not just a kitchen issue anymore."[4] At the time, federal officials ranked microbial hazards first among food safety issues, residues of animal drugs second, and new technologies (such as genetically modified foods) third. By 1994, more than 60% of consumers said they worried most about consuming rare beef, raw shellfish, and residues of animal drugs. In 1997, consumers and food editors said they were more concerned about food safety than they had been just one year earlier, and nearly all of them blamed meat and poultry producers—and government agencies—for not doing enough to prevent microbial pathogens in the food supply.[5]

To establish a basis for understanding the significance of such a profound shift in attitudes, this chapter begins with an introduction to the current status of microbial pathogens in the food supply. We will see that foodborne illness is more than a biological problem; it is strongly affected by the interests of stakeholders in the food system—the food industry, government (agencies, Congress, and the White House), and consumers. The present system of food safety oversight and its political implications are best understood in historical context. Thus, this chapter describes the origins of the century-old policies that govern federal actions to this day. In the case of meat safety, Congress designed those policies to prevent sick animals—not microscopic pathogens—from entering the food supply. As this chapter explains, efforts to modernize such policies do not come easily.

MICROBES IN FOOD: FRIENDS AND FOES

Thinking too much about the life we share with microbes can lead to paranoia. Microbes are everywhere: around us, on us, and in us. They inhabit soil and water, skin and digestive tract, and any place that provides favorable conditions for growth (and hardly any place does not). They are incredibly small, and incredibly numerous. All kinds—viruses, bacteria, protozoa, and yeasts—are ubiquitous in raw foods. Most are harmless. Some are even "friendly," helping to make bread, wine, vinegar, soy sauce, yogurt, and cheese, and keeping our digestive tracts healthy. Others are less helpful; left to their own devices, they rot apples, mold bread, and spoil meat. Some are decidedly unfriendly, and cause more than 200 known foodborne diseases.

To avoid getting food poisoning, we take precautions: we preserve foods and we cook them. Preservation methods—some ancient, some modern (among them salt, sugar, alcohol, acid, and freeze-drying)—all inhibit microbial growth. Refrigeration slows down growth, and freezing does so even more. Cooking, a brilliant invention, not only makes foods taste better but also kills microbial pathogens. Cooked

TABLE 3. The most frequent microbial causes of foodborne disease in the United States: estimated numbers of illnesses, hospitalizations, and deaths, 1999

Organism	Illnesses	Hospitalizations	Deaths
Bacteria			
Campylobacter Guillain-Barré syndrome (paralysis)	2,000,000	10,500	99
Clostridium perfringens	249,000	40	7
Escherichia coli O157:H7 Bloody diarrhea, kidney damage, hemolytic uremic syndrome	62,500	1,800	52
Escherichia coli, other	31,000	920	26
Listeria monocytogenes Spontaneous abortion, stillbirth, blood infection, meningitis	2,500	2,300	499
Salmonella species	1,300,000	16,000	556
Shigella species Dysentery	90,000	1,250	14
Staphylococcus species	236,000	2,100	2
Vibrio species Chills, fever	5,200	125	31
Yersinia entercolitica	86,700	1,100	2
Protozoa			
Giardia lamblia	200,000	500	1
Toxoplasma gondii Fever, swollen glands, liver and central nervous system complications, brain and eye damage in infants	112,500	2,500	375
Viruses			
Noroviruses (formerly Norwalk-like)	9,200,000	20,000	120

SOURCE: Mead PS, Slutsker L, Dietz V, et al. *Emerging Infectious Diseases* 1999;5:607–625.
NOTE: Illnesses generally include some form of gastrointestinal distress—diarrhea, vomiting, cramps— as well as the problems indicated. These figures continue to constitute the basis of prevalence estimates.

foods, however, do not remain sterile. Microbes in air, water, and other foods can recontaminate them, as can microbes on packages, plates, utensils, cutting boards, and hands. With common measures such as hand washing, dish washing, and other such basic precautions, we live with most food microbes in relative peace. Our digestive and immune systems take care of those that survive cooking. Mostly, we do not worry much about them.

Whether we *should* worry more about them is a matter of how we perceive risk. For most of us as individuals, an occasional episode of stomach upset—if not too severe—is tolerable. From a public health standpoint, however, the cost to society of such episodes is staggeringly high. Table 3 lists, for example, the most frequent causes of foodborne disease, along with estimates of their cost in illness, hospitalization, and death. Viruses cause most foodborne illnesses, but some bacteria and protozoa are also to blame. Nearly all induce highly unpleasant symptoms, usually mild but sometimes very severe. Table 3, however, lists only the best-known pathogens. The causes of the vast majority of episodes of foodborne illness remain obscure.[6] Furthermore, pathogenic microbes pervade the food supply. A *Consumer Reports* investigation in 1998, for example, identified *Campylobacter* in 63% of market chickens, *Salmonella* in 16%, and both in 8%. Pathogenic *Salmonella* can pass from chickens to their eggs. Because egg production is so enormous, a low rate of infection—one out of every 10,000 eggs, for example—means 4.5 million infected eggs each year. [7]

Counting Cases and Estimating Costs

If harmful microbes are widespread in food and if they make so many people sick, why isn't everyone—the food industry, health officials, and the public—doing something to prevent them from getting into food? One reason is that most episodes of food poisoning are not very serious. Another is that it is difficult to collect accurate information about the number of cases and their severity. Attributing a bout of diarrhea to food rather than to other causes is no simple matter. Most of us eat several foods at a time, several times a day, in several different places. How could we possibly know which food might be responsible for our getting sick, especially if there is a delay in the onset of symptoms? I cannot imagine bothering to call a doctor about a brief stomach upset. Even if I did, the doctor might not suspect food as the source of my problem. Busy doctors rarely report such suspicions to health authorities. It usually takes an "outbreak"—the severe illness or death of more than one person eating the same food—before health officials learn about a foodborne illness and attempt to trace its origin.

For these reasons, counting cases is a formidable undertaking, and to this day there is no national system for doing so. The current surveillance system, such as it is, evolved piecemeal. In the 1920s, the Public Health Service started tracking diseases carried in milk. In 1961, the Centers for Disease Control (CDC), an agency of what is now the Department of Health and Human Services (DHHS), took over that task and began to issue annual counts of illnesses transmitted by food and drinking water. Five years later, the CDC initiated a *voluntary* program of state surveillance of outbreaks, meaning that states could choose whether or not to participate.

As early as 1970 the CDC realized that its counts were way too low. Nearly half the participating states were reporting no outbreaks or very few, suggesting considerable underreporting. In 1985, several federal and private agencies began to make more serious attempts to estimate annual cases of foodborne disease, based on two assumptions: (1) an episode of diarrhea counts as a foodborne illness, and (2) the proportion of reported cases to those that are not reported ranges from 1 out of 25 to 1 out of 100 or more. The agencies understood perfectly well that diarrheal diseases could be due to causes other than foodborne illness, and that foodborne illness also causes symptoms other than diarrhea. Nevertheless, they multiplied the number of cases of diarrhea by 25 to 100 to estimate the "real" number of cases. During the next few years, these confusing assumptions led to widely varying guesses about the number of annual cases (6.3 to 81 million) and deaths (500 to 9,000), depending on how the assumptions were interpreted.[8]

In 1996, the CDC initiated a new surveillance program, FoodNet—the Foodborne Diseases Active Surveillance Network—in just a few states and for just seven microbial pathogens. In its first year, FoodNet identified 8,576 laboratory-confirmed cases of foodborne illness, of which 15% resulted in hospitalization. In 1999, the CDC used this and other information from its surveillance networks to suggest that *known* pathogens caused 14 million illnesses, 60,000 hospitalizations, and 1,800 annual deaths. When they added these estimates to those for cases caused by unknown pathogens, they arrived at the annual totals mentioned earlier: 76 million illnesses, 325,000 hospitalizations, and 5,000 deaths.[9] Because these estimates rely so heavily on diarrheal symptoms, and the reporting system is voluntary, these figures almost certainly underestimate the extent of foodborne illness. A 1998 report on food safety from the Institute of Medicine (IOM) in Washington, DC, for example, gave a higher estimate. It assumed that adults in the United States average about 1.4 episodes of diarrhea every year, and that food is implicated in about one-quarter of those episodes; these assumptions yielded an estimate of 91 million cases per year.[10] Some experts suspect that even this number may be too low.

Such uncertainty means that reported trends in foodborne illness must be interpreted with caution. In 2002, FoodNet data suggested that cases of infection from four key pathogens had declined markedly since 1996, but cases caused by some strains of *Salmonella* had increased.[11] Overall, the accuracy and significance of reported trends remain unclear.

If the extent of foodborne illness is uncertain, so must be estimates of its cost to society. Here are some examples of the wide range of figures reported from 1989 to 1998: $4.8 to $23 billion in 1989, $23 million to $6 billion in 1994, $5.6 to $9.4 billion in 1995, $12.9 billion (from illness caused by just six types of bacteria) in 1996, and $37.1 billion in 1998. Agricultural economists estimate that the costs of foodborne illness in children alone came to $2.3 billion in 2000.[12] Whatever the correct figure might be, it surely underestimates the costs to the victims in pain and inconvenience; to taxpayers in medical treatment for the indigent, higher health insurance premiums, public health surveillance systems, and investigations of outbreaks (estimated at $200,000 each); and to the food industry in plant closings, cleanup, and recalls as well as in legal fees, claim settlements, and higher insurance premiums.[8]

Raising the Stakes: Food Sources and Virulence

Regardless of the accuracy of cost and case estimates, one trend is clear: an increasingly broad range of foods is contaminated with harmful bacteria. Back in the 1970s, outbreaks of foodborne illness were most often traced to improperly stored turkey stuffing and deviled eggs prepared by home cooks.[13] Before examining how the food sources of contamination have expanded, we need to deal with one further complication: the distinction between cases and outbreaks. *Cases* refers to the number of individuals who become ill—whether or not they report the disease. In contrast, *outbreaks* always are reported; authorities discover them when more than one person gets sick from the same food source and doctors report the illnesses to health officials. It is easier to identify cases—and, therefore, report them—when an illness occurs right after the food is eaten. Cases that occur with a delay in onset are more difficult to attribute to specific foods and are much more likely to go unreported, even when they affect much larger numbers of people.

With these distinctions in mind, the tracking information indicates a change in the food sources of *outbreaks*: seafood ranks first, followed by eggs, fruits and vegetables (sprouts, lettuce, berries, cantaloupe), beef, poultry, and foods such as salads and sandwiches made with multiple ingredients. In part because so many more meals are consumed outside the home, foods other than those prepared by home cooks now account for 80% of the *outbreaks* (although not necessarily 80% of the *cases* of foodborne illness).[14]

The outbreaks have changed in one additional respect: they are getting nastier. Most used to be due to relatively benign species of *Salmonella, Staphylococcus, Clostridium, Shigella,* and *Vibrio,* but the more pathogenic strains observed since the 1990s are quite unforgiving. Among outbreaks of illness caused by *Listeria monocytogenes,* a particularly virulent species of bacteria, the death rate is 20% (table 3). For example, some years ago a carefully investigated *Listeria* outbreak among 142 people who had eaten a commercially produced unpasteurized soft cheese caused 48 deaths (of which 30 were fetuses or newborn children) and 13 cases of meningitis.[15] *Salmonella* infections can cause arthritis, and *Campylobacter* is a precipitating factor for up to one-fourth of reported cases of Guillain-Barré syndrome, a leading cause of paralytic disease.

Twenty years ago, three of today's worst bacterial pathogens— *Campylobacter, Listeria,* and *E. coli* O157:H7 (described below)—were not recognized as hazards. Also new are bacteria capable of flourishing under refrigeration (*Yersinia* and *Listeria*) or acidic or dry conditions (*E. coli* O157:H7). The alarming survival features of such bacteria undoubtedly evolved in response to changes in methods of food production and distribution that select for the hardiest bacteria and encourage their wide dispersal. Whereas undercooked hamburger and ground beef products used to be the only known source of *E. coli* O157:H7, other foods cross-contaminated by exposure to infected cattle or meat are now involved: apple cider, sprouts, and any number of vegetables. Outbreaks of the especially virulent *Salmonella enteritidis* used to be restricted to eggs; now they have been traced to carriers as unlikely as tomatoes, melons, and orange juice. As we examine the societal and commercial forces that foster these unwelcome trends, we need to understand a bit more about one of the three newly emergent pathogens, *E. coli* O157:H7.

Introducing E. coli O157:H7

E. coli O157:H7 merits special attention not only because of its exceptional virulence but also because it illustrates so well how changes in the food system and in society provide new opportunities for spreading microbial disease through food. When I first encountered the more common form of *E. coli* in a college biology class, instructors presented it as a harmless inhabitant of the digestive tracts of animals and humans, spread by accidental transfer of excreted material. It was known best as an indicator of fecal contamination of water supplies; if water supplies contained E. coli, they were likely to contain more dangerous bacteria. We now know much more about the biology of this organism. Like many bacteria, E. coli is able to accept genes from related bacterial species to form "stable variants" that can pass the borrowed genes along to other bacteria as they divide and multiply (see appendix). The E. coli variant known as O157:H7 is especially dangerous; at some point, it picked up a Shigella gene for a toxin that destroys red blood cells and induces a syndrome of bloody diarrhea, kidney failure, and death. This toxin is particularly damaging to young children.[16]

Other features of the O157:H7 variant are also noteworthy. Unlike common E. coli, this type resists heat; it grows at temperatures up to 44°C (111°F). It also resists drying, can survive short exposures to strong acid (pH 2.5), and sometimes resists radiation and antibiotics. For these reasons, controlling it is not easy. Worse, E. coli O157:H7 is infectious at very low doses. The normal digestive tract contains hundreds of billions of bacteria that compete for space and nutrients. In this environment, it takes thousands of Salmonella to induce symptoms, but the lowest infectious dose of E. coli O157:H7 appears to be less than 50—a minuscule number in bacterial terms. Control measures, therefore, must do more than just prevent growth; they must eliminate the very presence of these bacteria. Foods containing E. coli O157:H7 must be cooked at temperatures high enough to kill all of them. Table 4 presents recommendations for food-handling techniques to prevent problems with this microbe.

E. coli O157:H7 infections originate with farm animals, and such animals increasingly harbor this variant. Although earlier studies suggested that perhaps 10% of adult ruminant (cud-chewing) animals—mainly cows and cattle—were infected with E. coli O157:H7, the proportion now is as high as 28%, and may exceed 40% in slaughtered animals not yet processed. Young infected animals exhibit mild diarrhea, but most do not appear sick and go untreated. Deer, sheep, goats, dogs, birds, and flies also harbor the variant, almost certainly because they have come in contact with cattle feces. People pick up E. coli O157:H7 infections from direct contact with feces, from foods and water that have come in contact with feces, or from infected people who shed it in their feces and pass it along from unwashed hands—which is why hand washing is so important as a control measure. Uncooked foods derived from cattle (raw hamburger, for example) are the origin of most E. coli

TABLE 4. Recommendations for reducing the risk of infection from
E. coli O157:H7

Cook meat—especially ground meat—thoroughly to 160°F.*

Do not drink unpasteurized milk or juices.

Wash fresh fruits and vegetables thoroughly.

Wash hands thoroughly after handling animals, especially cattle, deer, goats, dogs.

Wash hands thoroughly after changing children's diapers or providing care to children or adults with diarrheal diseases.

Do not fertilize fruits or vegetables with manure from ruminant animals.

Avoid swimming in lakes or ponds used by cattle.

Do not drink surface water that has not been chlorinated, boiled, or otherwise treated to eliminate pathogens.

SOURCE: Buchanan RL, Doyle MP. *Food Technology* 1997;51(10):69–76.

*Bringing a food to 155°F is sufficient to kill these bacteria; recommended cooking temperatures provide a 5°F margin of safety. Pasteurization brings liquids to scalding temperatures (about 140°F) for short times; this process destroys most bacteria and delays the growth of those that survive.

O157:H7 outbreaks.[17] As we will see, fruits and vegetables that have come into contact with cattle feces or with contaminated raw meat also have become common sources.

E. coli O157:H7 is considered newly emergent because its recognition is so recent. The earliest case seems to have occurred in 1975, but the first reported outbreak occurred in 1982. Infections have now been observed in 30 countries on six continents. Outbreaks are increasing in frequency; there were 6 in 1997 but 17 in 1998. The infections are exceptionally serious; 82% of people infected with *E. coli* O157:H7 see a physician, 18% require hospitalization, and the mortality rate is 3–5%.[18] How *E. coli* O157:H7 emerged and spread throughout the food supply is a subject of considerable speculation. The most reasonable explanation involves the profound changes in society and food production that have taken place in recent years, matters to which we now turn.

REVOLUTIONIZING THE FOOD SYSTEM

Most of us imagine that the rapid advances in science and medicine of the last century would make microbial diseases a thing of the past, and we would hardly think agriculture to be a cause of medical problems. But alterations in the ways we produce food, choose diets, and live our lives have created conditions that favor the spread of pathogens into more foods consumed by more people. These changes foster the emergence of

TABLE 5. Modern developments in food production practices, dietary preferences, and demographics that favor the emergence and spread of foodborne illness

Food production practices
  Concentration and consolidation of production
  Transportation across long distances
  Centralized processing of food from many sources
  Use of low-dose antibiotics to promote animal growth
  Use of low-fiber animal feeds that promote growth of harmful bacteria
  Employment of a low-income workforce without health and sick-leave benefits
  Centralized production of prepared foods

Dietary preferences
  Emphasis on raw, partially cooked foods
  Use of prepared convenience foods
  Use of takeout foods, restaurant leftovers
  Demand for imported, year-round produce

Demographics
  Increased population of older and chronically ill people more vulnerable to infection
  Increased use of medications that suppress immune function

microbial pathogens that resist heat, cold, acid, and other preservation methods. They also encourage pathogens to develop resistance to treatment with antibiotic drugs. Refer back to figure 2 in the introductory chapter to see how the food system has changed from one based primarily on locally raised meat, fruits, and vegetables to one in which commodities like StarLink corn travel great distances—across many states and between different countries—before reaching supermarkets. Table 5 summarizes some of the developments in food production, consumer preferences, and demographics that favor foodborne illness. Because such developments involve consumers as well as food companies, they illustrate why food safety has to be a shared responsibility but also why it is difficult to determine accountability when outbreaks occur.

Concentrating Production

The most important trends favoring the growth and dispersion of microbial pathogens relate to methods of production, particularly the production of food animals. As a consequence of advances in technology, the globalization of food marketing, and economic imperatives, small farms raising multiple species of animals and crops have been replaced by incomprehensibly large "factory" systems. In the early 1970s, for example, many thousands of small farmers raised chickens; these were supplied by numerous feed mills and processed in thousands of local plants throughout the country. Today, just a few gigantic corporations control every aspect of chicken production, from egg to grocery store.

One measure of industry concentration is the proportion of an industry controlled by its four leading firms. The proportion of chickens slaughtered by the top four chicken-processing corporations increased from 18% in 1972 to 49% in 1998. Similarly, the top four hog-slaughtering firms controlled 32% of all hogs processed in 1972, but 43% in 1992, and the top four cattle-slaughtering firms increased their share from 30% in 1972 to 79% by 1998. Equivalent trends are seen in the dairy industry.[19] As a further example of such consolidation, Tyson Foods, "the world's largest fully integrated producer, processor and marketer of chicken and chicken-based convenience foods," merged with IBP, "the world's largest supplier of premium fresh beef and pork products," to create the world's largest provider of animal protein. This 2001 merger resulted in a company that controls about 28% of the world's beef, 25% of the chicken, and 18% of the pork.[20]

The most obvious effect of industry consolidation is to bring unimaginably large numbers of animals (or their meat) in close contact during production, transportation, slaughter, and processing. Raising large populations of chickens or cattle in one location means dealing with more manure than can possibly be contained or converted to fertilizer. Such practices have profound effects on the environment as well as on human health.[21] When farmers raise just a few animals, they can compost the waste, a process that usually generates enough heat to kill bacteria. In addition to the environmental problems brought on by excessive manure, the use of raw—rather than composted—waste to fertilize fields and orchards brings pathogenic bacteria into contact with grains, vegetables, and fruits not usually contaminated with such organisms.[22]

The concentration of cattle production means that animals are transported across long distances, crowded together in railroad cars. Unlike poultry, beef cattle are shipped from one location to another at various growth stages—between the U.S. and Mexico, for example—increasing the opportunity for bacteria to spread. Large holding pens also expose animals to common sources of food and water, meaning that a foodborne or waterborne infection can quickly reach large numbers of animals. Animals from many locations arrive at the slaughterhouse together and remain in close contact until killed; their carcasses remain in close contact until processed. Contact alone favors the spread of pathogens.

When it comes to processing, the implications of concentrated production are quite startling. Think, for a moment, about ground beef. To grind beef for hamburger, processors take beef from many sources—even from different states—mix it together and grind it. Packers regrind it, and grocers sometimes regrind it again. The result? Health officials estimate that just one infected beef carcass is sufficient to contaminate eight *tons* of ground beef. Even more remarkable, investigators once traced back the origin of a *single* lot of hamburger at one processing plant to slaughterhouses in six different states and to an almost unimaginable 443 individual animals.[23] It is difficult to imagine a system better equipped to promote the spread of disease—and to obscure the source of illnesses or outbreaks.

Single-source outbreaks, however, also illustrate the vulnerability of a centralized food supply. In the most dramatic instance, a *Salmonella* outbreak in 1994 affected more than 220,000 people in 41 states. Its source was a surprise: packaged ice cream. The ice cream was produced from a premixed liquid base delivered to the processing plant in a tanker truck that previously had carried unpasteurized liquid eggs.[24] Such incidents are fully preventable, as these chapters explain.

Abusing Antibiotics

The use of antibiotics in animal agriculture affects foodborne illness in ways that are especially troubling. Growers treat infected animals with antibiotics, of course, but they sometimes give antibiotics to whole herds or flocks as a preventive measure. Despite the questionable effects of this practice, what most alarms safety experts is the *routine* use of low-dose antibiotic drugs as growth promoters, a practice that began in the 1950s and seems impossible to stop. Antibiotics are chemicals that prevent bacteria from reproducing (see chapter 6), but for reasons poorly understood, animals grow faster and need less feed when low-dose antibiotics are added to their food or drinking water. This treatment kills some bacteria, but not all; those naturally resistant to the antibiotics survive and multiply. The unintended consequence of this practice is the proliferation of antibiotic-resistant bacteria. If antibiotic-resistant bacteria infect people and cause disease, the disease will be untreatable.

This possibility is not merely theoretical. By the mid-1970s, researchers *already* knew that such uses increased the population of antibiotic-resistant bacteria in farm animals as well as in their human caretakers. In 1977, alarmed by such findings, the FDA proposed to restrict the use of antibiotics in animal feed. Congress, however, overruled this idea under pressure from farm-state lawmakers, livestock producers, and the makers of the drugs. These groups all argued that such restrictions were unwarranted because they were not sufficiently supported by science.[25] This early blockage of safety regulations established a seemingly unshakable precedent.

In the following years, researchers reported that pathogenic bacteria resistant to *multiple* antibiotics could be passed from animals to humans. Every time the FDA attempted to restrict the use of the drugs, Congress again intervened, mainly as a result of drug industry lobbying and the invocation of "science" as an obstructive measure. Instead of taking action, Congress ordered the FDA to conduct further studies. By the early 1980s, the FDA stopped fighting this issue and instead proposed more relaxed standards, leading one Congressman to observe that the driving force behind the FDA's retreat on this issue was "protection of the health of the animal drug industry."[26]

In the mid-1990s, scientists demonstrated that *Campylobacter* resistant to high-potency antibiotics could be transferred from chickens to humans. The dangers of antibiotic-resistant foodborne bacteria were becoming more evident as more species acquired resistance to more and more antibiotics. Although calls for corrective action increased in urgency, a committee of the National Research Council (NRC) argued in 1999, "the use of drugs in the food-animal production industry is not without some problems and concerns, but it does not appear to constitute an immediate public health concern."[27] At least one critic viewed this surprisingly sanguine conclusion as just what one might expect when members of a scientific panel are "overwhelmingly associated with or linked to the drug industry."[28]

During this period, the European Union (EU) banned four animal antibiotics and proposed a total ban on the use of antibiotics as growth promoters. U.S. agencies finally developed plans for dealing with the problem in 1999 and 2000. These plans are already too little, too late. In 2001, the *New England Journal of Medicine* reported that up to 80% of meat packages—pork, chicken, or beef—collected from local supermarkets contained antibiotic-resistant bacteria. These bacteria survived a week or two in the intestines of people who ate them; if these people became ill, the antibiotics would not help.[29] Beef, pork, and poultry producers—and drug manufacturers—continue to oppose restrictions on the use of antibiotics in animal agriculture. Their arguments: antibiotics are essential to their industries, most animal producers use antibiotics prudently, and the dangers of transfer of antibiotic resistance from animals to people are unproven. By one estimate, nearly 25 million pounds of antibiotics are used in animal agriculture, whereas just 3 million are used to treat human infections. Altogether, nearly three-fourths of all antibiotics are used for nontherapeutic purposes in animals. On this basis, consumer groups, food-safety alliances, and some members of Congress have called for outright bans on use of antibiotics in farm animals, except for therapeutic purposes.[30]

Given the disproportionate use of antibiotics in animal agriculture, it is not surprising that the drug industry opposes any suggestion to ban their use and much prefers "judicious use and robust surveillance" as control strategies.[31] While the dispute rages on, the use of animal antibiotics continues. In this case, politics trumps science.

Two additional features of this situation are particularly compelling: (1) studies now indicate that induction of antibiotic resistance in bacteria is reversible, and (2) prevention of animal infections can be accomplished by means other than antibiotics. In 2002, Belgian researchers reported that banning certain antibiotics from use in animal feed decreases the prevalence of antibiotic-resistant bacteria and makes the drugs more effective in treating microbial illness in hospital patients. In part as a result of such findings, three large poultry producers in the United States announced in 2002 that they would reduce or eliminate the use of antibiotics in feed for healthy chickens.[32] This action—if diligently taken—is a useful step in reducing antibiotic resistance.

Another idea is to prevent the proliferation of E. coli O157:H7 in animals without using antibiotics by changing the way they are fed. Typically, producers feed cattle soy and corn to fatten the animals just before slaughter; these foods are low in fiber, reduce the acidity of digestive solutions, and promote the growth of unfriendly bacteria. In contrast, feeding high-fiber hay to ruminant animals selects for friendlier bacteria capable of breaking down cellulose to usable nutrients. Animals fed hay prior to slaughter generate less than 1% of the E. coli O157:H7 usually present in the feces of grain-fed animals, and they become free of the undesirable bacteria in just a few days. Adding certain strains of lactic acid bacteria—a friendly species—to cattle feed also interferes with the proliferation of E. coli O157:H7. The identification of E. coli O157:H7 infections in increasing numbers of farm animals makes such methods especially attractive as preventive measures.[33] Such low-tech approaches are unlikely to appeal to meat producers concerned about putting the maximum possible weight on their animals, however, or to drug companies eager to continue selling antibiotics to meat producers; billions of dollars are at stake. The government cannot intervene in this matter because, as the next chapter explains, USDA authority begins at the slaughterhouse; the agency has no authority whatsoever over farm practices.

Evolving Dietary Preferences and Demographics

Changes in society and in the behavior of consumers also contribute to the spread of harmful bacteria in food. Table 5 (page 43) summarizes them. Women left home to go to work, commuting distances increased, and work hours lengthened. As a result, convenience is a critically important issue in food choice. People eat more food outside the home and more food prepared in advance by others. Meals prepared in restaurants and other institutions account for roughly half of all national food expenditures. Centralized food production, of course, presents ample opportunities for spreading microbial pathogens from a common source.

Preferences for fresh fruits and vegetables—the object of much nutritional advice—also present such opportunities. Demands for strawberries and tomatoes in winter require fruits and vegetables to be imported from warmer countries in Asia, Latin America, and North Africa, where water quality and sanitation facilities do not necessarily meet U.S. standards. An unchlorinated water supply in a developing country is a good reason to avoid eating its vegetables raw, or its fruit unpeeled. Nevertheless, the United States imported nearly $1.4 billion worth of fresh vegetables (asparagus, cucumbers, peppers, tomatoes, and others) from one such country, Mexico, in 2000. Imported fruits and vegetables are supposed to meet U.S. sanitation standards, but sometimes do not.[34] Dealing with the safety of imported produce is politically sensitive on a number of levels. If we reject foods from a developing country, we hurt its economy. But if we accept them without more stringent controls, we make the foods more vulnerable to contamination or to threats of bioterrorism, as we will see in the concluding chapter.

Efforts to market fruits and vegetables in forms that require less preparation time and are more convenient for consumers also create opportunities for cross-contamination. Precut fruits and vegetables, preprepared salad mixes, salad bar items, and packaged juices all require handling, transport, and storage. Such foods increasingly become sources of outbreaks. Problems occur when the foods come in contact with animal feces prior to processing, with contaminated equipment during processing, or with infected people who handle them at any point.

Even when foods are cooked or pasteurized, they can be recontaminated. Foods prepared in supermarkets, restaurants, and convenience stores are often made in advance and stored for hours, allowing time for bacteria to proliferate. It was a relief to read about a 1999 investigation of New York City salad bars that found no trace of *E. coli* O157:H7. Investigators discovered that foods in some of these places exceeded allowable limits of *Salmonella*, however.[35]

The more people who handle foods between harvest and consumption, the greater the chance of passing along a foodborne illness. Thus, working conditions are critical factors in food safety. To pick just one example: when the rules in meatpacking plants restrict bathroom breaks, workers are forced, as one investigator puts the matter, to "urinate on the job."[36] Many jobs in food preparation and service pay minimum wages and provide no health care benefits or paid sick-leave—conditions that encourage people to work while they are ill. Workers in low-paying jobs are rarely trained in food safety. When such training is available, it usually requires proficiency in English. Workers who cannot understand food safety instructions or the importance of basic preventive measures (hand washing, for example) are not likely to follow safe procedures for food handling. A final factor is demographic. Because the population of the United States is aging rapidly, overall susceptibility to foodborne illness is increasing. From 1965 to 1995, the number of Americans aged 65 and over grew by 82%; one-fifth of the population is expected to be older than 65 within the next three decades. Immune function declines somewhat with age, but medications are a greater problem. Older adults often take multiple medications to treat whatever ailments they may have, and the drugs—paradoxically—sometimes compromise immune function and increase vulnerability to infectious agents.[37]

Arguing for a Historical Perspective

The trends summarized in table 5 interact to favor the emergence of new and more resistant bacteria able to make their way into a greater variety of foods and to inflict more damage on more people than formerly was possible. Because human factors such as improper food handling and depressed immunity influence the spread of foodborne illness, and because cooking kills most pathogens, the food industry and government have tended to downplay concerns about microbes that contaminate foods during production or processing. Instead, they blame outbreaks on consumers or on the people who prepare the food where it is served. This attitude should make us ask: why can't we expect meat and poultry—and, therefore, fruits and vegetables—to be free of harmful bacteria *before* the foods arrive in restaurants or home kitchens? And why doesn't government do a better job of controlling harmful bacteria in meat and poultry? Examination of such questions requires a look back in history as a basis for understanding the present relationships among the chief players in the food safety system—food producers, regulatory agencies, and Congress.

THE ORIGINS OF FEDERAL OVERSIGHT, 1875–1906

Prior to the late 1800s, the U.S. government took no responsibility for food safety. It was forced to do so by public demands elicited by the accounts of muckraking journalists who visited slaughterhouses and shared their unsettling experiences. Here, for example, is one of the *milder* passages from Lafcadio Hearn's 1875 report of his comparative visits to stockyards run by Gentiles and Jews:

> To describe one Gentile slaughter-house is to describe the majority . . .
> an impression of gloom and bad smells; daylight peering through loose
> planking; the head of a frightened bullock peering over the pen door;
> blood, thick and black, clotting on the floor, or oozing from the nostrils
> and throats of dying cattle; entrails, bluey-white and pale yellow . . .
> butchers, bare-legged and bare-armed, paddling about in the blood;
> naked feet encrusted with gore. . . . All this, however, is the brighter side
> of the picture—the mere background to darker and fouler things.[38]

The outrage generated by such accounts encouraged some meat packers to institute voluntary inspection programs. Furthermore, several countries in Europe refused to buy U.S. exports because they were suspicious about the safety of American beef. In what is still an endlessly recurrent theme, Congress acted to prevent meat safety from being used as a trade barrier. In 1890, it passed a Meat Inspection Act that authorized inspection of salt pork, bacon, and pigs intended for export.[39]

In addition to popular pressures to clean up meat production, Dr. Harvey Wiley (who headed the USDA's Bureau of Chemistry, which later became the FDA) relentlessly promoted reform laws to improve the safety of other foods. Nevertheless, federal involvement in food safety remained minimal.[40] This complacency ended abruptly in 1906 when Upton Sinclair published his dramatic exposé of the meat industry, *The Jungle*. Two years earlier, the editor of a Midwestern populist weekly had recruited Sinclair to do some investigative reporting on conditions in the Chicago stockyards. After a seven-week stay, Sinclair wrote up his findings, not—as might be expected—as an investigative report, but rather as a serialized work of fiction, chapter by chapter, in 1905. *The Jungle* came out as a novel the following year, and continues to be so germane to modern society that it has never gone out of print.

The book's longevity is particularly noteworthy because Sinclair was not especially interested in cattle, meat, or the food system. Instead, his explicit purpose in writing the book was political: to demonstrate the benefits of *socialism*. His novel is the story of poor European immigrants forced to take jobs in the Chicago stockyards and to endure the day-to-day anguish of "stupefying, brutalizing work." A few passages suffice to capture the spirit, power, and relevance of this book to current food safety concerns:

> The "Union Stockyards" were never a pleasant place. . . . All day long the blazing midsummer sun beat down upon that square mile of abominations: upon tens of thousands of cattle crowded into pens whose wooden floors stank and steamed contagion; upon . . . huge blocks of dingy meat factories, whose labyrinthine passages defied a breath of fresh air to penetrate them; and there were . . . rivers of hot blood, and car-loads of moist flesh, and rendering vats and soap caldrons, glue factories and fertilizer tanks, that smelt like the craters of hell.[41]

Sinclair's accounts of the production of ground meat and sausages were enough to turn the staunchest stomach: "The meat would be shoveled into carts, and the man who did the shoveling would not trouble to lift out a rat even when he saw one." Or this: "The workers fell into the vats; and when they were fished out, there was never enough of them to be worth exhibiting—sometimes they would be overlooked for days, till all but the bones of them had gone out to the world as Durham's Pure Leaf Lard!"

With respect to the behavior of government inspectors, Sinclair raised issues entirely relevant a century later.

> Before the carcass was admitted here, however, it had to pass a government inspector, who sat in the doorway and felt of the glands in the neck for tuberculosis. This government inspector did not have the manner of a man who was worked to death. . . . If you were a sociable person, he was quite willing to enter into conversation with you, and to explain to you the deadly nature of the ptomaines which are found in tubercular

pork; and while he was talking with you, you could hardly be so ungrateful as to notice that a dozen carcasses were passing him untouched.[41]

When ensuing investigations confirmed the worst of Sinclair's charges, Congress immediately passed two separate pieces of reform legislation: the Pure Food and Drugs Act and the Meat Inspection Act, both of 1906.[42] Congress designed these laws to prevent sales of "adulterated" foods, meaning those that were spoiled, altered in some way to make them unsafe, or labeled in some misleading manner. In accepting food safety as a federal responsibility, Congress assigned oversight entirely to the USDA, largely because that agency employed veterinary specialists who could recognize sick animals and keep them out of the food supply.[43] Because the two laws had different purposes, the USDA divided the oversight authority between two of its administrative units. It assigned responsibility for the Meat Inspection Act to its Bureau of Animal Industry, and it made the Bureau of Chemistry responsible for carrying out the provisions of the Pure Food and Drugs Act. This division established a dual system of rules and responsibilities that carries forward to the present—and still causes no end of trouble.

The Meat Inspection Act defined the regulatory system that continues to govern USDA actions. At the time of its enactment, the law required the USDA to appoint government inspectors, some trained as veterinarians, and install them in every one of the 163 slaughter and packing plants then in existence. It required Bureau of Animal Industry inspectors to examine all animals before and after slaughter and packing, and to reject and destroy animals that were "filthy, decomposed, or putrid." Inspectors were to examine *every* animal submitted for slaughter, set apart those showing symptoms of disease, and stamp the acceptable carcasses and meat as "inspected and passed." To decide whether an animal was free of disease, inspectors used their senses: sight, touch, and smell. These sensory methods, now categorized condescendingly as "poke and sniff," could identify most sick animals and allow inspectors to exclude them from the food supply. Indeed, diseases caused by animal illnesses (trichinosis from pork, for example) declined markedly. "Poke and sniff" methods, however, could only identify grossly sick animals; they could not possibly "see" invisible bacteria or infections that did not make the animals sick.[44]

The 1906 Meat Inspection Act limited the bureau's authority to regulate meat safety in other ways that make it difficult to deal with today's microbial pathogens. For one thing, the law specified that the department's authority began at the *slaughterhouse*. USDA inspectors had no right to examine animals on the farm, in transport, or at any other time before they arrived for slaughter. The law created a second serious impediment: the USDA had no right to recall meat once it left the plant. If USDA inspectors believed that a packing plant was producing tainted meat, their only recourse was to deny further inspection, in effect forcing the plant to close. Finally, the law placed the burden of guaranteeing meat as safe on government inspectors—whose inspection stamp implied wholesomeness—rather than on producers or processors. Whether the effects of its intentions were deliberate or not, the 1906 Congress established an oversight system that permitted the industry to rely on (and, therefore, blame) USDA inspectors for the most fundamental decisions about plant operations. Slaughterhouses and processing plants were to open when the inspector said they could and close when the inspector left for the day. If the inspector *said* that meat was safe, it was—and the producers and packers did not need to do anything else to ensure the safety of their products. As we will see, the modern consequences of these century-old congressional decisions continue to act as barriers to food safety reforms.

In sharp contrast, the 1906 Pure Food and Drugs Act did not require the USDA's Bureau of Chemistry to conduct continuous inspections. Instead, it instructed the Bureau to collect *samples* of foods and food products and determine whether they were "adulterated" or misleadingly labeled. If the bureau found a product to be unsafe or mislabeled, however, it could not block sales. Instead, it had to notify the manufacturer and request voluntary recall or hold hearings and take the company to court. Congress must have sensed that the differences in functions and procedures spelled out in the two laws would cause conflict because it also required the secretaries of the departments of Treasury, Agriculture, Commerce, and Labor to "make uniform rules and regulations for carrying out the provisions of this Act." The House wanted the Food and Drugs law to establish food standards that could serve as a basis for enforcement, but the more business-oriented Senate was "unalterably opposed" to this idea and agreed to pass the bill only if that provision were dropped.[45] As I discussed in my book *Food Politics,* the issue of food standards also has caused endless controversy during the intervening century.

Despite these limitations (and in contrast to the results of the Meat Inspection Act), the 1906 Pure Food and Drugs Act made food *producers* responsible for the safety of their products, and assigned government the role of enforcement. Food producers immediately objected to the enforcement aspects of the legislation and initiated lawsuits, thereby establishing a pattern that continues to this day. Dr. Wiley, who demanded much of the credit for enactment of the Pure Food and Drugs law, viewed his bureau's enforcement role as nothing less than a battle of the forces of righteousness against evil:

> For a third of a century, the fight for pure food has been waged and the end is not yet. . . . It was and is a struggle for human rights as much as for the Revolution or the Civil War. A battle for the privilege of going free of robbery and with a guaranty of health, it has been and is a fight for the individual right against the vested interest, of the man against the dollar. . . . The defeated squadrons . . . went to court, demanded executive action, resulting in an order that the Bureau bring no action. . . . It was a complete triumph for the hosts of Satan. . . . Inspired by a questionable zeal, I held on, hoping that . . . the spirit of service to the people might again enter into the heart of our high rulers.[46]

In subsequent years, amendments to both laws expanded the USDA's inspection authority but also increased the divergence of responsibilities between its two bureaus. For example, the 1906 Meat Inspection Act did not apply to poultry, which was then largely produced on small farms for local sale. As production grew in size and concentration, large flocks of chickens occasionally suffered from outbreaks of influenza. These illnesses worried consumers. To help the industry overcome fears that its chickens might transmit disease, the USDA encouraged voluntary inspection and certification programs. The department reasoned—correctly—that consumers were more likely to buy poultry when it was stamped "inspected for wholesomeness by U.S. Department of Agriculture." Legislation passed in 1957 and 1968 made these programs mandatory and required the USDA to inspect most chickens and turkeys sold to the public. Throughout the twentieth century, the USDA remained in charge of meat and poultry safety through a firmly entrenched inspection system now run by the department's Food Safety and Inspection Service (FSIS). Over the years, reorganizations of USDA agencies and amendments to the Pure Food and Drugs Act led to the creation of the FDA in 1930, its transfer *out* of USDA in 1940 and, eventually, its incorporation into the Department of Health and Human Services.[10] As we will see, meat inspections remained under USDA control, not only because the agency employed veterinarians, but also because meat and dairy producers, who did not hesitate to express themselves about the matter, much preferred its sympathetic stance on regulatory issues to the more rigorous enforcement approach of the FDA—a legacy of its founder, Dr. Wiley.

UNDERSTANDING FOOD SAFETY OVERSIGHT

A century later, the consequences of the division of food safety oversight are only too evident. The initial system worked well to keep sick animals out of the food supply but was poorly designed to deal with the challenge of microbes that affected a wider variety of foods. Congress passed subsequent amendments to the two 1906 laws without much concern about the need to coordinate oversight of the food supply as a whole. As one General Accounting Office (GAO) official explained to Congress,

> The federal regulatory system for food safety did not emerge from a comprehensive design but rather evolved piecemeal, typically in response to particular health threats or economic crises. Addressing one new worry after another, legislators amended old laws and enacted new ones. The resulting organizational and legal patchwork has given responsibility for specific food commodities to different agencies and provided them with significantly different regulatory authorities and responsibilities.[47]

Today, an inventory of federal food safety activities reveals a system breathtaking in its irrationality: 35 separate laws administered by 12 agencies housed in six cabinet-level departments. Table 6 lists these agencies and summarizes their areas of responsibility. At best, a structure as fragmented as this one would require extraordinary efforts to achieve communication, let alone coordination, and more than 50 interagency agreements govern such efforts. Among the six agencies with the broadest mandates, *all* conduct inspections and collect and analyze samples, and at least three—though not necessarily the same ones—have something to do with regulating dairy products, for example, as well as eggs and egg products, fruits and vegetables, grains, and meat and poultry. Until recently, the system had no mission statement (for whatever such statements are worth), and it still does not have consistent rules, clear lines of authority, a rational allocation of resources, or standards against which to measure success. With such a system, some issues—such as the use of animal manure to fertilize food crops—inevitably fall between the cracks and are governed by no rules whatsoever.[48]

The consequences of this system are famously absurd, and table 7 summarizes some of the more exquisite examples. The USDA, for example,

TABLE 6. The distribution of U.S. government regulatory responsibility for food safety, and annual budget allocations, 2000

Government Agency	Budget ($ million)
Department of Health and Human Services (DHHS)	
Food and Drug Administration (FDA)	$283
Regulates all foods (except meat, poultry, and processed eggs)	
Regulates animal drugs and feeds	
Centers for Disease Control and Prevention (CDC)	29
Surveys and investigates foodborne disease outbreaks	
U.S. Department of Agriculture (USDA)	
Food Safety and Inspection Service (FSIS)	712
Inspects meat, poultry, and pasteurized and processed eggs	
Agricultural Marketing Service (AMS)	13
Regulates safety of eggs and egg products	
Inspects egg, dairy, fruit, vegetable, meat, and poultry products	
Grain Inspection, Packers and Stockyards Administration (GIPSA)	*
Inspects corn, sorghum, rice for aflatoxin	
Animal and Plant Health Inspection Service (APHIS)	*
Protects animals and plants from diseases and pests	
Agricultural Research Service (ARS)	82
Conducts research on food safety	
Environmental Protection Agency (EPA)	171
Regulates pesticides and genetically modified plant pesticides	
Establishes pesticide tolerance limits	
U.S. Department of the Treasury	
Bureau of Alcohol, Tobacco and Firearms (ATF)	*
Regulates production, distribution, and labeling of alcoholic beverages	
(exception: FDA regulates wines containing less than 7% alcohol)	
Customs Service	*
Examines and collects food import samples	
U.S. Department of Commerce	
National Marine Fisheries Service	*
Conducts voluntary seafood inspection program	
Certifies seafood-based animal feeds and pet foods	
Federal Trade Commission (FTC)	*
Regulates advertising of food products	

SOURCE: Robinson RA. General Accounting Office (GAO-02-47T), October 10, 2001.
*Information not available, or amounts too low to record. The total federal food safety budget indicated here is just under $1.3 billion for fiscal year 2000.

TABLE 7. The illogical division of food safety oversight between
the U.S. Department of Agriculture (USDA) and the Food and Drug
Administration (FDA)

USDA Regulates	FDA Regulates
Hot dogs in pastry dough	Hot dogs in rolls
Corn dogs	Bagel dogs
Open-face meat and poultry sandwiches	Closed-face meat and poultry sandwiches
Soups with more than 2% meat and poultry	Soups with less than 2% meat and poultry
Spaghetti sauce with meat stock	Spaghetti sauce without meat stock
Pizza with meat toppings	Cheese pizza
Beans with more than 2% bacon	Beans with pork (no limit)

SOURCE: Robinson RA. General Accounting Office (GAO-02-47T), October 10, 2001.

oversees production of hot dogs in pastry dough; the FDA regulates hot
dogs in rolls. The USDA regulates corn dogs; the FDA regulates bagel
dogs. The USDA regulates pepperoni pizza; the FDA regulates cheese
pizza. And try to explain the one illustrated in figure 4: the USDA regulates beef broth, but the FDA regulates chicken broth; for dehydrated
broths, the agencies switch.[49]

Under the current system, a sandwich made with bread, ham, cheese,
lettuce, and tomato raises regulatory issues of terrifying complexity. If
the sandwich is made with one slice of bread, it falls under USDA rules;
if it is made with two slices, it is the FDA's responsibility. To protect the
safety of such a sandwich, three cabinet-level federal agencies—the FDA,
EPA, and USDA (including four major divisions of the latter)—oversee
its farm-to-table production. Because the USDA performs daily on-site
inspections but the FDA inspects plants under its jurisdiction only about
once every five years, any facility producing a food that involves both
agencies must deal with inspectors operating under two entirely different sets of guidelines and schedules. State inspectors add a third level of
inconsistent oversight.

These examples are amusing but unlikely to be dangerous. Four federal agencies, however, oversee one aspect or another of the safety of egg
and egg products, a situation that directly affects control of *Salmonella
enteritidis*. In the U.S., 45% of all egg-laying flocks are now infected with
this pathogen, which largely replaced less virulent forms of the bacteria
in chicken flocks during the 1960s. This replacement was not inevitable;

USDA Regulated   **FDA Regulated**

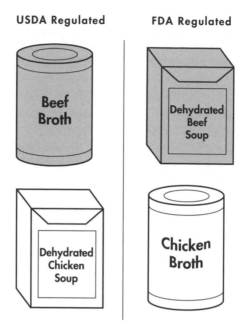

FIGURE 4. An example of the inconsistent and
illogical federal oversight of the safety of beef and
chicken broths. The U.S. Department of Agriculture (USDA) regulates beef broth and dehydrated
chicken soup, but the Food and Drug Administration (FDA) regulates dehydrated beef soup
and chicken broth. (Source: General Accounting
Office, GAO/RCED-92-152, June 1992.)

only five flocks infected with *S. enteritidis* have been identified in Sweden, for example, since 1987. Chickens infected with *S. enteritidis* do not
usually become sick, but they pass the bacteria along to their eggs and
to each other. Although the FDA is responsible for preventing transmission of foodborne illness from animals to humans, it inspects shell eggs,
not hen houses. Three USDA agencies have some responsibility for eggs.
The Animal and Plant Health Inspection Service (APHIS) oversees animal health but not egg safety—because the chickens are not sick. The
Agricultural Marketing Service (AMS) grades eggs for size and quality
but does not oversee their safety. The Food Safety and Inspection Service (FSIS) inspects liquid, frozen, and powdered egg products but not
shell eggs. Even though more than 10,000 cases of *S. enteritidis* infections are reported each year, and more than 600,000 cases are suspected,

these kinds of divisions impede cooperation, and none of the agencies has established a program to keep eggs free of a pathogen contributing to substantial illness in the population.[50]

Even with the best of intentions, it would be difficult to keep up with food safety problems given the changes in the U.S. food system since 1906. By the early 1980s, for example, the poultry industry had already expanded far beyond any reasonable inspection capacity. In 1975, USDA officials examined 14 billion pounds of birds at 154 plants; just six years later they had to inspect 29 billion pounds at 371 plants. The USDA has 7,000 inspectors or so, and they oversee 6,000 meat, poultry, and egg establishments—and 130 importers—that slaughter and process 89 million pigs, 37 million cattle, and 7 billion chickens and turkeys, not to mention the 25 billion pounds of beef and 7 billion pounds of ground beef produced each year. Today's poultry plants slaughter and process more than 90 birds per minute on production lines, and each USDA inspector must examine 35 birds per minute.[51] No matter how impossible such demands may be, current laws require USDA inspectors to examine every carcass, and they do so to the best of their abilities.

If anything, the demands on FDA are even more unreasonable. About 700 FDA inspectors must oversee 30,000 food manufacturers and processors, 20,000 warehouses, 785,000 commercial and institutional food establishments, 128,000 grocery and convenience stores, and 1.5 million vending operations. The agency also must deal with food imports, which comprised 40% of the country's supply of fresh fruits and vegetables and 68% of the seafood in 2000. The FDA's budget allocation for inspection purposes was just $283 million in 2000, minuscule by any standard of federal expenditure. It is not surprising that the FDA conducted only 5,000 inspections annually, visited less than 2% of the places under its jurisdiction, and inspected less than 1% of imported foods prior to 2001, when threats of bioterrorism temporarily forced improvements.[52]

Although the USDA has more than twice the budget and ten times the employees of the FDA, it regulates just 20% of the food supply, and foods under its jurisdiction account for just 15% of reported foodborne illnesses. A few years ago, Congress required the USDA to take its responsibilities more seriously, and the agency appointed an undersecretary for food safety. Within the arcane world of government, however, this official outranks the FDA commissioner, and the status differences add to coordination difficulties. The FDA chafes at the imbalance in budget and personnel resources, but has little clout with Congress. One

reason for its relatively low status is industry lobbying against regulations perceived as unfriendly. A more profound reason is rooted in the
history discussed here. Because the FDA began as a division of the USDA,
its budget allocations still come from congressional *agriculture* committees—not those concerned with health. Such committees view the FDA's
strictly science-based regulatory posture as unfriendly to agriculture and
to business (witness the FDA's unsuccessful attempt to regulate tobacco
as a drug), and they react accordingly.

Within FDA itself, the regulation of microbial hazards in food seems
less important than dealing with drugs or medical devices. In my six years
as a member of the FDA's Food Advisory Committee and, later, its Science Board, I often observed the agency's resistance to criticism—even
from groups supportive of its mission—and its apparent perception of
food issues as troublesome and unscientific rather than as challenging
problems demanding a high priority and focused attention. The FDA's
priorities, of course, also are shaped by budget restrictions and by congressional interventions, industry lawsuits, and intense pressures related
to other food issues under its domain: food labeling, health claims, dietary supplements, and—as I explain in part 2 of this book—genetically
modified foods.

Even this brief overview suggests why efforts to control foodborne
microbes are likely to prove contentious. Food safety politics involves
diverse stakeholders with highly divergent goals. In an environment of
food overabundance, food producers must compete for shares of the consumer's food dollar. One way to do this is by taking advantage of a divided, inconsistent, and illogical federal regulatory system. Food companies owe their primary allegiance to stockholders, and their principal
goal must be profit, not public health. Whenever safety measures raise
costs or intrude on autonomy, the affected industries mobilize their considerable political power to block actions perceived as unfavorable—even
when such measures are strongly supported by science (example: antibiotics). Government regulatory agencies also engage in competition,
in this case among themselves for scarce resources and territorial mandates. As we will see, they often appear to be more concerned about protecting their own turf—or that of the industries they regulate—than
about protecting the health of consumers. The public, unaware of such
disputes, simply wants food to be safe and assumes that both industry
and government share that goal and are doing everything possible to
achieve it.

In this environment, the various participants in the food system blame one another (but never themselves) when outbreaks occur. The costs of foodborne illness to individuals, to society, and to food companies should encourage everyone to collaborate in efforts to ensure safe food. That the groups do not collaborate is a curious consequence of food safety politics. In the remaining chapters in part 1 we will see how the initial distinctions in the legal mandates of the USDA and FDA affected their dealings with the food industries they regulate—particularly meat producers and processors—as the agencies attempted to protect the public against microbial illnesses transmitted through food.

CHAPTER 2

RESISTING MEAT AND POULTRY REGULATION, 1974–1994

IN CHAPTER 1, WE SAW HOW THE INITIAL DIVISION OF FOOD safety oversight between two federal agencies led to a system poorly equipped to deal with food pathogens. In this chapter and the next, we will see how century-old laws affected government responses to incidents caused by newly emergent pathogens, and how food producers used those laws to avoid having to change their practices. Because food animals are the ultimate source of pathogens, these chapters focus on disputes over meat safety, particularly those that involve attempts by the U.S. Department of Agriculture (USDA) to require the meat and poultry industries to control pathogens. Although meat includes pork and lamb as well as beef, and poultry includes turkeys as well as chickens, this chapter uses the phrase *meat and poultry* as shorthand for beef and chicken, and sometimes uses *meat* to refer to both.

I have two additional reasons for emphasizing meat safety. First, as I discussed in *Food Politics,* meat and poultry producers are especially adept at using the political system to their own advantage. They generously support both political parties, form close personal relationships with members of Congress and officials of regulatory agencies, and often use the so-called revolving door to exchange their executives' positions for those in government and vice versa. When meat producers complain about policies that appear unfavorable to their interests, government officials listen. As noted earlier, meat producers make little attempt to hide their lobbying activities, and their motives are transparent and readily documented. Second, as these chapters explain, the history of attempts to regulate the beef and chicken industries illustrates issues germane to other food commodities and products.

This chapter and the next recount events in the history of meat and poultry regulation from the early 1970s to the early 2000s. These events each illustrate one or more of the issues that make food safety political: (1) the weaknesses—grounded in past and present history—of the current governmental oversight system; (2) the close personal and professional relationships of meat and poultry producers with officials of Congress and regulatory agencies, particularly the USDA; (3) the consistent and often successful efforts of these industries to block regulations that might adversely affect their commercial interests; (4) the industries' denial of responsibility for outbreaks of foodborne illness; and (5) their invocation of science as a means to prevent unwanted oversight.

This chapter describes the events leading up to federal attempts to control microbial pathogens through development of the science-based preventive measures known collectively as *Pathogen Reduction: Hazard Analysis Critical Control Point (HACCP)*. Chapter 3 explains how the regulated industries reacted once the USDA and the Food and Drug Administration (FDA) finally required them to install and adhere to HACCP rules. We will see that HACCP systems hold great promise for protecting the food supply, especially when they require testing for microbial pathogens. To understand why meat and poultry producers—and their friends in Congress and the USDA—so resisted this approach, we must first examine the historical basis of the close working partnerships among these industries and government officials, committees, and agencies.

THE USDA'S HISTORIC MISSION: PROMOTING FOOD PRODUCTION

Congress created the USDA in 1862 for one principal purpose: to make sure that enough food was available at all times to feed the population. To accomplish this worthwhile goal, the department protected agricultural producers and promoted the marketing of American agricultural products. The USDA interpreted its mandate to include research and dietary advice to the public, and it established units devoted to such activities by the early 1900s. Much later, in the 1970s, Congress directed the department to provide food assistance to the poor and to take greater responsibility for issuing advice about nutrition. As I explained in *Food Politics*, these functions did not cause conflict as long as dietary advice encouraged people to eat *more* of U.S. agricultural products. When chronic diseases replaced infectious diseases among the leading causes of death, however, dietary advice shifted. Health officials began to recommend restrictions on the intake of fat, saturated fat, and cholesterol as a means to prevent heart disease. For the first time, following dietary advice meant eating *less*, and particularly less of foods containing fat and cholesterol: meat, dairy, eggs, and fried and processed foods. At that point, the purposes of the USDA came into sharp conflict. One branch of the department was advising the public to eat less of agricultural products promoted by other branches. Whenever such conflicts occurred, the USDA almost always chose to protect the interests of food producers.

Thus, the USDA's friendliness to food producers has a long history. Indeed, one reason for the friendliness is built into the system of governmental oversight. The USDA reports to congressional agriculture committees whose most powerful members frequently come from states and districts economically dependent on food processing and production. That in itself might not be a problem, but for decades, food producers, USDA staff, and members of the House and Senate agriculture committees constituted what was universally understood to be the "agricultural establishment." These groups firmly controlled farm policy through seniority appointments to agriculture committees that appeared to grant lifetime tenure. The classic example was that of Representative Jamie Whitten (Dem-MS), who chaired House agricultural appropriations committees for so long (1949 to 1992) that he was known as the "permanent USDA Secretary."[1] Although the overwhelming representation of industry interests on congressional agriculture committees lessened somewhat in recent years, the tradition continues. In 1991, for example, 90% of the members of the Senate agricultural committee came from states in which at least 20% of the entire labor force was employed in food production.[2] Such percentages alone explain why congressional committees might be more concerned about the interests of food producers and processors than about protecting public health and why they insist that the USDA follow this approach.

A second reason for the friendliness is the revolving door between government and industry. Job exchanges between industry lobbyists and the USDA are especially common, not least because 500 or so department officials are political appointees selected on the basis of party affiliation. As early as 1974, reports identified numerous USDA officials who were previously employed by the meat and dairy industries or who left the USDA to work for those industries. From 1980 to 1992, the secretaries of the USDA included in succession a hog farmer, a former president of a meat industry trade association, and a cattle rancher—all more likely to grant higher priority to the business concerns of meat producers than to the safety concerns of the public. The change in administration in 2001 continued this tradition. The new USDA secretary, Ann Veneman, appointed a lobbyist for the National Cattlemen's Beef Association as her chief of staff. The former USDA secretary, Dan Glickman, took a position with a law firm that lobbies for food and agriculture companies; although he may not personally have represented such clients, his presence in the firm gave an impression favorable to their interests.[3]

A third reason for the friendliness of the USDA to the industries it regulates has to do with congressional campaign contributions. The Center for Public Integrity, a group that tracks relationships between industry and Congress, provides lists of Senate and House members who receive the largest campaign contributions from various industries. From 1987 to 1996, contributions from meat and poultry groups seemed particularly well focused. Among senators, 18 of the leading 25 recipients of contributions from meat and poultry groups were members of the agriculture committee, and one was Senate majority leader. Of the 25 leading House recipients from such groups, 17 were agriculture committee members and one was the Speaker. The center reports similar patterns among contributions from grocery distributors, wholesalers, and retailers. It also notes that among 153 witnesses at House and Senate agriculture committee hearings during that decade, 59 were from industry while just 16 were from public interest groups. One reason for this imbalance may be that the committees do not enjoy hearing the complaints of consumer advocates about USDA's conflicts of interest or its failure to enforce reasonable standards of microbial safety. By one report, agricultural producers contributed nearly $25 million to presidential and congressional campaigns from 1999 to 2002.[4]

In the incidents that follow—each a milestone in the long road to better oversight of food safety—we will see how the interactions of government officials, meat and poultry producers, and Congress delayed the institution of measures to control food pathogens.

THE USDA REJECTS SAFE HANDLING LABELS:
APHA v. BUTZ, 1974

Our story begins in the early 1970s, by which time health officials were well aware of the dangers of pathogenic bacteria carried by meat. Officials of the industry, the USDA, and Congress knew that the poke-and-sniff inspection system could not identify contaminated meat, but did not seem too concerned. In 1971 the American Public Health Association (APHA) attempted to force the issue by taking the USDA to court. The APHA argued that the USDA's stamp of approval on meat—granted after inspection—was misleading. Meat, APHA said, often was contaminated with *Salmonella,* but because USDA inspectors did not use microscopes or analyze for bacteria, they could not possibly detect pathogens and had no right to assure the public that meat was safe. Instead, APHA argued, the USDA should place a warning label with cooking instructions on packages of raw meat and poultry.

The USDA chose to defend the industry with this rationale: because so many foods are contaminated with *Salmonella,* "it would be unjustified to single out the meat industry and ask that the Department require it to identify its raw products as being hazardous to health." Instead, the USDA countered by shifting responsibility; it argued that an education campaign for *consumers* would be more useful. In 1974, an appeals court ruled in favor of the USDA, but in a divided decision that causes arguments to this day. The court's majority agreed with USDA that "American housewives and cooks normally are not ignorant or stupid and their methods of preparing and cooking of food do not ordinarily result in salmonellosis." In the opinion of the majority, Congress did not intend the 1906 Meat Inspection Act or its subsequent amendments to mean that (1) the inspection stamp guaranteed meat and poultry to be free of *Salmonella,* (2) inspections should include microscopic examinations, or (3) bacterial contamination implied misbranding.

The USDA, according to the court, was entitled to choose consumer education over warning labels: "official inspection labels which are placed on raw meat and poultry products . . . and which contain the legend 'U.S. Passed and Inspected' . . . are not false and misleading so as to constitute misbranding, notwithstanding failure to warn against dangers of food poisoning caused by salmonellae and other bacteria. . . . No one contends that Congress meant that inspections should include such [microscopic] examinations."[5] The court did not consider what Congress might have done had its members known about microbial contaminants in 1906, nor did it suggest how consumer education might be achieved in the absence of warning labels.

Because some of the judges dissented, and because the presiding judge had his own opinion on the matter, the ruling turned out to be more ambiguous than it first appeared. The dissenting judges noted that "Congressional intent is not helpful in determining whether the labels are misleading; the relevant inquiry is the understanding of consumers." Furthermore, the presiding judge said he did "not read the Court's decision to preclude a new challenge if it develops that consumer education programs prove inadequate to provide realistic protection." USDA officials could have interpreted these comments to mean that they could warn consumers about microbial hazards and evaluate the effectiveness of the warning, but the agency chose not to pursue this interpretation. Instead, USDA officials said that the ruling in *APHA* v. *Butz* meant that because *Salmonella* and other pathogens are *inherent* properties of raw meat, the law prohibits the department from doing anything to control them. This interpretation favored the interests of the meat industry, which continued to pursue this line of reasoning in subsequent court actions, as we will see in chapter 3.

GENERAL ACCOUNTING OFFICE PROPOSES HACCP: "A RADICALLY DIFFERENT METHOD"

In the early 1980s, investigations by the General Accounting Office (GAO) revealed that USDA inspectors were no longer able to keep up with the recently increased line speeds in meat-processing plants, but the department had failed to do anything to solve that problem. The GAO investigators thought it was high time the USDA instituted a radically different method for keeping microbial pathogens out of the meat supply: Hazard Analysis and Critical Control Point, familiarly known as HACCP (and pronounced "hassip").[6] Despite its singularly obscure name, HACCP is a thoroughly modern and sensible method for keeping pathogens out of the food supply. Before proceeding further, we need to take a look at what it is and how it works.

The origins of HACCP date to the dawn of the space age. In 1959, the National Aeronautics and Space Administration (NASA) asked the Pillsbury Company to develop a food system for astronauts in outer space consisting of total meal replacements in the form of bars for foods and tubes for liquids. NASA demanded safety as the highest priority. The agency did not want its astronauts to come down with microbial food poisoning while on space missions—a difficulty likely to be especially unpleasant under conditions of zero gravity. Pillsbury scientists examined every stage of food production, transport, preparation, and storage, "from farm to rocket ship" (translation: they conducted a hazard analysis). They identified each of the steps—critical control points—at which microbial contamination might occur. They then developed meth-

TABLE 8. The seven principles of HACCP (Hazard Analysis Critical Control Point)

---

1. Conduct a hazard analysis: determine where microbial contamination is most likely to occur and identify measures for preventing such contamination.
2. Identify critical control points: locate the steps in processing where microbial contamination can best be prevented.
3. Establish critical limits or standards for each critical control point (temperature, for example).
4. Establish requirements for monitoring of standards at each critical control point (when and how temperature is to be measured, for example).
5. Establish corrective actions needed to maintain standards at each critical control point (for example, adjusting refrigerators or ovens).
6. Establish record-keeping procedures for monitoring standards and taking corrective actions.
7. Establish—and use—procedures for verifying that the HACCP system is working as intended.

SOURCE: USDA/FSIS. *Federal Register* 61:32053–32054, June 12, 1997.

ods to eliminate those possibilities (and accomplish pathogen reduction). The company designed this decidedly science-based process to *prevent* contamination at every stage of production and processing. The plan required supervisors to sample for microbial contaminants only when needed to prove that control measures were working. Later, Pillsbury used this system in its flour mills and processing plants, with great success.[7]

HACCP is simple in its basic concepts and can be highly effective when it is used correctly (we will soon see what happens when it is not). In addition to its demonstrable success in outer space, studies on earth also show that appropriate use of HACCP reduces foodborne illness. HACCP requires food companies to analyze production processes intelligently, anticipate safety hazards at appropriate critical control points, and establish effective prevention controls and standards. Table 8 outlines the seven principles of HACCP. These principles place the burden of ensuring safe food on its *producers*. Under HACCP, USDA inspectors would no longer poke and sniff animals or meat products. Instead, their job would be to examine control point records to make sure that companies were adhering to the HACCP plans.[8]

Figure 5 illustrates a typical HACCP plan for a cooked meat product. In this plan, the company takes temperatures and records them at three critical control points, and USDA inspectors check the temperature

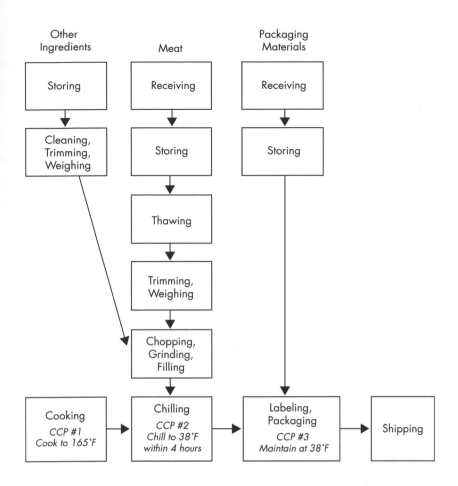

FIGURE 5. A Hazard Analysis and Critical Control Point (HACCP) plan for a cooked meat product. This plan depends on three critical control points (CCPs) to prevent growth of pathogenic bacteria. The product must be cooked to a temperature high enough to kill bacteria (CCP #1), then chilled quickly (#2), and packaged while cold (#3) to prevent bacterial regrowth. (Source: USDA/FSIS. *Federal Register* 61:32053–32054, June 12, 1997.)

records. Even so simple an example makes it evident that the effectiveness of any HACCP plan requires a major commitment from all parties concerned and entirely depends on (1) the diligence with which companies develop their plans, select critical control points, and monitor what happens at them, and (2) the diligence with which USDA inspectors oversee and enforce the plans.[9]

SCIENTISTS RECOMMEND HACCP:
A SCIENCE-BASED METHOD

With that understanding, we can now return to the history of attempts to require HACCP plans for meat production and processing. In the early 1980s when the General Accounting Office (GAO) first suggested reforms of meat inspection, the USDA agreed to study the matter. By that time, the department's Food Safety and Inspection Service (FSIS) was responsible for meat safety. In 1983, the FSIS asked the National Research Council (NRC), a private research organization often recruited to conduct studies on matters related to federal policies, to evaluate whether the poke-and-sniff inspection system had any scientific basis and, if not, to recommend ways to give it such a basis. The NRC's 1985 report pulled no punches; it said that the best way to reduce food pathogens was to require HACCP throughout the entire food chain—from production to final sale. In recommending HACCP, the NRC recognized that the USDA's underlying conflicts of interest could work against controlling what it euphemistically referred to as "aesthetic" problems in meat:

> The various federal meat and poultry inspection acts clearly give USDA
> multiple responsibilities with respect to the food supply. While FSIS
> has public health objectives, the laws also require that USDA assist in
> the marketing of products and that FSIS be concerned with aesthetic
> quality. . . . Neither law nor history provides FSIS with any good guide
> on which of these tasks—health protection, market assistance, or aesthetic
> control—should predominate, or how conflicts should be resolved.[10]

The NRC was quite correct about problems likely to be caused by USDA's conflicts of interest, as soon became evident.

Later in 1985, the NRC released a second report, this one dealing with microbial hazards in food. HACCP, it said, was remarkably successful in eliminating botulism in canned foods of low acidity, and should be extended to other food products. This report also noted food companies' lack of enthusiasm for HACCP but attributed the reluctance to "adversary attitudes and lack of cooperation between regulatory agencies and the food industry." It recommended the appointment of a multiagency commission to oversee federal food safety efforts, thus becoming one of the first groups to demand more government accountability for food safety—a call that resonates to this day.[11] Together, the two NRC reports revealed the extent to which the USDA's approach to food safety in the mid-1980s remained tied to 1906 laws and to the interests of industry. Both reports expressed concerns about the need to break through what food safety advocates later called "the closed society of meat inspection," in which the USDA and its inspectors viewed the industry they regulated as the group to which they owed primary allegiance.[12]

In 1987, partly in response to the National Research Council reports, Senator Patrick Leahy (Dem-VT) proposed the Safe Food Standards Act, to provide "farm-to-fork" protection against microbial pathogens. His bill would have required microbial testing of feed and animals, but it never reached the Senate floor, largely because "the very industries that the bill aimed to regulate owned the committees that had to pass it."[4] Industry lobbying groups such as the American Meat Institute strongly opposed the bill and continued to oppose similar bills introduced soon after.

In 1988, the USDA and the Food and Drug Administration (FDA)—in a rare moment of unity—appointed a joint committee to advise the agencies on how best to keep microbial pathogens out of the food supply. Like previous committees dealing with this problem, this one extolled the virtues of HACCP and provided detailed instructions about how to proceed with such plans. By the late 1980s, health officials understood HACCP to be the most sensible and scientifically grounded approach to reducing the risk of microbial food poisoning, but the regulated industry strongly opposed it.[13]

USDA TRIES "DISCRETIONARY" INSPECTIONS, 1986–1989

Despite the almost complete unanimity among scientists that properly developed HACCP plans could reduce pathogens, neither the industry nor federal agencies nor Congress promoted the idea. Instead, Congress passed a law in 1986 ostensibly designed to focus USDA inspection efforts where they were most needed. The law eliminated requirements for daily on-site inspections of meat-processing plants and gave the USDA the discretion to decide how often plants had to be inspected. This meant that the department could *reduce* the frequency of certain inspections. As part of the discretionary plan, the USDA proposed to "streamline" its inspection system by delegating some of the duties to the meat processors themselves (as would be done under HACCP).[14] The department tried out a preliminary version of this program in 1987 and 1988. Although this pilot study identified some problems, the USDA decided to expand discretionary inspection nationwide.

At this point, both consumer and industry groups charged that the USDA was deliberately choosing to ignore problems with discretionary inspection. Congress held hearings to review such complaints. At the hearings, meat inspectors raised vehement objections. With a graphic description worthy of Lafcadio Hearn or Upton Sinclair, Delmer Jones, the president of the inspectors' union, explained why his group believed that daily *visual* inspections of meat plants must continue. The problem, he said, is

> no control by industry of product that falls on the floor. . . . Product becomes a sponge when it falls to the floor. Many of the products are ready to eat. The problem . . . is because of chemical residues, fecal contamination, abscesses; the employees spit on the floor, blow their nose on the floor; they go in the bathrooms and track it back out into the plant and whatever they tracked into the plant, that is what you eat in cold cuts when you place that meat on a sandwich.

According to Mr. Jones, meat packers have a "stronger commitment to make money than to take care of sanitation and public health concerns." For this reason, he said, *more* visual inspection was needed, not less.[12]

Thomas Devine, the legal director of a government group that protects the rights of meat inspectors who blow the whistle on safety violations, raised yet another issue: harassment. In this early warning of the increasingly violent opposition of the meat industry to USDA safety requirements, Mr. Devine told the Congressional committee:

> The political climate is such that the special interest groups supporting the meat and poultry industry have won and now they have the ears of Washington. . . . The height of this program is an industry honor system . . . but I would like to tell you why we can't live with it because of what it will do to the plant employees who want to be whistle-blowers. They will be fired on the spot. . . . In fact, the bad news is so severe that plant management at some companies verbally and physically harass even the Federal inspectors. They have reported physical beatings that required hospitalization, death threats, letting the air out of their tires, chasing one inspector into the USDA office, trying to kick in the door, yelling, cussing, and generally keeping him a prisoner for a half hour.[12]

Soon after, the USDA withdrew its discretionary inspection plans for "further study," an action considered a sure sign that the idea had failed.[15] A year later, yet another National Research Council report, this time of the streamlined inspection system, concluded that such a system could not possibly protect the food supply unless "the reduced oversight by government inspectors is . . . compensated by a total commitment to product quality on the part of industry."[16] Such a commitment seemed unlikely.

E. COLI O157:H7 OUTBREAK INDUCES ACTION: JACK IN THE BOX, 1992–1993

If a single incident forced federal agencies to recognize the need for improvements in food safety regulation, it surely must be that of the disastrous December 1992 outbreak of *E. coli* O157:H7. Four young children in the Pacific Northwest died early in this outbreak. All were found to have eaten hamburgers at Jack in the Box restaurants. By February 1993, when the contaminated meat had been recalled and no new cases were emerging, Washington State alone had reported 400 cases and 100 hospitalizations, and another 100 cases had occurred in other states. Jack in the Box hamburgers were implicated in more than 90% of these cases.[17]

Despite the compelling circumstantial evidence, the source of the outbreak was not immediately apparent. The meat came from a California meat packer who said that his company had complied with federal regulations "and like other plants, has Federal inspectors who work on the premises" (translation: it's the USDA's fault).[18] Officials suspected that the meat had been contaminated in the slaughterhouse (it's the slaughterer's fault), but could not immediately confirm that suspicion.

Further investigation revealed that Jack in the Box restaurants had been following then-current FDA guidelines to cook hamburger to 140°F, a temperature too low to completely kill *E. coli* O157:H7. Six months prior to the outbreak, however, Washington State issued its own rules requiring hamburger to be cooked to 155°F, but Jack in the Box officials somehow missed that notification. The chain's president, Mr. Robert J. Nugent, was forced to admit that his 60 Washington State restaurants cooked meat below the 155°F standard. In testimony before a congressional committee, he explained that the company's procedures specified an internal temperature of 140°F but that the average cooking temperature in 1992 had been 154°F—a temperature just one degree below the state standard and high enough to kill most bacteria. Federal investigators, however, disputed that statement; they had found hamburgers cooked to just 120°F.[19] Despite such findings, Mr. Nugent also appeared to shift responsibility elsewhere—to meat processors and USDA inspectors—when he testified.

> Although our cooking procedures meet all Federal standards, we have increased cooking time and cooking temperature for our hamburgers and retrained our grill chefs. . . . We also have offered to pay the medical expenses of those who may have become ill after eating at one of our restaurants. But it is important to note that the contaminated meat that

was infected by the *E. coli* O157:H7 bacteria before delivery to our restaurants had passed all USDA inspections. Every one of our chefs had carefully followed all Federal food preparation standards.[20]

The consequences of the Jack in the Box outbreak were immediate. The parent company, Foodmakers, which earned two-thirds of its $1.3 billion in annual revenue from the chain, lost 30% of its stock market value. Despite attempting to shift blame elsewhere, the company offered to pay medical expenses for the victims and immediately recruited a nationally known expert to revamp its procedures. Eventually, its revised system set a food safety standard for the industry.

Perhaps as a result of the hearings, President Bill Clinton authorized the hiring of 160 more meat inspectors, although 400 positions still were left vacant as a result of budget cuts and deregulation. The president had just appointed Mike Espy, a former Democratic congressman from Mississippi, to be the new USDA Secretary. Mr. Espy soon met with meat inspector whistle-blowers to hear their complaints. In March, in a departure from the policies of previous administrations, President Clinton proposed to overhaul the meat inspection system, promised that modern biological tools would be used to evaluate pathogens in meat, and called for expanded use of irradiation for meat products (an issue discussed in chapter 4).[21] A *New York Times* editorial pointed out that the USDA had long been inclined to "put meat and dairy interests before public health," had "abdicated its duty to minimize the risk from contaminated products," and could have avoided the tragic deaths if the department had "stirred itself to contain the bacterial infection problem after a 1982 outbreak disclosed it." The *Times* considered the new administration's proposed policy changes a "refreshing break" in USDA's "traditional laxity in consumer protection."[22] In a further response to the Jack in the Box outbreak, the FDA recommended an increase in the minimal cooking temperature for ground beef from 140°F to 155°F (later, the FDA raised the recommended temperature to 160°F to provide an extra margin of safety for home cooks). The outbreak also stimulated calls for research to better identify microbial pathogens and find out how they get into the food supply.[23]

The Jack in the Box outbreak was by no means the first to involve *E. coli* O157:H7, but it was especially difficult for the public to accept. For one thing, children had died. For another, the source was hamburger—an American food icon. From then on, food companies and USDA officials would have a harder time convincing the public of the usual line of

TABLE 9. Advice from the Department of Agriculture: food safety
is everyone's responsibility

Farm
   Pathogens are found to some extent in all farm animals.
   Livestock operations should be separated from produce operations.
   Clean water should be used to irrigate produce.

Storage/Transport
   Keep products cold.
   Clean tanks between shipments.

Slaughter/Processing
   Apply HACCP preventive systems.
   New technologies can reduce the risk of pathogen contamination.

Consumer
   Clean: Wash hands and surfaces often.
   Separate: Don't cross-contaminate.
   Cook: Cook to proper temperatures.
   Chill: Refrigerate promptly.

SOURCE: Crutchfield S. *FoodReview* 1998;21(3):34 35.

reasoning: nothing can be done about pathogens, they are ubiquitous,
and the burden of food safety rests with home cooks. The responsibility
of producers, processors, and retailers was now apparent, as was that of
the government to make sure they met that responsibility.[24] Table 9
summarizes the USDA's subsequent and ongoing vision of how food
safety responsibilities are to be shared. It demonstrates that in 1998 the
department still could not require farmers or transporters to institute
HACCP plans, nor could it demand *performance standards*—maximum
levels of harmful microbes allowed as verified by testing—for reducing
pathogens.[15]

Any assumption that either the industry or the USDA would willingly
accept such responsibility was overly optimistic. Marian Burros of the
New York Times noted that USDA officials continued to deny two obvious facts: cases of food poisoning were increasing, and the meat industry had something to do with those cases. As she explained, "Blaming the victim takes the onus off the responsible government agency and
the meat and poultry industry. There are many ways the industry could
lessen the risks of food poisoning, but the Government does not require
any of those steps."[25]

Instead of taking such steps, industry groups employed damage control. They pointed out that *E. coli* O157:H7 infections were due to undercooking, not to the meat itself, and that consumers needed better education about food safety. They said the "recent outbreak sheds light on a nationwide problem: inconsistent information about proper cooking temperatures for hamburger."[4] They explicitly revealed their public relations objectives: "Our goal, first and foremost, is to stay out of the media spotlight. The coverage, so far, has focused on cooking procedures at the fast food outlets, not beef industry issues. Let's try to keep it that way."[26] Although actions beyond home cooking clearly were needed to ensure meat safety, industry leaders continued to deny responsibility. After the 1992 election, when safety advocates pressed the new political appointees at USDA for HACCP regulations to reduce meat pathogens, the industry encouraged its friends in that department to give lukewarm support to such efforts, if any.

PUBLIC PRESSURES OVERCOME INDUSTRY RESISTANCE: SAFE HANDLING LABELS, 1993

Twenty years after *APHA* v. *Butz,* at the peak of the Jack in the Box outbreak, consumer activist Jeremy Rifkin and parents of the children who died during the outbreak formed an advocacy group called Beyond Beef. In one of its earliest actions, Beyond Beef sued the USDA to require cooking and handling instructions on meat and poultry packages. This time, the outcome favored consumers. Although the new administration at the USDA was already considering such labels, the court ordered the department to "mandate labels regarding the handling and cooking of meat and poultry to minimize the chance that bacterial contamination will reach the consumer."[27]

Soon after, Secretary Espy announced that the USDA would institute "emergency rulemaking" to require safe-handling labels on all raw meat and poultry packages and, as the court required, would publish the rules by August 15, 1993. A representative from the American Meat Institute told the *New York Times* that its member companies had received "every indication from U.S.D.A. that these will not be warning labels. They will be care labels."[28] USDA officials said that package labels would explain that some meat might contain bacteria. Therefore, consumers should follow proper handling procedures and should "clean, separate, cook, and chill" (table 9). Meat producers found this proposal alarming. Despite their preference for consumer education above all other methods of pathogen control, they did not want package labels to suggest that anything might be inherently wrong with their products. The American Meat Institute complained that its members had not been given enough time to comment and that the proposal was unfair since only *ground* meat had been implicated in most food poisonings.

In response, the USDA agreed to limit its proposal just to ground meat and poultry. It permitted the industry to delay labeling of all other uncooked meat products (except ground meat) from October 15, 1993, until April 15, 1994. Three industry groups, one of them led by John Block, a former USDA secretary in the administration of President Ronald Reagan, thought this delay not nearly long enough. They sued the USDA in a Texas federal court to block safe handling labels on a technicality—the agency's "emergency rulemaking" had not permitted the amount of time mandated by Congress for the industry to respond to regulatory proposals.[29]

On October 14, the day before the rule for *ground* meat was to take effect, the federal court in Austin, Texas (Judge James Nowlin, presiding), issued an injunction that blocked the labeling plan, saying that the Jack in the Box outbreak was insufficient to justify any "departure from the normal rule-making procedures." Industry groups hailed the injunction as "a victory of fairness over bureaucracy."[30] That very week, however, three children in Texas died from eating ground meat contaminated with *E. coli* O157:H7, tragically demonstrating why such labels might be essential.[31] Nevertheless, the appeals court refused to lift the injunction and scheduled a hearing for January 1994—three months after the labeling rule for ground meat was to take effect and a full year after the onset of the Jack in the Box outbreak.

Rather than wait three more months for a hearing of uncertain outcome, the USDA chose to revise its proposals and provide the mandated period for public comment. As one indicator of how much the new administration was changing USDA policies, a spokesman for the trade group led by former USDA secretary Block, the National American Wholesale Grocers Association, told the *New York Times*: "Quite frankly, we are wondering if Mr. Espy is taking all this too personally. . . . Mr. Espy is making safe handling a bit of a crusade." Janet Riley, a spokeswoman for the American Meat Institute, said: "Warning labels really frighten the public. . . . If consumers follow safe handling procedures, there's no need to scare people about what is really a very wholesome and nutritious product."[31] In the end, industry protests caused critical delays but failed to prevent the USDA from requiring

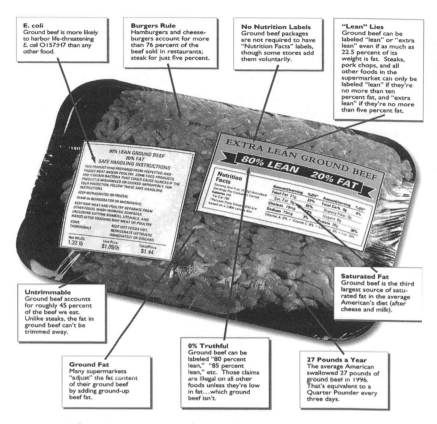

E. coli
Ground beef is more likely to harbor life-threatening *E. coli* O157:H7 than any other food.

Burgers Rule
Hamburgers and cheeseburgers account for more than 76 percent of the beef sold in restaurants; steak for just five percent.

No Nutrition Labels
Ground beef packages are not required to have "Nutrition Facts" labels, though some stores add them voluntarily.

"Lean" Lies
Ground beef can be labeled "lean" or "extra lean" even if as much as 22.5 percent of its weight is fat. Steaks, pork chops, and all other foods in the supermarket can only be labeled "lean" if they're no more than ten percent fat, and "extra lean" if they're no more than five percent fat.

Untrimmable
Ground beef accounts for roughly 45 percent of the beef we eat. Unlike steaks, the fat in ground beef can't be trimmed away.

Saturated Fat
Ground beef is the third largest source of saturated fat in the average American's diet (after cheese and milk).

Ground Fat
Many supermarkets "adjust" the fat content of their ground beef by adding ground-up beef fat.

0% Truthful
Ground beef can be labeled "80 percent lean," "85 percent lean," etc. Those claims are illegal on all other foods unless they're low in fat...which ground beef isn't.

27 Pounds a Year
The average American swallowed 27 pounds of ground beef in 1996. That's equivalent to a Quarter Pounder every three days.

FIGURE 6. The U.S. Department of Agriculture's safe-handling instructions for raw meat products, as annotated by the Center for Science in the Public Interest (CSPI). This illustration appeared in *Nutrition Action Healthletter*, September 1999. (Courtesy of Michael Jacobson. Reprinted with permission.)

warning labels. Figure 6 illustrates the label that caused all this trouble. This label is now in use on supermarket meat products in the United States.

THE POULTRY INDUSTRY VERSUS PERFORMANCE STANDARDS: A USDA SECRETARY'S DOWNFALL, 1993–1994

Whether or not Mr. Espy's support for food-handling labels indeed constituted a personal crusade, the industry's actions to oppose his efforts illustrate some of the less savory aspects of food safety politics in action. As noted earlier, President Clinton had appointed Mr. Espy, then a fourth-term member of the House of Representatives (Dem-MS), as USDA Secretary in 1993. Mr. Espy's measures to overhaul the inspection system for meat and poultry appeared quite serious, and they worried the industry. Beef producers objected and, among other complaints, accused the USDA of favoring chicken producers by holding that industry to less stringent safety standards. Perhaps in response, the USDA moved to require freshly killed poultry to be treated with sterilizing solutions of trisodium phosphate and acids before chilling the meat. The USDA was also working on rules that would require poultry companies to test for microbial pathogens. As might be expected, the poultry industry opposed both suggestions.[32]

Soon after Mr. Espy took office, his staff warned him that federal conflict-of-interest rules applied more strictly to agency officials than to members of Congress or Mississippi legislators, and that he must be especially careful not to accept gifts or favors from people working for companies that might be affected by USDA regulations. This warning derived from interpretations of provisions of the 1906 Meat Inspection Act, designed originally to prevent corruption of meat inspectors. The law made it a federal crime to do anything to exert undue influence on an inspector. A later law, the Bribery, Graft and Conflicts of Interest Act of 1962, set penalties for anyone who offered "anything of value" with the intention of influencing a public official. Although *intention* was the crucial issue, federal lawyers have interpreted this law to mean that officials of government agencies should refuse *any* gifts—no matter how seemingly inconsequential—from representatives of companies with matters under USDA regulatory review.

Despite the warnings, Mr. Espy accepted a variety of favors from lobbyists for Tyson Foods, then the world's largest chicken-processing company (and now the largest producer of beef as well). Early in 1994, federal investigators accused Mr. Espy of violating the Meat Inspection Act by accepting—or permitting a companion to accept—airline travel, tickets to sporting events, a small scholarship, and other gifts worth about $12,000 from Tyson Foods, plus similar gifts from other meat and poultry companies. The results of that investigation forced Mr. Espy to resign from his position as USDA secretary, and a later investigation by a special prosecutor led to his indictment by a federal grand jury. Eventually, Mr. Espy was acquitted of all charges, largely because the prosecutor could not convince a jury that the gifts were *intended* to influence the USDA. Although it is difficult to imagine what other purpose the gifts might have served, the Supreme Court also ruled that Mr. Espy was entitled to accept them because they were not directly linked to regulatory matters.[33]

Federal prosecutors also accused Mr. Espy's chief of staff, Ronald Blackley, of interfering with USDA attempts to regulate poultry safety. A USDA staff member told a reporter that Mr. Blackley had been surprised to learn that the agency was working on poultry rules: "He said to take [them] out of the computer. . . . We were a little shell shocked . . . wondering if we had all heard what we thought we'd heard. We put a stop to all poultry activity."[32]

At the time, the scandal made the USDA's ongoing efforts to improve poultry safety much more difficult. Some critics charged that the department's proposed rules for poultry inspection were simply "an effort to prove that . . . Espy was not beholden to poultry interests."[34] When the agency decided not to go forward with the plan, officials had to deny that they had made this decision just to please the poultry industry. The Espy scandal, neither the first nor the last of its kind, was unusual only in that the favors were so visible and the issues so important. This particular USDA secretary had the opportunity and the ability to convert his department's century-old inspection system to one better equipped to deal with microbial pathogens. Tyson Foods' donation of tickets to sporting events demonstrated that even small favors produce substantial benefits if given at the right time, in this case just when the USDA was trying to get poultry producers to test for *Salmonella* and other pathogens. If nothing else, it worked greatly to Tyson Foods' advantage to keep Mr. Espy preoccupied with responses to legal challenges from a special prosecutor. As if the political nature of this situation were not transparent enough, one of President Clinton's last acts in office was to grant presidential pardons to Mr. Blackley and six food company executives and lobbyists who had been convicted of attempting to corrupt Mr. Espy. Reportedly, the White House *invited* defense lawyers to request the pardons, and granted them just hours before George W. Bush took office as president in January 2001.[35]

USDA REQUIRES PATHOGEN TESTING:
E. COLI O157:H7 IN GROUND BEEF, 1994

By the early 1990s, USDA officials had argued for two decades that the decision in *APHA* v. *Butz* meant that the department did not have legal authority to set limits on microbial contaminants in meat and poultry because pathogens like *Salmonella* were "inherent" in raw meat. As late as 1993, the administrator of USDA's Food Safety and Inspection Service (FSIS), H. Russell Cross, explained to a congressional committee: "At the present time, meat and poultry inspection laws do not define raw meat and poultry containing bacteria as adulterated."[36] As noted earlier, the USDA could have interpreted *APHA* v. *Butz* as giving the department considerable latitude to do whatever seemed necessary to protect the public, including setting performance standards—allowance limits verified by testing—for pathogens in meat. While Mr. Espy's legal difficulties were front-page news, he chose Michael Taylor to become administrator of FSIS. Mr. Taylor, a lawyer, moved to the USDA from the FDA; there, his previous employment with Monsanto raised conflict-of-interest questions about his role in setting policy for regulation of genetically modified foods (see chapter 7). His actions at the USDA raised no such questions. In late September 1994, six weeks after assuming leadership of FSIS, Mr. Taylor gave his first public speech in his new job to an annual convention of the American Meat Institute. He said that it was high time for everyone involved in meat production and processing "to be driven as much by public health goals as by productivity concerns." FSIS intended to take advantage of "the tools of microbiology to ensure that preventive controls are in place to reduce the risk of harmful contamination and to verify that those controls are working." He announced that FSIS would soon propose regulations requiring installation of science-based HACCP systems in every meat and poultry plant. "Raw ground beef contaminated with *E. coli* O157:H7," he said, "poses a serious risk to public health, and contaminated lots should be excluded from commerce." The USDA intended to require the destruction or reprocessing of contaminated meat and "we expect companies who encounter contaminated lots of raw ground beef . . . to take similar action."[37]

If that challenge was not enough to bring his audience to rapt attention, he explained that FSIS would be taking these actions on the basis of the department's revised interpretation of *APHA* v. *Butz:*

> To clarify an important legal point, we consider raw ground beef that is contaminated with *E. coli* O157:H7 to be adulterated within the meaning of the Federal Meat Inspection Act. We are prepared to use the Act's enforcement tools, as necessary, to exclude adulterated product from commerce. Finally, we plan to conduct targeted sampling and testing of raw ground beef at plants and in the marketplace for possible contamination with *E. coli* O157:H7. This sampling program . . . will serve as an example and an incentive for those commercial enterprises that produce, process, and market raw ground beef to control their processes and conduct their own tests.[37]

Furthermore, because *E. coli* O157:H7 is infectious at very low doses, FSIS would consider *any* level of contamination of ground beef with these bacteria to be unsafe, adulterated, and subject to enforcement action. The agency, however, would restrict this "sample, test, and destroy" approach to just this one pathogen, *E. coli* O157:H7, and to just this one product: ground beef.[38]

Food safety advocates admire Mr. Taylor for his courage in delivering this speech to an audience expected to be unsympathetic if not downright hostile. They also appreciate his skill in shifting USDA food safety policies to those more favorable to public health, especially at a time when the department's leadership was in such deep trouble. Indeed, he needed courage. His speech caused consternation in the cattle, meatpacking, and grocery industries. Meat producers and processors understood that if the USDA considered *E. coli* O157:H7 an "adulterant," they would break the law if they sold foods containing this pathogen. They would be vulnerable to criminal prosecution. As a representative of the American Meat Institute told the press, "the new USDA policy has the perhaps unintended consequence of creating rampant, irresponsible, criminal litigation."[39] Industry lawyers instructed their clients not to do their own testing of ground beef for *E. coli* O157:H7 because finding it would expose them to legal liability. Rosemary Mucklow, then the executive director of the Western States Meat Association, said, "How can FSIS treat *E. coli* in hamburger meat as an adulterant subject to enforcement strategies, while not applying the same standard to salmonella in broilers. . . . Automated chicken lines allow birds to leave the plant as Inspected for Wholesomeness with . . . grossly unacceptable defects. . . . Such gross policy interpretation favoring the poultry industry and disfavoring the beef industry is a travesty indeed."[40] We will encounter further commentary from Ms. Mucklow later in these pages.

In the meantime, the American Meat Institute—which had opposed the safe-food-handling labels—now used them to complain that the proposed testing program would *cause* food safety problems. Microbial testing would "mislead consumers with promises of a safer food supply, and as a result they may relax their own cooking and handling standards."[4] The Food Marketing Institute also shifted responsibility to consumers in its argument against the initiative: "It is essential that nothing dilute the consumer message that the proper cooking of meat eliminates food-borne pathogens."[41] The two trade associations and five others quickly filed suit to block the pathogen testing plan, based on this wonderfully convoluted argument: because the USDA had done nothing to control

E. coli O157:H7 since the first outbreak in 1982, the present situation could hardly be considered an emergency. This transparently self-serving argument prompted the *New York Times* to note the industry's "odd way" of promoting public health: "Trying to give their obstructionist lawsuit a respectable veneer, the plaintiffs voice concern that the spot-inspection program could mislead consumers into relaxing their own safe handling and cooking practices. . . . It is not consumers the lawsuit seeks to protect but the industry's right to sell tainted beef."[42]

Among the many ironic aspects of this dispute, the trade associations' lawsuit turned out to be heard by the very same Texas district court judge, James Nowlin, who had ruled against the USDA's proposals to require food-handling labels on procedural grounds just a year earlier. This time, the court surprised observers by ruling in favor of the USDA. Its rationale: because ordinary cooking temperatures could not kill *E. coli* O157:H7, the USDA had good reason to consider these bacteria as adulterants and test for them. This decision at last permitted the USDA to redesign its ancient food inspection system and start testing for this one harmful pathogen. Industry groups, however, saw the decision as mandating a program that "fails to protect consumers, wastes tax dollars and violates the law," and they vowed to "maintain our course of legal action to stop it."[43]

The trade associations' lawsuit had one additional—and unanticipated—consequence. It mobilized the families of children killed by *E. coli* O157:H7 to form their own group—Safe Tables Our Priority (STOP)—to lobby for more rigorous meat regulations. The group picketed a meeting of the American Meat Institute and held a press conference to accuse meat producers of obstructing safety efforts: "My 6-year-old son Alex deserves to be alive today. . . . I hold the meat institute personally responsible" and "It's time to stop blaming consumers for not cooking and give them a clean product."[44] Another consumer group, the Safe Food Coalition, proposed a "simple household solution" to the problem of the industry's intransigent refusal to test for *E. coli* O157:H7 and its persistent avoidance of accountability: obtain proof of responsibility. "Tired of being a victim? . . . Weary of subjecting your family to a game of Russian Roulette every time you buy a package of hamburger meat? . . . [When] unpacking groceries, tuck the supermarket receipt and a small lump of hamburger in a ziplock bag. Toss this in the freezer. . . . In five seconds, at virtually no cost, you've got accountability. . . . This simple act gives control back to you and tells industry loud and clearly that we're not going to take it any more."[45]

In this instance, the political context permitted the USDA to hold its position and test one product (ground meat) for one pathogen (*E. coli* O157:H7). When the department attempted to extend testing requirements to other forms of meat and other pathogens, it again met with fierce resistance, as chapter 3 will reveal.

USDA POISED TO PROPOSE HACCP, 1994

By the early 1990s, the long history of collusion between meat producers, Congress, and the USDA seemed to have entered a new phase in which public interests held greater influence. Meat producers' protection of the century-old inspection system no longer seemed credible. Although the industry contended that testing for microbes is unnecessary because so few samples are contaminated, this argument ignored a key point: even a small level of contamination can do great harm when the number of animals is large. For example, if just 0.2% of cattle are contaminated with *E. coli* O157:H7, 74,000 beef carcasses might be infected and, therefore, hundreds of thousands of pounds of hamburger.[46] For this reason alone, the pathogen reduction component of HACCP (which necessarily includes performance standards and testing for microbes) seems thoroughly warranted.

USDA's historical reluctance to change its inspection and pathogen control systems derives directly from the agency's conflicting mandates: to ensure the safety and quality of foods under its jurisdiction and, at the same time, to promote their marketing and consumption. The long-term collusion between the department and the meat industry impedes progress. Over the years, the breakdown of the agricultural establishment, the emergence of new food pathogens like *E. coli* O157:H7, and the appointment of USDA officials interested in the health effects (as well as the economic effects) of agricultural products, paved the way for more vigorous efforts to institute HACCP with performance standards for controlling pathogens.

In the 20 years between 1974 and 1994, resistance to HACCP with pathogen reduction came from many sources: federal agencies unwilling to confront powerful constituents, industry groups willing to accept HACCP only without government oversight (especially of pathogen levels), consumer groups suspicious of the industry's commitment to safety standards and the government's ability to enforce them, and inspectors unwilling to change the nature of their work. By 1994, advocates feared that more lives of children would need to be sacrificed before Congress, the USDA, and the industry would take action to keep dangerous bacteria out of meat. Even the threat of financial liability did not seem severe enough to induce industry action. The institution of HACCP rules appeared inevitable to all but the most determined segments of the meat industry, but whether the rules would include requirements for pathogen performance standards and testing remained open for debate. Chapter 3 explains how that debate developed.

CHAPTER 3

ATTEMPTING CONTROL OF
FOOD PATHOGENS, 1994–2002

DESPITE THE BARRIERS DISCUSSED IN CHAPTER 2 AND THE objections raised by businesses likely to be affected by the new regulations, government agencies were eventually able to institute HACCP (Hazard Analysis and Critical Control Point) systems designed to prevent harmful microbes from getting into food. This chapter describes how that happened, mainly with respect to HACCP controls for beef. Beef industry protests were more vehement and often more effective than those of other industries, and interactions of beef trade associations with the U.S. Department of Agriculture (USDA) and with Congress left more visible traces. Because most outbreaks of microbial illness derive from foods regulated by the Food and Drug Administration (FDA), this chapter also explains how the FDA tried to require the industries under its jurisdiction to institute HACCP plans, how those industries opposed the plans, and how that agency's systems—once in place—operated in practice. Opponents of HACCP often framed their objections in scientific terms: because cooking kills most food microbes, government intervention is unnecessary. When outbreaks did occur, food producers, processors, and retailers accused each other of causing them, and all blamed government inspectors and consumers. We will see that food companies were not alone in their objections to HACCP requirements. Meat inspectors opposed the new regulations because HAACP changed their work from examining animals to examining paper. In addition, some food safety advocates agreed with the inspectors' contention that HACCP gave too much control of production to industry and allowed foxes to guard chickens, as it were.

To gain some insight into the basis of this conflict, I wanted to observe a HACCP system in action. Shortly after the USDA's final HACCP rules for meat went into effect in the late 1990s, the owner of a meat-packing plant in New York State agreed to let me visit as long as I did not identify the plant by name.

His company cooks meats under HACCP plans similar to the USDA model illustrated in figure 5 (page 69), and his plant illustrates both the strengths and weaknesses of HACCP systems. Production practices followed the prescribed plan to the letter (a strength), but HACCP plans require mountains of paperwork and the attention of a full-time employee (at considerable added expense). Because some of the products include vegetable as well as meat ingredients, they fall under the regulatory requirements of three agencies: the FDA, the USDA, and New York State. Inspections vary in frequency—the USDA daily, New York State four times a year, and the FDA once a year—and are conducted according to the unique rules and reporting requirements of each agency. In practice, the multiple authorities mean that plant officials must fill out three distinct sets of reporting forms (a time-consuming and expensive nuisance). The on-site USDA inspector I met at the plant checked temperature records but seemed entirely uninterested in the production process (a serious weakness, as I will explain). One plant employee confided to me— shades of Upton Sinclair—that "someone could be butchering a dog in front of them [the inspectors], and they wouldn't have a clue."

Because the first of the three critical control points was to measure the temperature of products after they were cooked (see figure 5), the managers learned that the ovens were not heating properly. They identified a succession of faults in the engineering of the ovens and tinkered with them until the problem was fixed (a strength). After the products were cooked, however, they were immediately transferred to open racks in a refrigeration room and chilled—uncovered—by cold air blasted in from a ceiling unit. The temperature of the products dropped quickly, as required by the plan (a strength). Unfortunately, the plan did not account for the ability of harmful bacteria like *Listeria* to flourish at cold temperatures in the cooling system and to contaminate the uncovered products *after* they were cooked (a weakness). The plant managers seemed unaware of the potential hazard. Because they followed the HACCP plan so scrupulously, they did not think the uncovered products posed problems (a further weakness). Within weeks of my visit, the company had to recall thousands of pounds of products because some had been found to be contaminated with *Listeria*.

From this experience, it seemed obvious that HACCP plans can prevent contamination but that diligence in following them is not enough; the plans also must be thoughtfully designed and overseen, and verified by testing. The role of the on-site USDA inspector was particularly striking. He was not involved in promoting the plant's microbial safety. As a 20-year USDA veteran, he had been trained to inspect animals, not paperwork, and was unaware of the peculiar characteristics of newly emergent bacterial pathogens. He seemed much in the tradition of the inspector described in *The Jungle* a century earlier, as we have already seen.

With this understanding of HACCP systems in action, we can now return to the political battles of the mid-1990s that eventually enabled federal agencies to require some industries to follow HACCP plans. By late 1994, with the legal obstacles out of the way, federal agencies could begin the formal—and glacially tedious—rule-making process to require HACCP controls for one food industry or another: proposing rules in the *Federal Register;* requesting, collecting, and dealing with public comments; rewriting the proposals; and, eventually, issuing final rules that would go into effect some years later. The USDA proposed rules for meat and poultry, and the FDA proposed rules for some of the foods under its jurisdiction. The two agencies approached the task in quite different ways, particularly in their decisions about whether HACCP plans, performance standards, and requirements for pathogen testing should be required or voluntary. The FDA was the first to place its notices in the *Federal Register,* and we begin with this agency's approach to HACCP rules.

THE FDA TRIES HACCP, ONE FOOD AT A TIME

Although up to 80% of outbreaks are caused by foods regulated by the FDA, this agency has had a difficult time figuring out what to do about them. The FDA first proposed to develop HACCP controls for seafood in January 1994 and, in late summer of 1994, asked for public comment on whether and how HACCP might be extended to "land foods." In approaching HACCP regulation in this manner, the FDA was responding not only to the need to control pathogens but also to its own internal difficulties. The resource constraints on the FDA's food safety program seemed unlikely to improve. It also seemed unlikely that the agency would ever be able to inspect, sample, and analyze more than a tiny fraction of the foods for which it was responsible. In deciding how to regulate food safety without funds or personnel, the FDA floated a trial balloon:

Although the agency has reached no final conclusions about how its regulatory programs should be revised to make food as safe as possible, FDA has tentatively concluded that the improvements in the agency's current food safety assurance program should be based on a state-of-the-art, preventive approach known as HACCP. . . . The agency has tentatively chosen a HACCP approach because HACCP addresses the root causes of food safety problems in production, storage, transportation, etc., and is preventive.[1]

The FDA was careful to note that it expected to engage in further conversations with industry and other groups and that it planned to work closely with the USDA to make sure the rules of the two agencies were consistent. It asked for public comment on whether HACCP should be mandatory for all of the food industries under its jurisdiction or just for certain segments of those industries. It also asked for input on how mandatory HACCP plans might apply to the entire chain of food distribution, from production to retail sale.

As a further reflection of this cautious approach, the FDA asked companies to *volunteer* to develop pilot HACCP systems. The idea was to study the plans and use them as a basis for deciding how to proceed further. As it turned out, several firms agreed to be guinea pigs for this purpose: Alto Dairy, Campbell Soup, ConAgra, EarthGrains (Sara Lee), Pillsbury (General Mills), and Ralston Foods. Their pilot plans—which involved products such as cheese, frozen dough, breakfast cereals, salad dressing, fresh and pasteurized juices, bread, and flour—demonstrated that HACCP controls worked well to help companies identify safety problems and correct them. This was only to be expected given Pillsbury's experience 30 years earlier. Furthermore, the companies reported a decline in the frequency of product recalls (also to be expected with reduced contamination), along with unanticipated benefits in improved production efficiency, employee "ownership" and participation, and customer satisfaction. None of the volunteers, however, included microbial testing as a component of their plans. The pilot plans demonstrated that HACCP would reduce pathogens and be good for business but also suggested that companies would not test for harmful bacteria unless forced to do so.[2]

While these studies were underway, the FDA proposed HACCP rules for a few additional foods that seemed especially hazardous. It began with HACCP for seafood and shellfish (proposed in 1994 to take effect in 1997), for raw sprouts and eggs (to take effect in 1999), and, as discussed below, for fresh juices (2000). The FDA also initiated another voluntary

HACCP experiment, this time for dairy products, and it proposed safe-handling instructions for eggs: "Eggs may contain harmful bacteria known to cause serious illness, especially in children, the elderly, and persons with weakened immune systems. For your protection: Keep eggs refrigerated; cook eggs until yolks are firm; and cook foods containing eggs thoroughly."[3] But by 2009, the FDA required HACCP only for seafood. For all its other foods, HACCP was *voluntary*. The FDA's food-by-food approach to HACCP, its lack of requirements for microbial testing, and its scarcity of inspectors left industries with many opportunities to avoid installing such plans or adhering to them. For example, only 44% of seafood processing firms had implemented HACCP plans by 1999, and more than half of all inspections revealed serious problems with the plans five years after their implementation. By 2001, the shellfish industry's chief safety strategy—education of consumers—had failed to reduce the illnesses and deaths caused by eating raw products, and neither the industry nor its FDA regulators had imposed preventive measures. This experience reinforced suspicions that voluntary approaches would not work.[4]

USDA'S POLITICAL BATTLES

In contrast, and rather a surprise in view of its past history, the USDA moved quickly to introduce HACCP under the more consumer-friendly leadership appointed by President Bill Clinton. By the mid-1990s, some segments of the meat industry were asking the department to institute HACCP regulations, if for no other reason than to reassure the public that meat was safe. The Food Safety and Inspection Service (FSIS) began to develop HACCP rules for meat and poultry through a method previously unimaginable for this agency: it openly consulted stakeholders. The FSIS held information briefings, scientific conferences, public hearings, federal and state conferences, agency meetings, and a professional forum to listen to points of view. Its 1995 proposed rules differed from those of the FDA in several critical respects, most notably in their emphasis on requirements for pathogen testing. Indeed, the department called the plan *Pathogen Reduction: HACCP*—a critical distinction. The USDA plan established performance standards and required the companies to prove by daily sampling and testing that pathogenic contaminants did not exceed levels specified in the standards.[5]

True to form, some meat industry groups objected. An official of the Armour company, for example, told a congressional committee that HACCP was an imperfect system that did not address the real problem—

consumer education: "There is a concern that HACCP has been over-sold and public expectations may be unrealistically high. In particular, HACCP cannot guarantee the absence of enteric pathogens on raw meat or poultry. . . . Food safety is a shared responsibility involving industry, Government, and consumers. Public education on safe handling of foods continues to be a key factor in preventing foodborne illness."[6]

Untrue to form, the American Meat Institute petitioned the USDA to require HACCP for all meat and poultry plants: "We believe so strongly in HACCP's benefits for meat and poultry safety that we think it should be mandated for our segment of the industry." This group's unexpected support of HACCP is explained by its assumption—erroneous, as it happened—that *industry* inspectors would replace those of USDA. Later, when meat industry associations realized the implications of pathogen testing—that products found contaminated would be considered adulterated and unfit to sell—they tried to block the proposals. Meat producers and processors much preferred a "virtual" safety system: HACCP without pathogen reduction and entirely voluntary compliance.[7]

Congress Demands "Negotiated Rulemaking," 1995

Before proposed regulations become final and go into effect, they are supposed to be held open for a specified period of time for public comment. The comment period for the proposed Pathogen Reduction: HACCP rules occurred at a time when especially conservative Republicans had taken control of Congress and were attempting to reduce regulatory burdens on industry. Meat and poultry lobbyists took advantage of this favorable situation to urge Congress to block the proposed rules. They used the usual argument: home cooks are responsible for most episodes of foodborne illness, and oversight of industry is unnecessary. Despite the false premise (most outbreaks derive from foods prepared outside the home), the lobbying succeeded in several respects. First, Congress extended the comment period to give the industry more time to organize opposition. Next, industry lobbyists convinced some members of Congress to amend the appropriations bill to delete funding for HACCP implementation. Finally, while discussions of this funding amendment were in progress, the lobbyists also convinced Congress to order the USDA to participate in "negotiated rulemaking," a process that would require the department to work closely with meat producers to make the regulations mutually acceptable. To observers offended by the idea that the industry would define its own regulations, the purpose of negotiated rulemaking seemed clear—to postpone or eliminate HACCP. Representative George Brown (Dem-CA), explained: "The House Agriculture Committee would like to write more industry-friendly legislation and cut the USDA regulations off at the pass."[8]

The congressman who introduced the anti-HACCP funding amendment, James Walsh (Rep-NY), chaired the appropriations subcommittee for agriculture. Mr. Walsh seemed to be acting on behalf of the meat industry—a lawyer for the National Meat Association had participated in drafting his amendment.[9] In a further action, Senator Robert Dole (Rep-KS), then majority leader and already campaigning for president, introduced a regulatory reform bill that would require federal agencies to review new regulations likely to cost industry more than $50 million annually, and to demonstrate that the benefits of such regulations would outweigh their costs. One purpose of the Dole bill was to stop government from regulating food safety. It contained provisions to (1) eliminate rules for pathogen testing, (2) postpone seafood inspection, (3) repeal the Delaney clause in the Food, Drug, and Cosmetic Act (which precluded use of carcinogenic food additives), (4) permit use of some carcinogenic pesticides, and (5) privatize approvals of food additives.

Such blatantly consumer-unfriendly legislation was ripe for satire, and figure 7 presents one such pointed commentary, in this case, from political cartoonist Garry Trudeau. Consumer advocate Ralph Nader observed that the Dole bill represented nothing less than a "big business takeover of the U.S. government in its health and safety responsibilities." Nevertheless, after contentious debate, the Senate passed various amendments to the Dole bill as part of the Republicans' Contract with America. As if to soften the bill's evident purpose, one such amendment expressed "the sense of the Senate that nothing in the bill is intended to delay the timely promulgation of any regulations that would meet a human health or safety threat."[10]

Mr. Walsh's industry-driven appropriations amendment was also under consideration, but the *New York Times* urged opposition: "By voting to defeat Mr. Walsh's amendment today, the Appropriations Committee would send a welcome signal that it cares more about protecting constituents' health than about pleasing the meat and poultry industries." Consumer advocates from the Washington, DC–based Center for Science in the Public Interest (CSPI) wrote that the Walsh proposal was "just a smoke screen to give businesses free rein to do business as usual—even if that means killing innocent children."[11]

Late in June, the House committee passed the Walsh amendment,

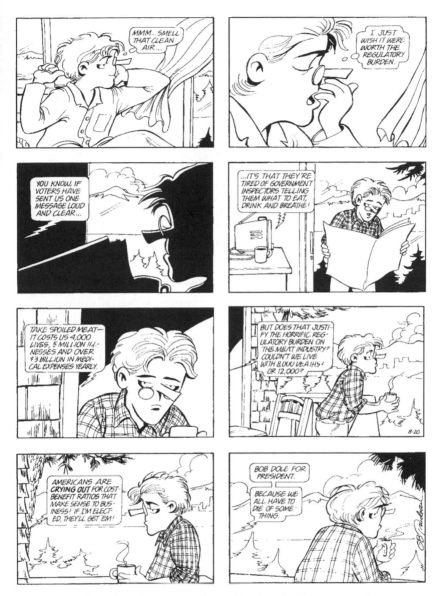

FIGURE 7. The political cartoonist Garry Trudeau had this to say about Senator Robert Dole's attempt to deregulate the meat industry. Mr. Dole was expected to run for president in the next election. (Doonesbury, August 20, 1995, © 1995 G.B. Trudeau. Reprinted with permission of Universal Press Syndicate. All rights reserved.)

making it clear that it was doing so to give "meat packers a chance to win relief from new food-safety regulations."[12] This meant that if the Senate also passed the amendment, the USDA would not be able to issue HACCP rules until it completed its "negotiated rulemaking" conversations with meat and poultry processors. This possibility inspired further editorial comment in the *New York Times*:

> Two things will happen to anyone who takes a close look at the way meat is processed and inspected in this country: they will wonder how it is that even more people are not made sick by tainted meat, and they will get sick to their stomachs themselves. . . . Naturally, the meat industry and its stooges in the Republican Party have ganged up on the Agriculture Department (and the American consumer) to make sure the new inspection system never sees the light of day. . . . [Negotiating rulemaking] is like negotiating prison rules with convicts. . . . Children will continue to die in excruciating pain because the meat they ate was contaminated, and because unscrupulous Republicans in Congress fought aggressively to keep it that way.[13]

At this point, Mr. Walsh suddenly withdrew his amendment, attributing this surprising retreat to a revelation that Congress could in fact work out its differences with the USDA: "We got the personal commitment of the secretary to create the dialogue we sought."[14] Alternative explanations seem more likely, however. Pressure from advocacy groups was surely a factor, especially a campaign organized by the families of children who became ill or died after eating contaminated hamburger. Advocates took credit for the amendment's withdrawal as a "resounding victory for public health and an unmasking defeat of good ol' boy politics." This last was a reference to press accounts that Mr. Walsh had accepted $66,000 in donations from meat and agricultural interests.[15] It also seems likely that members of Congress, not wanting to be viewed as destroyers of public health and killers of innocent children, suggested that Mr. Walsh would face a difficult floor fight if he pursued his anti-HACCP agenda. Ultimately, the Dole bill also failed to pass. Thus, one unanticipated—and positive—result of Mr. Walsh's amendment was to unite food safety advocates and encourage them to press for an independent food agency that would not be subject to such crass political pressures, an issue discussed in greater detail in chapter 4.[16]

The Last Attempts to Derail HACCP, 1995–1996

With the demise of the Walsh amendment, the USDA released the nearly 200 pages of "final" rules for Pathogen Reduction: HACCP for meat and poultry products. As with the earlier drafts, these would need to be made available for public comment before going into effect in July 1996. The rules required large firms to develop, install, and implement HACCP plans by the beginning of 1998, small firms by 1999, and very small firms by 2000. To help companies figure out how to proceed, the department created 13 model plans and provided detailed instructions for developing and using them (figure 5 in chapter 2 is based on one such model).[17] The published Pathogen Reduction: HACCP rules revealed that political pressures succeeded in achieving at least one compromise. Although the USDA originally wanted meat and poultry companies to be responsible for *Salmonella* testing, it now said that federal inspectors would test for *Salmonella* "on an unannounced basis." Companies would have to test for the *generic* form of *E. coli* (as a marker of fecal contamination) in just a small number of samples: 1 out of every 300 beef carcasses, 1,000 hogs, 3,000 turkeys, and 22,000 chickens.[5]

This time, meat processors used the comment period to press Congress to eliminate requirements for *Salmonella* testing. Their congressional sympathizers introduced an amendment to the Farm Bill that would create an "independent" oversight panel of food, meat, and poultry scientists with broad powers to review FSIS decisions on HACCP procedures, standards, and practices. The amendment required the USDA to submit proposed rules to the panel and then allow 90 days for public comment. At the very least, this plan would further delay the regulations. The policy director of the House Agriculture Committee explained that the purpose of the panel was *scientific:* "The H.A.C.C.P. rule is purported to be science-based, but it seemed clear that some of the regulatory decisions have no scientific validity. The regulations should never have gotten to this stage."[18] Reporters, however, viewed the panel as yet another political tactic to allow the meat industry to avoid having to test for pathogens. Eventually, this amendment failed to get enough votes to be included in the final bill.

Sorting out the political forces for and against Pathogen Reduction: HACCP is especially complicated because USDA inspectors also opposed the regulations. They had experienced a huge increase in "tasks not performed" just since the year before, meaning that their workloads had increased to the point where they could not complete assignments. One inspector, for example, complained that he was supposed to inspect 16 meat plants within a six-hour period. Once HACCP went into effect, workloads would be reduced (a benefit), but the inspectors did not like the idea that their jobs would change from inspecting animals and meat products—useless for preventing microbial contamination as that might be—to inspecting paperwork. The on-site USDA inspector at the meat-packing plant I visited, thoroughly disenchanted with having to deal with that paperwork, was counting the days until he could retire. Old-time inspectors quipped that because HACCP minimizes risk but can never assure absolute safety, its initials really should stand for "Have a Cup of Coffee and Pray."[19]

The General Accounting Office (GAO), however, continued to press for HACCP, also invoking science as the rationale. For years it had been issuing reports urging Congress to require oversight of food safety based on science (meaning assessment of hazards at critical points and evaluation by microbial testing) rather than sensory perception (poke-and-sniff). GAO officials complained that federal agencies repeatedly ignored their warnings and were still inspecting foods by obsolete systems that could not possibly address modern microbial hazards.[20]

In the case of meat and poultry regulation, reason eventually won out over politics, the benefits of HACCP prevailed, and the USDA issued its final set of regulations in July 1996—an election year in which the political climate had shifted to one more friendly to consumer interests. Perhaps as a sign of that change, the White House Office of Management and Budget (OMB), which typically opposed expansion of government regulations, praised the new rules: "For years, we have had the Government doing the work, the inspectors in the plants, and you hear stories of cursory checks and that's it. . . . This is an attempt to get away from Government micromanaging the process and instead saying to the regulated entity, 'you figure out how to do it, you're responsible, and we'll do some testing to make sure there are performance standards.'"[21]

An alternative reason for the OMB's blessing may have been financial. USDA economists calculated that the economic benefits of Pathogen Reduction: HACCP would outweigh its costs even under the most conservative estimates. Although the new rules were expected to cost industry more than a billion dollars over a 20-year period, the economic benefits to society would exceed that amount even if just 5% of foodborne illnesses could be prevented. Economists thought that if HACCP could achieve a 90% reduction in illnesses caused by just the six most common food pathogens, the 20-year savings in medical costs and lost productivity would be $170 billion or more.[22] Furthermore, the meat and poultry industries would share financial benefits in the form of reduced recalls and liability, enhanced consumer confidence, and robust sales.

By mid-1996, the HACCP schedule was in place. The E. coli O157:H7 testing of ground meat proposed in 1994 was due to start in January 1997. Large companies were to install Pathogen Reduction: HACCP plans by January 1998, and smaller companies by January 2000. From then on, all meat and poultry companies were to follow such plans and test for generic *E. coli*, endure USDA testing of ground meat for *E. coli* O157:H7 and spot-checking for *Salmonella*, and meet performance standards for pathogen reduction. Food safety would depend on how carefully they designed and implemented the plans, and how well the USDA enforced them. For most foods regulated by the FDA, however, HACCP remained voluntary. As we will now see, events soon revealed serious gaps in the regulations, and indicated additional needs: for extension of HACCP rules to all food products at all stages of production, for federal authority to recall contaminated products, and for ways of countering the culture of entrenched resistance to government oversight so prevalent in the meat industry.

THE PRODUCT GAP: ODWALLA APPLE JUICE, 1996

In October 1996, an outbreak of *E. coli* O157:H7 made it clear that *all* foods needed to be produced under Pathogen Reduction: HACCP because lapses could be catastrophic, not only for the victims, but also— temporarily, if not permanently—for the companies responsible for them. This outbreak put about 70 people in hospitals, made 14 children dreadfully ill, and resulted in the death of one child.[23]

The unexpected feature of the outbreak was its source: apple juice. Investigators used genetic techniques and diet histories to trace the infections to freshly bottled apple juice produced by Odwalla, a California company specializing in "natural" foods. The company included windfall apples, those that had fallen off the trees onto the ground, among the lots pressed to make the juice, and investigators suspected that the fallen apples must have come in contact with animal manure containing *E. coli* O157:H7. Although apple juice is naturally acidic, its acids are not strong enough to kill this hardy microbe. Odwalla did not pasteurize its juices; its managers believed that temperatures high enough to kill most bacteria would alter the flavor of the juice and reduce vitamin content (which pasteurization does, but only slightly). The managers also believed—gravely in error—that the acidity of the solutions used to wash the apples and of the juice itself would kill harmful bacteria.[24]

Investigators made other disheartening observations. Just before the outbreak, the company had relaxed its standards for accepting blemished fruit. It overruled warnings from its own in-house inspector not to use the batch of apples responsible for the outbreak without special precautions. At the time, Odwalla was expanding rapidly and having difficulty meeting production demands. Its stock price was declining. These pressures also contributed to the company's failure to follow its own established procedures.[25]

To their great credit, Odwalla officials quickly took full responsibility for the failure of their safety systems and issued a recall. They paid medical expenses for the people who had become ill and an indemnity of about $250,000 to the family that had lost a child. Eventually, they settled more than a dozen civil suits at a cost of more than $12 million— just for the families of the five children who had been most injured. They also paid in other ways. In the first criminal conviction recorded in a large-scale outbreak of foodborne illness, Odwalla officials pleaded guilty to violating federal food safety laws, paid a $1.5 million fine, and were placed on probation for five years.[26]

Odwalla's corporate policy includes an explicit statement of social responsibility to employees and customers. Its officials immediately admitted wrongdoing and wrote checks. They also took action to improve production practices. Odwalla now flash-pasteurizes its juices (high temperature, short time), uses a HACCP plan, and actively promotes its quality-control efforts. These actions restored consumer confidence. By 1999, sales had almost returned to former levels, and by 2001 the company was comfortably profitable. The actions also restored investor confidence. In 2000, Odwalla merged with Fresh Samantha, another fresh juice company. A year later, ironically, this producer of fresh, "healthy" juices was purchased by Coca-Cola, the world's largest soft drink company, in a deal said to be worth $181 million.[27]

Among the many lessons of the Odwalla outbreak is the vulnerability of the nation's supply of fruit and vegetables to cross-contamination from infected animals, pointing even more forcefully to the need to prevent foodborne illness at its source. The Odwalla incident induced the FDA to demand a warning label on unpasteurized juices. Manufacturers would have to prove that their production practices achieved a "5-log" (100,000-fold) reduction in the number of dangerous contaminants in their juice products. Otherwise, juice labels would have to display this statement: "WARNING: This product has not been pasteurized and, therefore, may contain harmful bacteria that can cause serious illness in children, the elderly, and persons with weakened immune systems."[28]

Makers of unpasteurized juices, however, objected to the warning requirement. They argued that health risks posed by apple cider are too low to need a warning label: such labels are discriminatory (the FDA requires no such warnings for fruit, eggs, melons, or seafood); and the statement is frightening, confusing, and misleading. As the chairman of Odwalla explained: "The regulation issue is a 'very sensitive' one for the natural-food industry. Fresh food, and especially fresh produce, is very hard to regulate."[29] Despite industry complaints, the FDA required the warning statement, and also issued HACCP regulations for domestic and imported juices in 2001.[30]

The Odwalla outbreak provided convincing proof that unpasteurized and uncooked "natural" foods could contain the same pathogens as meat and poultry if they had the bad luck to come in contact with contaminated animal manure or meat. For the industry, the lessons were mixed. If food companies failed to reduce pathogens, their liability costs could be substantial—in money, time, legal penalties, and reputation—but these problems could be temporary and soon overcome. From a regulatory perspective, the Odwalla outbreak illustrated the universal need for Pathogen Reduction: HACCP, but an additional lesson was that the FDA was only likely to require such plans for the foods it regulated when confronted with disaster.

THE RECALL GAP: HUDSON FOODS, 1997

The Odwalla outbreak also had implications for the livestock industry. Although beef industry officials were relieved to learn that fruit and vegetables could also be sources of *E. coli* O157:H7, meat products continued to cause outbreaks and unfavorable press. The USDA responded to the Odwalla outbreak by extending its generic *E. coli* testing requirements to include meat from goats, ducks, geese, and other animals but, in accordance with provisions of the old laws governing such matters, only after the animals had arrived at slaughterhouses.[31]

Limitations on USDA authority became even more evident as a result of yet another *E. coli* O157:H7 outbreak, this one beginning in July 1997 as a case of bloody diarrhea in a supermarket employee who brought ground meat home from his store. The employee remembered eating a lightly cooked hamburger from a lot that was still stored in his freezer. Investigators quickly traced other patties from that lot to a Nebraska plant owned by Hudson Foods. Eventually, 16 people became ill as a result of eating meat processed at the Hudson plant.[32]

At first, Hudson Foods officials told investigators that the contaminated lot included 3,400 pounds of meat that had been "reworked" into 20,000 pounds of hamburger the next day. They explained that their usual practice was to mix any meat left over from one day's production into the next day's batch of hamburger. This meant that if leftover meat contained harmful bacteria, the contaminated meat could get mixed into the next day's production. Plant officials neglected to tell USDA investigators that meat continued to be reworked from one day to the next, meaning that once a contaminated lot of meat got into the system, it would be mixed sequentially into all subsequent lots. Thus, the plant could not guarantee that *any* subsequent lot would be free of harmful bacteria. Because the Meat Inspection Act does not authorize the USDA to recall contaminated products, the department's only recourse was to withdraw inspectors, thereby forcing the plant to close. Faced with this possibility, Hudson began a "voluntary" recall that eventually included 25 million pounds of potentially contaminated meat.[33]

Meat industry officials complained that the forced recall was excessive in relation to the actual problem, as none of the 16 victims had died. Instead, they thought the USDA should pay more attention to practices in slaughterhouses and retail stores. A Nebraska Chamber of Commerce official defended Hudson Foods: "There's always somebody out there trying to downgrade the meat industry. . . . I'm sure the people—veggies, is that what they call them—I bet they're rejoicing right now."[34]

At the end of August, Burger King placed full-page ads in major newspapers announcing that its franchises would no longer use Hudson's meat: "Although there was absolutely no indication that any of the beef Hudson Foods supplied to us was unsafe, we issued the recall anyway, because the trust and confidence you need to have in us every time you visit one of our restaurants is more important than any loss of business." Because Burger King flame-broils its hamburgers to temperatures much higher than those needed to kill bacteria, the business press criticized its action as "impossible to explain in scientific terms. . . . The company's fulminations about *E. coli* are thus pure public relations."[35]

Hudson's bad luck was to receive a shipment of contaminated meat from one of its seven supplier slaughterhouses. Any other processing plant could have had the same problem, as *all* of them typically rework leftover ground meat or poultry into the next day's production, and do so day after day. On this basis, an American Meat Institute official blamed the USDA for the problem because its on-site inspectors did not challenge the reworking: "To my knowledge . . . the USDA doesn't consider that to be an unsafe practice or against any regulations."[36] This critique may have been accurate under the circumstances, but it did not speak to the need to prevent contamination at an earlier stage of production or to give USDA the authority to recall contaminated products.

In September, the USDA reported that hamburger meat from the Hudson plant was contaminated on more dates than previously thought but the company had failed to disclose that information: "The department was originally told by Hudson that only 20,000 pounds of meat was involved and had to find out from other sources that far more was at stake." For misleading the USDA, a federal grand jury indicted Hudson and two of its employees, a decision considered unfair by Hudson Foods officials. The former chairman of the company told a reporter: "The overreaction of the U.S.D.A. in Washington in this incident destroyed my company's good name." Late in 1999, a federal jury in Nebraska agreed, and found Hudson officials *not guilty* of lying to government inspectors. Hudson closed the plant after the outbreak, but it was soon bought by Tyson Foods and reopened. As noted earlier, Tyson Foods was then the largest producer of chickens in the world and was soon to become the largest producer of beef as well. Of the 25 million pounds of hamburger recalled, 10 million pounds were recovered, an amount significantly *higher* than for most recalls. For example, a late 1990s recall of E. *coli* O157:H7-contaminated hamburger from Beef America recovered only 400 of 443,656 pounds. Furthermore, the average percentage of product recovered in recalls fell from 40% in 1997 to 17% in 2000.[37]

In 2002, ConAgra "voluntarily" recalled 19 million pounds of ground beef after 19 people became ill with E. *coli* O157:H7 infections. The company produced the meat over a period of three months at a plant cited frequently for violations of safety codes. This incident provided further evidence that the USDA enforcement program was not working. A leaked GAO investigation of such matters was said to conclude that the USDA was taking more than a year (average: 566 days) to enforce standards in plants with high rates of *Salmonella* contamination, and some members of Congress complained about the USDA's "sluggish" pace of investigating deadly outbreaks.[38]

For food safety advocates, the contamination at the Hudson and ConAgra plants, and the USDA's inability to recall unsafe meat, illustrated the "linked failure of federal food safety programs and mismanagement by [the] food industry."[39] For USDA officials, it provided further evidence of the need for recall authority. As one official told a reporter during the Hudson controversy:

This enforcement gap gets downright absurd. . . . We can use fines to protect farmers and ranchers from unfair trading practices. Abuse a circus elephant, sell a cat without a license, market a potato that's too small, keep bad records on watermelons, fail to report to the union committee—fine, fine, fine, fine, fine. Yet if you produce unsafe food—the only one of these items that puts people's lives at stake—there is no civil penalty.[40]

On the other hand, the meat industry interpreted the Hudson recall as a further example of excessively intrusive federal rules: "The statutory authority sought by the USDA is not necessary and would be contrary to sound public policy. . . . Frankly, to take away a company's limited right to discuss with the agency the scope and depth of its recall would likely lead to less co-ordination and more litigation."[19] And Rosemary Mucklow of the National Meat Association charged that the ConAgra recall "may be an effort that is not justified" because the meat had already been in circulation for three months.[38] For the industry, the Hudson recall provided another opportunity for finger-pointing. Retailers such as Burger King blamed Hudson, while Hudson blamed the slaughterhouses and USDA inspectors. Everyone blamed the unregulated cattlemen, and not without reason. Investigations of cattle-rearing practices found *E. coli* O157:H7 in feeding troughs, where the bacteria can survive in sediments for four months or more; in one instance, 40% of the troughs had not been cleaned in a year.[41] The bacteria also survive in manure for months, and many animals are found to be shedding them at the time of slaughter.[42] Despite these and other safety concerns, nobody in Congress or the administration wants to take on the cattlemen, leaving food safety advocates in the USDA without much in the way of political support for controlling pathogens on farms and feedlots, let alone in slaughterhouses, packing plants, or grocery stores.

THE TESTING GAP: "NONINTACT" BEEF, 1999

Chapter 2 described how, as a result of the Jack in the Box outbreak, the USDA identified ground beef contaminated with *E. coli* O157:H7 as a public health risk, declared such beef "adulterated" under the terms of the Meat Inspection Act, and required the industry to reprocess or destroy it. It also described how the meat industry went to court to oppose— unsuccessfully, in that case—the USDA's 1994 imposition of a sampling and testing program for just this one pathogen (*E. coli* O157:H7) in just this one product (ground meat). Five years later, the USDA said it wanted to extend the definition of "adulterated" beyond just ground beef to include other forms of "nonintact" meat—meat that has been pounded, tenderized, or injected. Such procedures can introduce bacteria into the interior of the meat where they are unlikely to be cooked to as high a temperature as bacteria that contaminate outer surfaces. The USDA, however, continued to restrict its definition of "adulterated" to *E. coli* O157:H7. It excluded *Listeria* or *Salmonella* from this definition because these organisms are more easily killed during cooking. The department was not concerned about intact meat such as steak or chops because cooking or searing raises their surface temperatures high enough to kill bacteria.[43] Although USDA officials said they would not test nonintact meat other than ground beef and veal, industry officials did not believe them and reacted with "shock, disbelief, and anger," viewing the new policy as nothing more than an attempt to divert public attention from current political concerns. According to Rosemary Mucklow, who by then had become executive director of the National Meat Association: "This will be an extraordinarily confusing issue. . . . This is just another step in this administration's obfuscation of the impeachment activities."[44]

Ms. Mucklow's connection of *E. coli* O157:H7 testing to the then-current scandal involving President Clinton and a young White House intern, Monica Lewinsky, might seem a stretch for any group less relentless and self-serving than the beef industry. USDA Secretary Dan Glickman said he was "deeply and personally offended by this statement. USDA's efforts to improve food safety are grounded in science and a steadfast commitment to protecting public health."[45] The industry, however, continued to oppose the USDA's plans to test for *E. coli* O157:H7. Indeed, some thought that extending the testing requirements might backfire because companies would have an even stronger disincentive to do their own testing: "Given the serious financial ramifications of a positive test—the product would have to be recalled and then cooked or destroyed—it could be in the industry's best interest not to know."[38]

Over the next year or so, the USDA opened the nonintact beef policy for public comment, held a public meeting, issued a position paper on *E. coli* O157:H7 testing, and dealt with opposing opinions in *Federal Register* notices. The meat industry's position on pathogen testing remained fixed: microbes are inherent in raw meat, testing would put companies out of business, and testing is ineffective. Instead, meat officials argued, the USDA should gather more data on risk before taking action, and consumers and farmers should take more responsibility for food safety. Furthermore, they said, the policy discriminates against beef because pork and poultry are similarly contaminated.[46] Overall, the reactions to this proposal demonstrated that the beef industry was determined to oppose any expansion of pathogen testing, no matter how limited or beneficial to the public.

THE LEGAL GAP:
LAWSUITS AGAINST PATHOGEN REDUCTION: HACCP

As the consequences of Pathogen Reduction: HACCP for recall or destruction of contaminated products became increasingly evident, the beef industry went to court to force the USDA to adhere to the intent of the 1906 Meat Inspection Act: protect the public against sick animals, not bacteria. Two cases in the late 1990s illustrate the degree to which the industry would invoke that law, leaving to consumers the responsibility for avoiding bacterial contaminants.

Supreme Beef v. USDA

The lawsuit brought by Supreme Beef Processors in Dallas illustrates how the industry used the courts to block the USDA's imposition of *Salmonella* testing. When HACCP regulations for small meat-processing firms went into effect in 1999, companies had to meet this performance standard: testing must find no more than 7.5% of sample products to contain (give "positive" results for) *Salmonella*. During that first year, 20% or so of Supreme Beef's ground beef tested positive on two occasions. When a third round of testing also showed that the company's meat exceeded the 7.5% standard, the USDA withdrew its inspectors and forced the plant to close. The USDA must have been especially concerned because this company supplied nearly half the ground beef distributed to schools participating in the national school lunch program. Supreme Beef immediately sued the USDA. The department, it charged, had acted in an "arbitrary and capricious" manner because it did not have legal authority to regulate *Salmonella*. The suit also charged that because cooking kills *Salmonella*, these bacteria do not threaten public safety and cannot be considered adulterants.

Four meat trade associations supported the suit for the usual fingerpointing reasons. Rosemary Mucklow of the National Meat Association told reporters: "Supreme Beef . . . is experiencing the consequences of a requirement that we think has some serious problems. It would have been better if U.S.D.A. had tried to work it out" and "Poor sanitation at ground-beef plants is seldom to blame for salmonella contamination. . . .

It would be more effective to enforce performance standards at packing plants or feedlots and farms."[47] The USDA, as Ms. Mucklow surely must have known, has no enforcement authority over feedlots and farms.

At this point, a U.S. District Court judge in Dallas, A. Joe Fish, ruled that the USDA did not have the authority to close the Supreme Beef plant since doing so could irreparably harm the company. Instead, he issued an injunction against the USDA, forcing its inspectors to continue stamping the meat "USDA Inspected and Passed." The USDA dealt with this frustrating setback in its ability to enforce Pathogen Reduction: HACCP by canceling the department's school lunch contract with Supreme Beef.[48]

Furthermore, the USDA continued to test Supreme Beef's ground meat for *E. coli* O157:H7. Just two weeks after the Dallas court decision, USDA tests identified this pathogen in one sample of ground beef and again forced a "voluntary" recall, this time of 180,000 pounds. To the USDA, this finding proved that Supreme Beef's safety procedures were faulty and its lawsuit unjustified. The company, however, maintained that this recall was unrelated to the previous one because *Salmonella* "has nothing to do with the safety of the meat we produce."[49] In May 2000, the same Dallas judge (A. Joe Fish) who had supported Supreme Beef's position on *Salmonella* testing, extended his ruling to other plants in northern Texas; they also would not need to test for *Salmonella*. The *New York Times* found this ruling startling:

> Under the judge's strange reasoning, a plant that produces Supreme Beef's dismal salmonella test results might still be perfectly clean. The judge was troubled by the idea of penalizing a plant when the meat may already have been contaminated when it arrived there. . . . As a matter of logic and science, the excessive presence of dangerous salmonella in any meat turned out by a plant should be deemed evidence that conditions at the plant are unsanitary.[50]

In the months following those decisions, Supreme Beef again failed its *Salmonella* tests but could not be forced to close because of the court ruling. The president of the company, Steve Spiritas, characterized USDA's actions as an "all-out assault by the federal government on our small business." He charged USDA with "manipulating the testing results, suppressing critical information, . . . [and] using bullying tactics to support a position that a federal court has told it has no legal, logical, or scientific basis."[51] He also pointed out that meat supplied to Supreme Beef bore the stamp "USDA Inspected and Passed," meaning that USDA had certified its safety.

Some legislators attempted to introduce bills granting USDA the authority to impose limits on *Salmonella,* but these bills failed to pass. The USDA tried other approaches; it cited Supreme Beef for violating sanitation standards and initiated *daily* testing of ground meat for *E. coli* O157:H7. These actions caused Mr. Spiritas to complain that his small business was being held to unreasonable, discriminatory, and retaliatory standards. Eventually, he gave up, declared bankruptcy, and threatened to sue the USDA for its harassing tactics. The USDA tried to have the case declared moot because of the bankruptcy, but the courts denied this request. Supreme Beef, with the support of the National Meat Association and other meat industry groups, continued to pursue the case, as so much was at stake. If the USDA could shut down plants producing meat contaminated with *Salmonella,* as much as *half* the meat supply would be considered adulterated and subject to recall or destruction.[52]

In December 2001, a three-judge federal appeals court in New Orleans ruled that the USDA's *Salmonella* performance standards conflicted with the "plain language" of the 1906 law, which defined adulterated meat as "prepared, packed, or held under insanitary [*sic*] conditions whereby it may have become contaminated with filth, or whereby it may have been rendered injurious to health." The court referred to the 1974 decision in *APHA* v. *Butz* to argue that "*Salmonella,* present in a substantial proportion of meat and poultry products, is not an adulterant *per se*. . . . This is because normal cooking practices for meat and poultry destroy the *Salmonella* organism."[53] This ruling essentially overturned the pathogen reduction portion of HACCP. The beef industry welcomed the decision: "Using a relatively infrequently encountered pathogen such as salmonella as an indicator organism that can objectively measure a processing plant's performance is not scientifically warranted. . . . Supreme's brave lawsuit and the court's ruling against imposition of these flawed standards stands as a shining moment for the meat industry, a momentary triumph of reason over regulation."[54]

Less self-interested observers, however, did not see it that way. The *New York Times* called the court's decision "misguided" and its logic "seriously flawed," saying, "It ignores both the government's broad discretion under the law to police unsanitary conditions in meat plants and the serious danger, unresolved by proper cooking, that arises when contaminated raw meat and poultry come in contact with cutting boards, utensils and other foods, such as fruits and vegetables."[55]

The USDA's response to the decision was to announce that it planned to continue to conduct microbial testing to ensure food safety. The court's ruling eliminated our ability to take enforcement action based solely on salmonella standards. The ruling doesn't prevent the department from using salmonella standards to verify a plant's ability to address food safety hazards. Salmonella standards alert us that there may be a problem in a plant and that the whole plant needs to be examined, not just one piece of meat.[56]

Food safety–conscious senators and representatives introduced bills to give the USDA greater authority to regulate meat safety but, as noted by the *New York Times,* "These proposals have so far attracted no Republican co-sponsors. Even more troubling, the noises from the Agriculture Department suggest that the administration is more interested in satisfying industry's wish for lax regulation than in restoring the government's power to shut unsanitary plants. The Supreme Beef Processors decision has left a hole in the inspection system, putting consumers everywhere at increased risk."[57]

Lending further support to this charge, the USDA announced that it would not appeal the ruling, enforce *Salmonella* standards, or ask Congress to intervene. Under the administration of President George W. Bush, USDA officials appeared to be withdrawing support of HACCP, despite its evident effectiveness. Instead, the USDA would continue to test for *Salmonella,* but would use the results only as a basis for further inspections—not for closing plants or recalling products. These decisions "disappointed consumer advocates and [drew] praise from industry."[58] In response, Senator Tom Harkin (Dem-IA) introduced legislation that in effect would *order* USDA to follow its own rules for microbial contaminants. He said that he hoped the USDA had "not ceded the fight for safer food to the meat and poultry industry. . . . We must make it clear, once and for all, that the U.S.D.A. has the authority to set and enforce standards to reduce pathogens."[59] Whatever the outcome of such cases or legislation, they thoroughly expose the politics of food safety and the glaring gaps in federal regulatory authority.

USDA Inspectors versus "HACCP-Based Inspection Models"

In June 1997, the USDA asked for comments on how the department might develop new ways of inspecting meat in slaughterhouses and processing plants "in a HACCP environment." Inspectors were still examining every carcass, but the department thought they would be better employed checking for fecal contamination, sampling for microbial pathogens, and monitoring meat that left the plant. The department proposed to try out a HACCP-Based Inspection Models Project (HIMP) that would substitute such activities for examination of every meat and poultry carcass coming off the production line.[60] This time, the objections came from federal meat and poultry inspectors. The inspectors, their union (the American Federation of Government Employees), and a consumer advocacy group, the Community Nutrition Institute (CNI), sued the USDA to prevent the department from trying to do anything other than the carcass-by-carcass inspection required by the 1906 law. The inspectors' motivation is best expressed by the mission statement given on the union's Web site: "The-Inspector.com has been established in support of the thousands of dedicated Food & Consumer Safety Inspectors, working on the front lines of the meat, poultry & egg products industries, usually under miserable conditions, safeguarding the American food supply." At the time (it has since been sold), the Community Nutrition Institute published *Nutrition Week,* a newsletter that tracked current events in food and nutrition. Both were run by Rodney Leonard, long an outspoken advocate of improved food safety. Mr. Leonard's otherwise inexplicable role as a plaintiff in this anti-HACCP lawsuit reflected his view that the meat industry could not be trusted to conduct its own inspections or testing and that this responsibility properly belonged to government. A U.S. appeals court agreed. It chided the USDA for attempting to reinterpret the Meat Inspection Act.

> The government does not deny that in the ninety or so years since passage of the [1906 Act] . . . "inspection" has been taken to mean an organoleptic examination of the carcass, an inspection, that is, using the senses. Now the government has discovered another meaning. A "federal employee has performed an inspection of a carcass," the government tells us, "when he has watched a plant employee conduct the kind of examination, organoleptic or otherwise, that is necessary to determine whether the carcass is fit for human consumption." . . . In other words, the government believes that federal employees fulfill their statutory duty to inspect by watching others perform the task. One might as well say that umpires are pitchers because they carefully watch others throw baseballs.[61]

The decision against USDA left the future of HACCP uncertain. *Nutrition Week* called it "a great victory for consumers. . . . USDA is no longer allowed to abdicate its responsibility for food safety," and quoted a representative of the inspectors' union: "The court found what we have maintained for years—allowing industry to inspect itself is a violation of the law."[62] USDA responded by modifying the pilot system so that inspectors would continue to monitor carcasses. In January 2001, a federal court permitted the USDA to implement the proposed revisions, but the plaintiffs said they would appeal that decision. They argued that USDA's changes were insufficient and that the true purpose of the new system was to deregulate the meat industry.[63]

While the court case was in progress, Congress asked the General Accounting Office (GAO) to evaluate the effectiveness of the model inspection system. After a nine-month investigation that involved close examination of records from 11 model inspection projects in chicken plants, interviews with numerous participants, a survey of more than 200 inspectors, and visits to similar projects in Canada and Australia, the GAO produced a lengthy report of its findings in December 2001. Its conclusion: "a risk-based inspection system—such as the one that USDA is pilot-testing at chicken plants and is starting at hog plants—has merit in concept and is consistent with the existing risk-based framework for HACCP." GAO investigators, however, thought that the design of the projects was so flawed that it was impossible to determine whether the new system performed as well as the one it was supposed to replace. In particular, they noted that the results of *Salmonella* testing were worse at nearly half the plants using the modified inspection system. Nevertheless, they said,

> This report reiterates our previous recommendation for legislative revisions aimed at reducing the potential for further legal challenges by providing USDA with a clear authority to modify its inspection system. . . . We continue to believe that . . . Congress should consider revising the Meat and Poultry Acts . . . to provide FSIS with the flexibility and discretion to target its inspection resources for the most serious food safety risks. Such revisions would eliminate the requirements that USDA has traditionally implemented through continuous carcass-by-carcass government inspection and replace them with a risk-based inspection system that includes government oversight and verification. [64]

In response, the USDA said, "No food safety or non-food safety defects are acceptable to FSIS. While no system is perfect, the models project is an effort to reduce and eliminate defects that pass through traditional inspection."[65]

Although further court action allowed the USDA to continue to test alternative inspection methods, studies continued to reveal serious flaws in food safety at the plants using the model systems. The USDA's own studies showed that 13 of 16 plants had higher rates of *Salmonella* contamination under the new system (but lower rates of problems with *E.*

coli O157:H7).[66] The most obvious interpretation of such dismal results is that neither the plants nor the USDA nor its inspectors were sufficiently committed to doing what is necessary to protect the public and reduce foodborne illness.

No matter how the model projects and court cases eventually resolve, they reveal how strongly HACCP conflicts with entrenched views. Inspectors worry about protecting their jobs; some consumer groups distrust the industry's willingness to develop and monitor HACCP controls appropriately; the USDA is caught between Congress, the industry, and the courts; and each component of the meat and poultry food chain—producers, processors, retailers, and consumers—believes that responsibility for food safety belongs elsewhere. If nothing else, the legal battles over HACCP implementation make it clear that nothing less than a complete overhaul of the existing food safety system can fix the problems and provide adequate oversight.

THE CULTURE GAP: MEAT INDUSTRY VERSUS INSPECTORS

The persistence of some segments of the meat industry in opposing pathogen testing can be explained by economic interests, of course, but also by the cultural tradition of individualistic, antigovernment attitudes reflected in images of cowboys riding herd on cattle in remote areas of the West. The industry culture also reflects what the meat industry itself is about—the slaughter of animals for food. As Upton Sinclair so graphically explained, much of the work of this industry is "stupefying and brutalizing." Despite reforms, more recent observers like Eric Schlosser continue to find this work repetitive, filthy, and terribly dangerous.[67]

Although meat producers and inspectors both oppose one or another aspect of USDA regulations, their common opposition does not unite them. On the contrary, the inspectors despise the industry for supporting self-inspection (albeit without testing for pathogens), and the industry does little to discourage—worse, actively encourages—open hostility, not only to the USDA regulations, but also to the individual inspectors who enforce them. In June 2000, in an extreme example of such hostility, the owner of the Santos Linguisa sausage factory in San Leandro, California, opened fire on four state and federal meat inspectors, wounding three of them; he then reloaded and killed three of them execution style with shots to the head. HACCP requirements for the plant had taken effect that January, and inspectors subsequently identified repeated failings of temperature control points and other problems. The plant's owner,

Stuart Alexander, was known to have threatened the meat inspectors. He posted their photographs in the plant and displayed this sign outside its walls: "To all our great customers, the U.S.D.A. is coming into our plant harassing my employees and me, making it impossible to make our great product. Gee, if all meat plants could be in business for 79 years without one complaint, the meat inspectors would not have jobs. Therefore, we are taking legal action against them." Evidence presented to a grand jury included a video of the shootings and electronic mail messages from Mr. Alexander. One example: "I'm taking action against these government slime balls. . . . They messed with the wrong guy this time, baby."[68]

This incident, isolated as it was, appeared to be just the tip of the cowboy-culture iceberg. Meat inspectors told USDA officials that "threats from business owners upset over citations or what they perceive as unfair investigations are commonplace. . . . It's intimidating when you go into an office of some individual who is violating the codes and he has a pistol sitting on his desk." Verbal abuse was *normal* in the course of their duties, they said. At one meeting, 40% said they had been threatened, and 10% said they had been physically attacked—sometimes with knives or guns.[69] In the wake of the shootings, an Internet newsletter for meat processors published a series of articles on the industry's relationships with inspectors. The articles reported humorous accounts of the incident ("Jokes about the murders sprang up like poison mushrooms") and quoted a ground beef producer in New York City, referring to an article about the shootings on his wall: "'Oh, we have that there as a joke. . . . Those guys—meaning the inspectors—can really aggravate you.' 'I tell my inspectors they're next,' laughed another." The articles noted that inspectors had the power to make life miserable for companies: "Some inspectors—not all, of course, but some—seem to take advantage of this power with particular relish. . . . Worse, the retribution may be endemic to the federal inspection program. . . . Administrators at FSIS seem powerless—or too weak-willed—to stop it."[70]

USDA officials asked meat industry leaders to tone down the hostile rhetoric, called a series of meetings on workplace conflict and violence, issued directives on how to handle violent incidents, and encouraged employees to report incidents to a hotline. The number of hotline reports increased from 62 in 1999 to 161 in 2001 and affected every inspection district. Overall, the USDA documented 252 incidents of workplace violence against inspectors in 2001.[71]

Changing such ingrained patterns of hostility among meat industry employees will not be easy. The laws require what everyone agrees is a "unique regulatory framework. . . . In no other industry are regulators required to be continuously present in order for the regulated facility to operate," and "a certain segment of the population harbors strong animosity toward authority in general and the federal government in particular."[72] The primary activity of the meat industry is the killing of animals for food, and some level of "stupefying, brutalizing" callousness is only to be expected.

From the incidents discussed in chapters 2 and 3, we see that the politics of food safety early in the twenty-first century involves multiple elements. Microbial outbreaks are due to new and more dangerous organisms that affect an increasing number of foods. Federal agencies issue regulations for reducing pathogens for some—but nowhere near all—foods vulnerable to contamination. Government oversight remains mired in century-old laws, fragmented between two agencies with conflicting missions and rules. Both agencies lack adequate resources, political will, and industry support. The regulated industries resist pathogen controls as impositions, blame government or consumers for safety problems, and tolerate occasional legal liability as a reasonable price for conducting business as usual—even if doing so results in completely avoidable illness and death. As we will see in the next chapter, food companies much prefer consumer education or food irradiation to Pathogen Reduction: HACCP, and they continue to oppose any genuine strengthening of a federal role in food safety.

CHAPTER 4

ACHIEVING SAFE FOOD

ALTERNATIVES

AS CITIZENS, WE NEED TO UNDERSTAND THAT PRODUCING SAFE food is not impossibly difficult. Food scientists proved years ago that HACCP systems prevented foodborne illness in outer space. Those systems should work just as well on earth. Sweden, Denmark, and the Netherlands have reduced foodborne illnesses by instituting control systems at every stage of production, starting on the farm. They set testing standards to reduce pathogens, limit antibiotics in animal feed, prevent infections in transported animals, test for microbes at slaughterhouses and supermarkets, and provide incentives to the industry to comply with safety rules. Our government could also take such actions. That it does not is a result of an entrenched political system that allows federal regulators to avoid enforcing their own rules, and food companies to deny responsibility and blame each other, the regulators, or the public whenever outbreaks occur. Rather than collaborating to reduce foodborne pathogens, the agencies and companies shift attention to consumer education as the best way to ensure safe food. Failing that, they call for foods to be irradiated or pasteurized. This chapter examines the education, irradiation, and pasteurization alternatives along with two others: using the courts to impose legal liability for foodborne illness, and reorganizing government to consolidate and improve oversight of food safety.

Before addressing these alternatives, we need to deal with one further issue: food imports. Pathogen Reduction: HACCP applies to domestic food production. The countries from which we import fruits, vegetables, and other foods do not necessarily follow such rules. Because food imports are influenced (if not governed) by international trade agreements, methods to ensure food safety must also take such agreements into consideration.

IMPORTING SAFE FOOD: THE POLITICS OF FOOD TRADE

We live in a global economy with a global food supply. If we insist on having fresh strawberries and tomatoes in January (beyond those grown in our southern states), we have to buy them from countries with warmer climates. In 2000, the United States imported fresh and processed foods worth nearly $49 billion (including about $8 billion worth of fruits, vegetables, and juices), many of them from places with lower standards of water quality and sanitation. Imported foods have caused notable outbreaks: Hepatitis A from Mexican strawberries, *Vibrio* from Thai coconut pudding, *E. coli* O157:H7 from French semisoft cheeses, *Staphylococcus* from Chinese canned mushrooms. That we do not experience more episodes of illness is nothing less than miraculous, a tribute more to our healthy immune systems, the benefits of cooking and food preservation, and plain good luck than to federal oversight.[1]

Any system for grappling with the safety of imported food must deal with the usual two agencies, neither with anywhere near the resources required for this task. The USDA samples about 20% of imported meat and poultry products and rejects those from countries that do not meet our safety standards; it holds the "right of equivalency." In contrast, the FDA does not have this right and cannot reject imported foods that fail to meet our standards. This enforcement gap is not for lack of trying. FDA Commissioner David Kessler specifically requested the right of equivalency in 1993, and the General Accounting Office (GAO) called on Congress to grant it in 1998. Until recently, the FDA inspected less than 1% of the imported foods under its jurisdiction, down from 8% in 1992. In response to concerns about "homeland security," the level doubled—to 2%—in 2002. The FDA's challenge is daunting: in the late 1990s, it employed just 113 inspectors to examine 3 million food shipments flowing through 309 ports of entry to the United States. Yet at the Laredo, Texas, crossing point alone, 1.3 million trucks from Mexico enter the country each year. In 1997, Congress allotted $41 million to improve food inspection across the *entire* nation. At the same time, it granted $230 million for narcotics control, just for the Southwest border with Mexico. Food safety has never been a Congressional priority and, as we will see in the concluding chapter, it still is not.[2]

Trade works both ways; we exported about $54 billion worth of food products in 2000. Food exports represent 20% of the value of U.S. agricultural production and about one-third of our total harvest. The ability to sell agricultural products abroad is a critically important factor in our economy. If Congress gave the FDA the authority to reject foods from countries with lower safety standards, countries with higher standards might refuse to accept *our* products. The result: trade problems. Other countries, after all, can exercise their own rights of equivalency. In 2002, for example, Russia temporarily banned imports of U.S. poultry, saying the chickens carried influenza, had been treated with antibiotics, and were contaminated with *Salmonella*. The ban affected nearly one-quarter of the more than 1 million tons of frozen chicken (worth $640 million) expected to be exported to Russia that year. U.S. officials argued that the Russians were more worried about protecting their own chicken production than about safety. Trade negotiators worked for three weeks to resolve the dispute.[3] Regardless of the agencies' need for more inspection resources, any additional regulatory authority over imported foods might backfire if trading partners refused our exports.[4] Hence, politics.

International trade issues related to food safety are resolved through a commission of the United Nations known as Codex Alimentarius (Latin for "food code"). The commission's purpose is to "promote the elaboration and establishment of definitions and requirements for foods, to assist in their harmonization and, in doing so, to facilitate international trade."[5] With respect to food safety, this goal places the commission in potential conflict of interest; the Codex promotes safe food on the one hand, but trade on the other. As it turns out, trade issues almost always take precedence, perhaps because of the commission's composition. Among the nearly 2,600 individuals who participated in Codex meetings in the early 1990s, for example, 25% represented industry while only 1% represented public interest groups (the others were government officials). Among delegates from the United States at that time, nearly half (49%) were drawn from industry.[6] That imbalance continues.

The Codex commission asserts that its safety standards are science based. If so, it can—and does—demand that members view its requirements as legitimate protections rather than trade barriers. In practice, the commission's efforts to "harmonize" the differing food safety regulations of member nations appear as pressures to *lower* standards: "Members shall ensure that any sanitary and phytosanitary measure is applied only to the extent necessary to protect human, animal, or plant life or health, is based on scientific principles and is not maintained without sufficient scientific evidence."[5] Because scientific proof of safety is difficult to attain, and the results of most (if not all) scientific studies are subject to interpretation, the Codex criteria leave much room for trade disagreements in which science is invoked in the self-interest of one country or another.

A 1997 U.S. outbreak of *Cyclospora* attributed to Guatemalan raspberries illustrates how difficult it can be to sort out such disputes. Until the mid-1980s, Guatemala did not grow raspberries. Then, during the country's campaign against leftist guerrillas, the U.S. Agency for International Development promoted development of "nontraditional agriculture" and encouraged farmers to grow exotic foods for North Americans as cash crops rather than continuing to grow corn and beans for themselves. Production grew rapidly. In 1992, Guatemala produced less than 4,000 pounds of the berries, but in 1996 it shipped 700,000 pounds.

Guatemalan raspberries become ripe and are ready to ship in April and May, when there is no competing source. Spring rains, however, encourage the growth of *Cyclospora*, a common cause of diarrhea among Guatemalan children and of illness among raspberry pickers. During the outbreak in the United States, investigators from the Centers for Disease Control and Prevention (CDC) found *Cyclospora* in the feces of people who had eaten Guatemalan raspberries. They did not, however, find the bacteria in the raspberries. Nevertheless, as a measure of prudence, they advised the public not to eat Guatemalan raspberries. Guatemalan growers were understandably distressed by unproven assumptions that their raspberries had caused the outbreak. They voluntarily suspended shipments but also "kicked the C.D.C.'s field investigator off their farms [and] denounced the American scientists as snipers fighting a trade war on behalf of the growers' California competitors." Reports quoted a spokesman for the berry growers: "Last year the guerrillas were in the fields asking my workers about their conditions . . . and this year it was the C.D.C. The C.D.C. is killing us. They kill us every time they open their mouths." The growers charged the United States with unfair trade practices: "Cyclospora? . . . They can't find it. . . . Protectionist forces find bugs or whatever to protect their market. It's a commercial war."[7]

To add to such complexities, some countries do have food safety standards higher than ours, which is one reason they resist imports of our genetically modified soybeans and corn, as discussed in part 2 of this book. As we will see, such disputes fall under the purview of the multinational World Trade Organization, a higher-level international entity that takes precedence over the Codex Commission. As is often the case with food safety, the ability of U.S. regulatory agencies to ensure the safety of imported foods is influenced by politics—in this case, global politics. With that said, we can now return to the measures we might take—as individuals and as a society—to promote food safety at every stage of production, from farm to table.

ALTERNATIVE #1: EDUCATE

When it comes to food safety, the public bears all of the health risks. But does that mean that we also must bear the entire burden of preventive measures? Of course, home cooks should follow basic principles of food safety, especially because doing so is not difficult and is almost always effective. Cooking kills most microbial pathogens, and cooked food remains relatively free of them when refrigerated or stored properly. Surveys, however, frequently find that home cooking practices violate the FDA's manual of food safety rules, the *Food Code*. This should be no surprise; hardly anyone has heard of it. Furthermore, the code is easy to violate; one merely needs to wipe a counter with an old sponge, use a dish towel more than once, store fresh and cooked foods on the same refrigerator shelf, or forget to wash hands. Even so, home code violations cause much less illness than those made by out-of-home food preparers who did not follow food safety rules.[8]

Nevertheless, addressing food safety in the home is now a primary goal of national public health policy. In 1980, when the Department of Health and Human Services (DHHS) established its first ten-year plan to improve health practices, officials estimated that nearly 75% of foodborne infections originated in restaurants, institutional food services, or processing plants. The plan mentioned washing hands and proper food handling as useful educational measures for workers in the food industry. Ten years later, DHHS assigned home cooks their own food safety objective: "Increase to at least 75 percent the proportion of households in which principal food preparers routinely refrain from leaving perishable food out of the refrigerator for over two hours and wash cutting boards and utensils with soap after contact with raw meat and poultry. (Baseline: for refrigeration of perishable foods, 70 percent; for washing cutting boards with soap, 66 percent; and for washing utensils with soap, 55 percent, in 1988)."[9] This meant that by the year 2000, 75% of home cooks should be routinely washing cutting boards with soap, as compared to 66% in 1988. The 1988 baseline figures indicated that a sizable proportion of the population *already* followed safe food-handling practices fairly often—or at least said they did.

In 2000, with foodborne infections increasing in frequency and severity, DHHS assigned an entire section to food safety in its ten-year plan for 2010. The overall goal, to *reduce foodborne illnesses*, includes three objectives dealing with pathogens—reduce infections, reduce outbreaks, and prevent antibiotic-resistant *Salmonella*. Another objective calls for an increase to 79% in "the proportion of consumers who follow key food safety practices." Because baseline data from a 1998 survey confirmed that 72% of consumers already did so, the goal recognizes that home code violations are not the principal cause of outbreaks. For this reason, DHHS added a "developmental" objective—one for which no baseline information is available—to "improve food employee behaviors and food preparation practices that directly relate to foodborne illnesses in retail food establishments."[10] Taken together, these objectives continue to place the responsibility for food safety on food handlers, not on food producers or processors.

The phrase *key food safety practices* refers to elements of an education campaign jointly organized by the USDA and DHHS through an entity called the Partnership for Food Safety Education, an "ambitious public-private partnership created to reduce the incidence of foodborne illness by educating Americans about safe food handling practices."[11] Additional members include the U.S. Department of Education, an association of food and drug officials, seven food trade associations, two consumer organizations, and one individual—the outspoken food safety advocate Carol Tucker Foreman, a partnership entity unto herself.

Because Ms. Foreman appears again in these pages, she deserves a more formal introduction. In 1999, she became distinguished fellow and director of the Food Policy Institute of the Consumer Federation of America, but her previous career reflects the revolving door between jobs in government, industry, and the public interest sector. From 1973 to 1977, she directed the Consumer Federation. Under the administration of President Jimmy Carter, she served as USDA assistant secretary for Food and Consumer Services, where she was a strong advocate of consumer-friendly policies in dietary guidance, food assistance, and food safety. Subsequently, she founded the Safe Food Coalition, which advocated overhaul of the USDA's meat and poultry inspection system. For 18 years, she headed a Washington, DC–based consulting practice that included corporations such as Monsanto, the agricultural biotechnology company, among its clients. Because she lobbied on behalf of Monsanto in its successful attempt to win FDA approval of a bioengineered cow growth hormone (see chapter 6), some groups question her reliability as a food safety

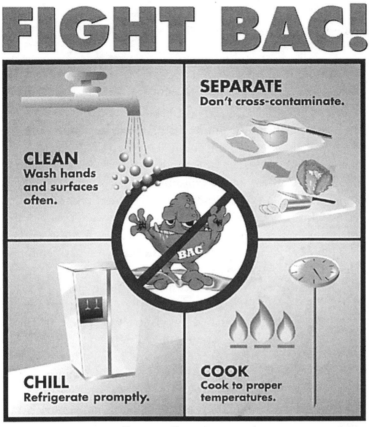

FIGHT BAC!

CLEAN
Wash hands and surfaces often.

SEPARATE
Don't cross-contaminate.

CHILL
Refrigerate promptly.

COOK
Cook to proper temperatures.

Keep Food Safe From Bacteria™

FIGURE 8. The Partnership for Food Safety's Fight BAC! campaign. This public-private partnership places the burden of food safety responsibility on the public rather than focusing on food production, processing, or service, which are more prevalent sources of food-borne illness.

advocate.[12] On the issue of food safety, her record speaks for itself; her forceful lobbying for Pathogen Reduction: HACCP has been unwavering, as will soon be evident.

To return to the partnership: its principal contribution to food safety education is a campaign called Fight BAC! Keep Food Safe from Bacteria. Fight BAC! promotes the four food safety actions described in table 9 (page 75) and illustrated in figure 8: clean, separate, cook, and chill.[13] The partnership produces this illustration and related materials—brochures, posters, public service announcements, and refrigerator magnets—in English and Spanish.

In addition to its role in the partnership, USDA's Food Safety and Inspection Service (FSIS) offers its own Food Safety Education (FSE) programs. These encourage consumers to cook ground beef to temperatures high enough to kill harmful bacteria and to use cooking thermometers to check such critical control points. Its materials emphasize the scientific nature of such practices: "A unique aspect to the FSE programs is their basis in sound science, as well as education theory and market research. The safe handling advice consumers get from FSIS educational programs and the USDA Meat and Poultry Hotline is based on the latest scientific information available."[14] Large food corporations also promote home food safety. ConAgra, for example, developed a campaign in 2000, "Home Food Safety . . . It's in Your Hands," in partnership with the American Dietetic Association.[15]

Although the advice given in such campaigns makes perfect sense, the education alternative hardly appears adequate to deal with problems of food safety, especially when focused exclusively or primarily on consumers. Scientifically based or not, the educational programs of the partnership, the USDA, and food corporations are directed toward a minor source of foodborne illness at the very end of the food chain. If anything, food producers, processors, and servers are the groups most in need of education about food safety. If, for example, meat and poultry producers better understood their role in the safety of the food supply, they might be less hostile and more receptive to the value of Pathogen Reduction: HACCP. They might understand why it is so important to institute healthier working conditions and more comprehensive training programs for employees. As noted earlier, food handlers typically earn the minimum wage, receive no sick leave or health benefits, and may not have obtained much education. Many workers in meat and poultry processing plants are illegal immigrants with even less access than others to such benefits.[16] These labor issues affect food safety because they lead to unsafe handling practices such as washing hands infrequently, staying on the job while sick, and failing to obtain treatment for intestinal infections. Education of employees would help, but education alone is not enough to ensure safe food. If we as a society are serious about preventing foodborne illness, we need to make certain that everyone who handles food is educated, is paid adequately, and, when needed, obtains sick leave and health care.

ALTERNATIVE #2: IRRADIATE

Because regulatory approaches to food safety are endlessly obstructed, and educational approaches do not address underlying causes, the food industry and some health officials urge more immediate action: irradiate foods to kill pathogens. Here is how Dr. Michael Osterholm, a leading national expert on foodborne illness, explains the meaning of the Hudson ground beef recall discussed in chapter 3:

> The current recall reinforces the impression that government can fully protect us against contamination of our food supply, and that when problems do occur, they'll quickly be fixed. The truth is quite the opposite. . . . Routine testing of the product will not provide us with a reliable way to detect every single episode of contamination. . . . There is one major step we, as a society, can take toward producing safer food. The answer is irradiation.[17]

Dr. Osterholm and many others fully agree that irradiation kills unwanted microbes. It uses the elements cobalt-60 and cesium-137 or electric current as sources of gamma rays, x-rays, or electron beams to bombard foods. These rays disrupt the genetic material (DNA) of cells in proportion to the intensity of the source element and the length of exposure. Lower or shorter bouts of radiation reduce the number of microbes on a food; higher and longer exposures can kill all of them.

Contrary to the belief of some critics, irradiation does not cause the foods themselves to become radioactive, and its physical effects on food are not so different from those induced by cooking (which also disrupts cell structures). High-intensity irradiation induces minor losses of nutrients as well as slight changes in color, flavor, and odor, particularly in fatty meats. Whether these changes matter depends on point of view. Proponents of irradiation view taste disadvantages as minor in comparison to the ravages of E. coli O157:H7. From the perspective of science-based risk assessment, the benefits of food irradiation far outweigh taste considerations.[18]

The sterility induced by irradiation, however, is usually incomplete and temporary. The foods must be irradiated in intact packages; once the packages are opened or damaged, foods can become recontaminated. Thus, irradiated foods must be handled like fresh foods and may need to be refrigerated to retard bacterial growth. Even so, this process confers substantial advantages to food producers and processors. They no longer need to be concerned about *preventing* contamination, because irradiation takes care of whatever pathogens are present. It also extends shelf life; irradiated strawberries, for example, can last 22 days on the shelf instead of the usual 3 to 5 days.[19]

Despite such advantages, the process is highly controversial and has been slow to gain acceptance. The very idea of irradiation induces dread and outrage, not least because it involves radiation, a foreign and personally uncontrollable technology. It also cannot guarantee sterility, and it treats rather than prevents safety problems. At best, irradiation is an end-stage technological fix.

The controversy is best understood in historical context. During World War II, the U.S. Army discovered that irradiated ground beef stayed fresh longer. Companies developed methods for commercial use by the late 1950s, but a congressional act in 1958 classified irradiation as, of all things, a food additive. This meant that companies had to prove the safety of irradiated foods before the FDA would authorize their sale. Because the companies thought the public would not accept such foods, they did not bother to press for approval.

In the early 1960s, the FDA began to authorize irradiation for limited use, one food at a time: first wheat and wheat flour; then spices, dried vegetable seasonings, pork, and chicken products for the general public; and then steak and turkey for astronauts. In turn, the USDA authorized irradiation for pork, poultry, and beef. Both agencies work to expand this list. In 2002, for example, the USDA proposed to permit Hawaii to export irradiated peppers, eggplants, mangoes, pineapples, squash, and tomatoes to the mainland.[20] Overall, more than 35 countries have approved irradiation as a means to preserve more than 50 different kinds of foods. Numerous national and international organizations have endorsed the process, among them health and food technology associations and—most enthusiastically—groups representing irradiation companies.

In the United States, the FDA requires irradiated foods to be labeled "treated with (or by) radiation" and to display the international symbol of irradiation—the radura—printed in green. As shown in figure 9, the radura symbol resembles the logo of the Environmental Protection Agency (EPA) and is meant to reassure the public that irradiated foods are ecologically correct, or "green." As we will see, supporters of irradiation say that any disclosure of the process is contrary to the public interest, and they consistently demand more favorable labeling requirements or—preferably—none at all.

Because fears of public disapproval inhibited development of the irradiation industry, the first multipurpose commercial food plant did not open until 1991. In 1994, Isomedix, a New Jersey company with 16 plants

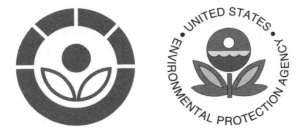

FIGURE 9. The friendly radura symbol of irradiation used on food package labels is shown on the left. Perhaps by coincidence, its color (green) and design resemble the logo of the U.S. Environmental Protection Agency, shown at right.

that irradiate medical devices and food packaging materials, petitioned the FDA to authorize irradiation of raw beef and lamb. Cattlemen strongly supported the petition and discussed the matter with their friends in Congress. Congress, in turn, pressured the USDA and FDA to come to a rapid decision. In 1997, during the period when USDA Secretary Dan Glickman was attempting to convince the Senate agriculture committee that his department should be allowed to issue mandatory recalls of contaminated meat, the senators "reacted skeptically, saying the plan would impose unnecessary new regulations when the focus should be on emerging technology like irradiation."[21]

Other groups also advocated approval of irradiation, charging that opposition to it was antiscientific. For example, Elizabeth Whelan of the industry-supported American Council on Science and Health (ACSH), proposed a much friendlier euphemism for the process in an article in the *Wall Street Journal:*

> Pasteurization through irradiation is safe and effective and is used in other countries and in the U.S. for pork, poultry, and other foods. . . . Antitechnology advocates . . . are circulating unfounded claims that irradiation poses a health hazard. . . . It is time for all of us to stop responding to the scaremongers. We must listen, instead, to scientists, who are unanimous in their conclusion that food irradiation—not more government regulation—will make America's food supply even safer.[22]

The Produce Marketing Association, an industry trade group, also supported irradiation for reasons of both science *and* values, in this case the value of "consumer choice": "Sound science must be the basis for decisions about all food issues. . . . Irradiation has been deemed to be a safe and viable technology . . . providing consumers the choice in the marketplace." Such statements, as we have seen, mistakenly equate safety (a scientific concept) with acceptability (a social concept). Meat industry officials, while lobbying for approval of irradiation, wanted to make sure that using it would not increase their accountability for foodborne illness: "Irradiation . . . is particularly important for ground beef . . . but the ultimate responsibility for food safety still rests with the food handler and preparer."[23]

The FDA delayed approval of irradiation for beef and lamb, not only because its approval processes are always slow, but also because its staff still needed to evaluate the effects of the process on meat from sheep as well as cattle and on fresh cuts as well as those that had been refrigerated and frozen. While the FDA was plugging along on its proposals for these rules, Congress passed the Food and Drug Administration Modernization Act of 1997 which, among other things, restricted the agency's ability to regulate irradiated foods: "No provision . . . shall be construed to require on the label or labeling of a food a separate radiation disclosure statement that is more prominent than the declaration of ingredients," and "FDA must act on petition within 60 days of enactment or provide to House and Senate an explanation of the process followed . . . and the reasons action on the petition was delayed."[24] Congress, therefore, insisted that the FDA allow food labels to disclose irradiation in very small type and approve irradiation requests within months rather than years.

Under that kind of pressure, the FDA immediately authorized irradiation of beef and lamb, explaining that the process "will not present a toxicological hazard, will not present a microbiological hazard, and will not adversely affect the nutritional adequacy of such products." The American Meat Institute hailed the approval as "a victory for consumers and the red meat industry."[25] Rodney Leonard of the Community Nutrition Institute (CNI) offered a different opinion. Although he firmly opposed HACCP (as noted in chapter 3), he also opposed irradiation:

> In addition to blaming the victim, government and industry are proposing a quick fix—food irradiation—to a problem of official neglect and industry abuse. . . . Bombarding contaminated foods with gamma rays will not improve public health, however, because it does not remove the feces of cattle and poultry. . . . The treatment is the only measure which government and industry can adopt which will not require the food supply to be cleaned up.[26]

Food safety advocate Carol Tucker Foreman succinctly reinforced this last point in a comment to *Consumer Reports:* "After all, sterilized poop is still poop."[26]

Despite such opposition, pressures to hide irradiation from consumers continued. In 2002, Congress passed the Farm Security and Rural Investment Act, mostly to authorize $190 billion in price supports for basic farm commodities, but also to equate irradiation (a radiation process) with pasteurization (usually understood as a heat process). The act requires the FDA to allow food labels to use *pasteurized* for any process that reduces pathogens in meat and poultry and to substitute this term for irradiation. This creative idea originated with Tom Harkin (Dem-IA), chair of the Senate agriculture committee, and a representative of the state housing the nation's largest irradiation plant for ground beef.[27] Even with such legislation, it is not clear whether the public will accept irradiated foods. Some experts believe that people will simply refuse to buy irradiated products; this possibility makes food producers so nervous that they all "want to be second to try it."[28] Some companies deliberately appeal to distrust of irradiation by advertising their products as nonirradiated. Fears of consumer resistance easily explain why the industry and its supporters pressed so forcefully for more attractive euphemisms such as "ionizing pasteurization" or "cold pasteurization." Will euphemisms convince people to buy irradiated products? Surveys reveal that at least half of consumers do not like *any* term for irradiation.[29]

Other surveys, however, report the public to be relatively unconcerned about this process, leading its proponents to reassure the food industry that consumers will readily accept irradiated foods. One report to industry (costing $75 a copy) promises readers that most consumers think irradiation will prevent foodborne illness and reduce disease risk (85–90%) and that most would buy irradiated products even if they were labeled as such (80%). The report quotes the president of the Food Marketing Institute: "Food irradiation is one safety tool whose time has come! . . . As an industry, we must also have the courage to support irradiated food products in the marketplace. . . . We must not let those who are afraid to let consumers make their own judgments use misinformation and scare tactics to win arguments they would lose on the scientific merits of the issues."[30]

Cost considerations, however, are likely to influence levels of outrage about this method, as may euphemistic labels so small as to be unnoticeable. Food technologists believe that when informed of the benefits of irradiation, the public will buy treated foods even if they cost more, as they most certainly will. Irradiation is expensive because of the equipment, the labels, and the transport from centralized facilities; the higher costs will be passed along to consumers. In 1997, USDA economists estimated that the cost to the beef industry alone could range from $28 million to $89 million annually, or from about 1.6 cents to 5 cents a pound. Although the costs to society of foodborne illness greatly exceed such amounts, and the additional price seems too small to make any difference to individual consumers, market comparisons suggest that a 10% premium for irradiated products would cause the proportion of people who might choose them to drop from 43% to 19%.[31]

This experiment is now underway. As irradiated foods increasingly enter the marketplace, the degree of acceptance by industry and the public will soon become evident. Furthermore, irradiation companies are using the anthrax scare of fall 2001 (discussed in the concluding chapter) to "do something they've been unable to do themselves: sell consumers on their controversial germ-zapping technology."[32] Even if consumers do opt to buy irradiated foods, the process is unlikely to solve food safety problems. On this point, I defer to Rodney Leonard:

> All irradiation will do is add partially decontaminated fecal matter to the American diet, a practice that is likely to cause food poisoning cases to skyrocket when bacteria develop the survival tactics to resist irradiation. All past efforts to "eradicate" microbial organisms . . . have succeeded only in creating new generations of super bugs, and irradiation will be no different. . . . *The solution to the food safety problem is to produce safe food* (emphasis added).[33]

Like many other food safety matters, irradiation raises issues of societal values that extend beyond the scientific. To questions about costs and benefits must be added others about the safety of those employees who work with and transport hazardous radioactive materials, and the environmental effects of discarding surplus sources of gamma rays. From a value-based perspective, irradiation is a techno-fix: a short-term corrective to a late-stage contamination problem that should be addressed much earlier in the chain of production.

ALTERNATIVE #3: PASTEURIZE

Technical solutions to food safety problems are linked, as we have seen, to conflicts between science and other kinds of value systems. The Odwalla company's corporate policy valued "fresh" and "natural," and it took a lethal outbreak to convince its managers to apply basic principles of microbiology to production processes; the company now pasteurizes its juices (in the old sense of the term). Many of my friends who are chefs or specialty food producers strongly believe that the sensory and cultural values of traditional raw or undercooked foods far outweigh the small risk of acquiring a foodborne infection. Raw (unpasteurized) milk—and cheeses made from it—have become rallying points for such views. For years, raw milk foods have caused rare but occasionally lethal outbreaks of *Listeria, Salmonella, E. coli* O157:H7, and other pathogens. The catalog of foodborne outbreaks maintained by the Center for Science in the Public Interest (CSPI) reported just 11 from raw milk and 8 from cheeses made with raw milk during the 11-year period from 1990 to 2001.[34] These numbers seem excessively high to the people who became ill from eating the foods, to the families of those who died, and to safety officials who want such foods pasteurized. The number of outbreaks appears minor, however, to people who prize such foods for their taste subtleties and cultural traditions and who believe that such benefits outweigh what seems like an occasional risk. In the case of raw milk foods, the choice is voluntary, and the foods generate little dread or outrage.

The risks are not equally distributed, however. Raw milk and soft cheeses such as the Mexican *queso fresco* are implicated most often; these are particularly dangerous when contaminated with *Salmonella* or other bacteria resistant to multiple antibiotics.[35] Harder domestic and foreign imported cheeses also have caused outbreaks and such incidents—rare though they may be—invariably elicit demands for mandatory pasteurization and restricted import of raw milk cheeses. As explained by an Oregon food safety expert, Dr. William Keene:

> Even after almost 100 years of effort, medical and public health experts have been unable to eliminate raw milk consumption. Raw milk has been and continues to be a staple in the epidemiological literature, linked to a long list of diseases. . . . There is no mystery about why raw milk is a common vehicle for salmonellosis and other enteric infections; after all, dairy milk is essentially a suspension of fecal and other microorganisms in a nutrient broth. Without pasteurization or other processing to kill pathogens, consumption of raw milk is a high-risk behavior.[36]

Dr. Keene points out that the aging and drying processes required to make many kinds of cheeses will kill most pathogens, but soft cheeses are "well documented hazards." Defenders of raw milk cheeses, who would be appalled by his characterization of dairy milk as a broth of fecal bacteria, seize on the protective benefits of the aging and drying processes. They argue that problems caused by raw milk cheeses are due to flagrant lapses in good manufacturing practices such as leaving raw milk unrefrigerated overnight or washing the equipment with water from a backyard garden hose (as was the case with the *queso fresco* harboring antibiotic-resistant *Salmonella*). Furthermore, requiring milk to be pasteurized might have prevented the *queso fresco* outbreak, but pasteurized milk also can become contaminated if it is handled carelessly.[37] The CSPI outbreak catalog lists just as many incidents due to pasteurized milk or cheeses (or to products of unspecified pasteurization status) as to those attributed to raw milk products. Foods made from raw milk still carry a higher risk, however, as fewer of them are on the market.

The American Cheese Society, a trade group representing the makers of specialty "artisanal" cheeses, advises its members to institute Pathogen Reduction: HACCP. With HACCP plans seemingly taking care of the science, the society also opposes mandatory pasteurization for reasons of values—democracy and individual rights:

> The American Cheese Society supports the continued democratic option to use both pasteurized and unpasteurized milk to produce America's cheeses. . . . We support the rights of individuals in all countries to enjoy their own great cheese historically made with unpasteurized milks. . . . We believe that mandatory pasteurization places an unnecessary hardship on those cheesemakers dedicated to safe and healthy practices. . . . We will ensure that our cheesemakers' options to use pasteurized and unpasteurized milks are both heard and understood.[38]

I like the cheeses produced by the members of this society, and I enthusiastically support the work of artisanal cheese makers. Many of them make superb products, whether from unpasteurized or pasteurized milk. I am happier eating them, however, when I know that the maker of the cheese is following a carefully designed Pathogen Reduction: HACCP plan that includes microbial standards verified by testing. No matter how rarely an unpasteurized cheese causes an outbreak, its makers and consumers are taking a gamble—and one with unknown odds.

Good manufacturing practices can reduce the odds to practically nothing, however. On a trip to Italy in 2002, I visited a producer of handmade pecorino and ricotta cheeses derived from raw sheep's milk (*latte crudo*). The owner employed a full-time microbiologist to test every batch of cheese for *Salmonella, Listeria, E. coli* O157:H7, and several other potential pathogens. He also insisted that his milk suppliers do such testing, and aged his cheeses beyond the time the FDA requires for imports. With this level of care, raw milk cheese raises minimal safety concerns.

To generalize from this example: Pathogen Reduction: HACCP should reduce foodborne illness when manufacturers follow the plan and monitor pathogen levels in the products. Failure to do so can cause severe illness in consumers (and severe liability for manufacturers). It may be true that only an occasional child gets sick or dies from eating contaminated food, but that event becomes a personal tragedy rather than a statistical matter if the child is *yours*. Whether eating raw foods is worth the risk is a matter of personal values when—and only when—all parties understand and take responsibility for what is at stake. Education of consumers or techno-fixes cannot protect against illness when the problems originate at the production or processing level, which is why Pathogen Reduction: HACCP and monitoring of performance standards are essential for producers of all foods, artisanal as well as corporate.

ALTERNATIVE #4: LITIGATE

It might seem reasonable to think that the cost of outbreak judgments in the tens of millions of dollars would be enough to make companies leap to put effective HACCP plans in place, required or not. That they fail to do so is in part a result of the shared responsibility for food safety among producers, processors, retailers, food service providers, and the public. USDA officials explain the behavior of meat and poultry producers in these terms:

> When consumers cannot trace an illness to any particular food or even be certain it was caused by food, food retailers and restaurateurs are not held accountable by their customers for selling pathogen-contaminated products and they, in turn, do not hold their wholesale suppliers accountable. This lack of marketplace accountability for foodborne illness means that meat and poultry producers may have little incentive to incur costs for more than minimal pathogen and other hazard controls.[39]

As we have seen, criminal charges in food-poisoning cases are rare, especially in comparison to the number of cases of illness and outbreaks. In 2000, about 20 of the nation's 6,000 meat processors pleaded guilty to violations of meat inspection regulations. In 2001, the Sara Lee company admitted to charges that it sold *Listeria*-contaminated meat responsible for the deaths of at least 15 people in 1998. Furthermore, the penalties can be quite light. In 2002, one of the owners of a Texas salvage food operation was fined $2,000, ordered to pay a $100 fee, and placed on probation for three years (including 120 days of home confinement) for selling rodent-contaminated meat.[40]

The typical corporate culture of "it's not my fault" is one reason for the lack of accountability, but another is the difficulty of assigning direct responsibility for an outbreak to one or another link in the chain of food production and consumption. A 1999 outbreak of *E. coli* O157:H7 illustrates this problem. The outbreak occurred among people who attended a state fair in upstate New York. Investigators recorded more than 1,000 cases of illness, 65 hospitalizations, and two deaths, one of a child and the other of an elderly man. They traced the source to drinking water from a well at the fairgrounds. A recent deluge of heavy rains had flooded the fairgrounds and allowed contaminated water, first thought to have come from manure from nearby barns, to leak into the well. Later, they discovered a nearby sewage pit that belonged to a fairgrounds dormitory run by a Cornell Cooperative Extension 4-H program. The well water was not chlorinated. In a situation like this, who is liable? Contributing to the outbreak were the fairgrounds, the cow barns, the dormitory, and the rain (an "act of God"). Eventually, suits were filed against Cornell Cooperative Extension on behalf of some of the sick children.[41]

Even if liability could be assigned easily, it is not clear that damage payments would be much of an incentive to food producers to be more careful. In a 1998 report on food safety, a committee of the National Research Council (NRC) pointed out that the risk of bad public relations is likely to be a much greater motivating force, as "the public is quick to shun whole categories of food products alleged to be tainted."[42] This reaction certainly was true of the Jack in the Box and Odwalla outbreaks, but in these cases it was short-lived. Both companies recovered customers and sales. Filing lawsuits is an expensive proposition—in time and emotion—for the victims of outbreaks and is another end-stage solution to a problem that should have been prevented in the first place.

ALTERNATIVE #5: REORGANIZE

Political problems require political solutions, which is why people without a vested interest in the current system—and some who have such an interest—support an entirely different approach to food safety: creation of a single independent government oversight agency. The idea is hardly new. A White House nutrition conference implied this need in 1969, and the National Research Council explicitly recommended creating such an agency in 1979. In 1988, the Food Marketing Institute, a conservative trade organization representing retailers and wholesalers, proposed that "the government's role can be accomplished if authority and responsibility for food safety are assigned to a single federal government agency. . . . It is vital that those agencies that currently have food safety responsibility be given sufficient resources to do the job properly and to ensure public confidence."[43]

The congressional watchdog agency, the General Accounting Office (GAO), has urged creation of a single food agency for years, despite the evident political barriers. In 1992, for example, the GAO told Congress that in a food safety system as entrenched as this one, "reaching agreement on such a major structural change would be difficult, at best."[44] Nevertheless, it continued to press Congress on this point. In 1993, it said, "In our view, creating a single food safety agency is the most effective way for the federal government to resolve long-standing problems, deal with emerging food safety issues, and ensure the safety of our country's food supply."[45] In 1999, the GAO again said:

> During the past 25 years, we . . . made numerous recommendations for change. While many of these recommendations have been acted upon, improvement efforts have fallen short, largely because the separate agencies continue to operate under the different regulatory approaches implicit in their basic authorities. Consequently, it is unlikely that fundamental, lasting improvements in food safety will occur until systematic legislative and structural changes are made to the entire food safety system.[46]

Despite such urgings from impartial investigators, Congress has failed to follow this advice. Government agencies, rather than taking whatever steps they can to unify the system, tend to protect their own resources. In 1993, for example, FDA commissioner Dr. David Kessler agreed on the need for a comprehensive food safety policy but insisted that *his* agency take the lead in federal safety efforts and that any new initiatives should be designed to strengthen the FDA's role in this area.[47]

As a result of political pressures, federal leadership on food safety appears unfocused. In 1997, President Clinton announced a budget of $43 million for early detection and prevention of foodborne microbial outbreaks; of that amount, more than half would go to the FDA for seafood inspection. Instead of a single agency, he created the Food Safety Initiative—a joint effort led by the chief administrators of USDA, DHHS (the FDA's parent agency), and the Environmental Protection Agency (EPA). He asked these officials to work with industry and consumer groups to recommend improvements in food safety research, inspection, and education.[48] As is customary in such situations, the group issued a report— this one designed to improve the *separate* programs of each agency. Its one concession to joint efforts: a proposal for a plan to "make the best use of each agency's limited resources, with no mention of a single food agency."[49]

Later that year, Senator Richard Durbin (Dem-IL) introduced legislation to replace the current system with an independent food safety and
inspection agency, but his bill did not get very far. President Clinton asked
Congress for a $101 million increase in spending for the Food Safety Ini-
tiative to bring the total federal expenditure for this purpose to $817 mil-
lion. This, he said, would "take the agencies that deal with food inspection from the 19th century to the 21st century."[50] Relatively small as these
amounts might be, Congress did not want to grant them. Agriculture
committee members said that until the day federal agencies could define
precisely how much it would cost to reduce foodborne illness, "they won't
get any more money. . . . Some of the Food and Drug Administration's
duties [should] be delegated to states and local governments."[51] GAO
investigators continued to press two points: (1) the USDA wasted most
of its food safety budget on archaic inspections of slaughtered carcasses,
and (2) the Food Safety Initiative failed to address fundamental weaknesses in coordination. Such arguments proved irrelevant when Congress
provided only limited funding that year.[52]

In 1998, the National Research Council (NRC) issued *Ensuring Safe
Food*, a report commissioned by Congress at a reported cost of $420,000.
The NRC committee must have been uneasy about how its work might
be received, because it repeatedly emphasized the report's scientific un-
derpinnings. Its purposes, said the committee, are to "determine the *scientific* basis of an effective food safety system," "identify *scientific* needs
and gaps," and "[recommend] *scientific* and organizational changes in
federal food safety activity needed to ensure an effective *science*-based
food safety system" (emphasis added).[42] Although Rodney Leonard described this report as "one of the most expensive term papers ever written,"[53] the committee's scientific defensiveness is understandable, as it
took considerable courage to recommend

> a unified and central framework for managing federal food safety pro-
> grams, one that is headed by a single official and which has the responsibil-
> ity and control of resources for all federal food safety activities. . . .This
> recommendation envisions an identifiable, high-ranking, presidentially
> appointed head, who would direct and coordinate federal activities and
> speak to the nation, giving federal food safety efforts a single voice. The
> structure created, and the person heading it, should have control over the
> resources Congress allocates to the food safety effort; the structure should
> also have a firm foundation in statute and thus not be temporary and easily
> changed by political agendas or executive directives. . . . The most viable
> means of achieving these goals would be to create a single, unified agency
> headed by a single administrator.[42]

In arguing for one accountable official, the NRC deliberately rejected two other leadership options, one of them a joint coordinating committee like the one in charge of the Food Safety Initiative. President Clinton, however, ignored this advice. Instead of appointing a *czar,* he did something even less likely to be effective. He appointed a *troika*—a President's Council on Food Safety led by three people: the secretaries of USDA and DHHS and a high-level science advisor. A spokesman for the National Food Processors Association seemed delighted that the program would not be led by a single person holding considerable power and said, apparently without irony: "When you have a czar, that would probably create a new bureaucracy. . . . It is important to keep politics out of food safety."[54]

In its formal announcement of a National Food Safety Initiative, the troika produced this cheerfully optimistic vision statement:

> Consumers can be confident that food is safe, healthy, and affordable. We work within a seamless food safety system that uses farm-to-table preventive strategies and integrated research, surveillance, inspection, and enforcement. We are vigilant to new and emergent threats and consider the needs of vulnerable populations. We use science- and risk-based approaches along with public/private partnerships. Food is safe because everyone understands and accepts their responsibilities.[55]

To support this vision, Congress allocated a budget of $370 million for the *entire* surveillance, coordination, inspection, risk-assessment, education, and research components of the initiative for fiscal year 2000. This figure amounted to about $1.50 per person and was about the same size as the advertising budget of Burger King that year. One full year after release of the NRC report, officials of the FDA and USDA seemed in no hurry to make progress on its recommendations. Instead, the troika of the Council on Food Safety, now joined by the secretary of commerce as a *fourth* member, was at work on yet another report. When released early in 2000, the report made no specific recommendation for structural change but instead suggested a range of options for consideration: (1) tweaking the current system so that it would speak with a "single voice"; (2) tweaking it to make one agency (but not necessarily the same one) responsible for chairing the council, leading the efforts, or overseeing everything having to do with specific food products such as pizza or sandwiches; (3) giving one unit within each agency full responsibility for all of that agency's food safety functions; or (4) creating a stand-alone, cabinet-level food safety agency.[56]

Perhaps because the council listed the single agency as the last option, food industry groups praised its science-based approach and its lack of enthusiasm for erecting "a monolithic super bureaucracy that would do little to reduce the risk of foodborne diseases."[57] To food safety advocates, however, the plan was nothing but "platitudes"—federal agencies protecting themselves—because it provided no timelines, deadlines, or budgets. In defending the plan, an FDA official said that he understood why people might view the agency's insistence on science-based approaches to regulation a "stall," as the FDA would always need more data on which to base decisions. Nevertheless, he said, the FDA intended to make the plan "real."[58]

The council's strategic plan, released a year later, in January 2001, analyzed the various options and unsurprisingly concluded that improvements in coordination and consolidation were necessary but not sufficient to improve oversight. Although a stand-alone agency could eliminate perceptions of bias or competing missions, it "might create new problems and inefficiencies in the oversight of dietary supplements and other food-related issues not included in the new agency." Thus, the council recommended "efforts to strengthen agency coordination . . . and the development of comprehensive, unifying legislation, followed by the development of a corresponding organizational reform plan by allowing *risk-based* allocation of resources and utilization of *science-based* regulation, enforcement, and education" (emphasis added).[56] The strong emphasis on a science-based regulatory approach—always requiring more studies and more reports—provided little ground for optimism that reforms would come soon.

As soon as President George W. Bush took office in January 2001, he issued a number of antiregulatory executive orders, including one delaying the USDA's imposition of performance standards for *Salmonella* and *Listeria* in meat and poultry. The American Meat Institute used the delay to argue for a complete review of the rules, while consumer groups urged the newly appointed USDA Secretary, Ann Veneman, to move them forward. One month later, the USDA released the rules, reportedly because Secretary Veneman convinced the White House to grant an exception to the executive order. Industry groups were not pleased and complained that the rules were unfair because they singled out meat and poultry for testing when other foods were equally contaminated.[59] Nevertheless, weaknesses in the system remained evident. In March, newspapers reported frequent violations of safety procedures in meat-producing plants in New York and New Jersey; they also headlined flagrant lapses in retail meat inspection throughout the Northeast. These reports

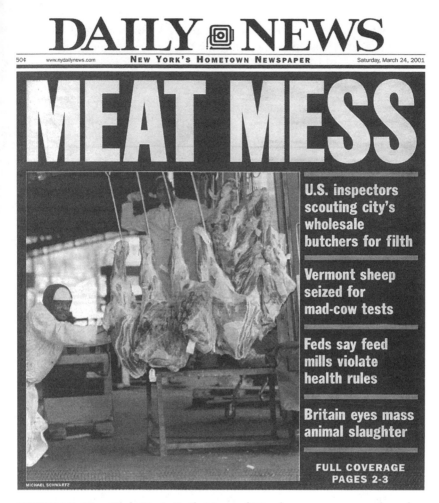

FIGURE 10. New York City's *Daily News* of March 24, 2001, summed up the complicated local, national, and international politics of meat safety in two words: "Meat Mess." (© 2001 New York *Daily News* L.P. Reprinted with permission.)

only added to concerns about meat safety, then driven by the highly publicized epidemics of mad cow disease and foot-and-mouth disease among cattle in Great Britain and Europe. Together, the problems amounted to what the New York *Daily News* characterized as a "Meat Mess" worthy of front-page attention, as shown in figure 10.

Adding to this mess, the administrator of USDA's Agricultural Marketing Service announced that testing for *Salmonella* in beef served in the federal school lunch program (the cause of the problems with Supreme Beef discussed in the previous chapter) was no longer necessary and schools could now serve *irradiated* beef instead. This suggestion elicited surprised comments from Senator Richard Durbin (Dem-IL), who viewed it as another attempt by corporations to circumvent safety regulations under an administration so friendly to industry that it had already reduced standards for the levels of arsenic permitted in drinking water: "The school lunch program is a very sacred budget in our program, and a lot of senators and congressmen don't feel it's a political issue. . . . First, it was arsenic in drinking water. Now it's salmonella in school lunches. Where will it end?" Apparently, the suggestion also surprised USDA Secretary Veneman. The next day, she said that she had not approved the change and would withdraw it, a turnaround that caused Senator Durbin to comment, "Someone in the department got caught with their hand in the hamburger."[60]

This incident revealed the alarming increase in outbreaks of foodborne disease among school children eating contaminated meat served in school lunch programs. The *Chicago Tribune* identified dozens of such outbreaks, some of them affecting thousands of students; it attributed them to inadequate cooking of badly contaminated frozen meat shipped from careless and uncaring packers. The packers did the usual denying and blaming, along with one unusually creative response: "The real problem . . . is America's strict food safety laws. The more we battle these so-called pathogens, the more problems we're creating. . . . Our immune systems here are in pathetic shape. . . . We're not able to deal with elevated levels of bacteria that people in other parts of the world can deal with because we are in such a sterile environment."[61] The *Tribune's* disturbing reports made it clear that state inspectors could not be counted on to do their jobs adequately, thereby strengthening the case for stronger federal oversight.

The GAO supported this case a few months later when it told Congress that at least 292 outbreaks from school meals—affecting more than 16,000 children—had occurred since 1990. Such outbreaks were clearly increasing, but no federal agency monitors the safety of school meals or issues special security measures to protect school children. The GAO said that closing this safety gap would require "addressing the overarching problems that affect the nation's federal food safety system as a whole."[62] In 1992, Michael Taylor (the former USDA administrator introduced in chapter 2) proposed specific legislative actions that might be taken to achieve that goal.[63] Table 10 summarizes some of his suggestions, along with some others derived from the ideas discussed in these chapters.

TABLE 10. Suggestions for legislative actions to ensure safe food

Congress should provide the mandate, authority, and funding necessary to achieve:

- A single agency accountable for providing consistent and coordinated oversight of food safety, from farm to table

- Revision of the 1906 safety inspection laws to permit oversight of microbial pathogens

- Institution of Pathogen Reduction: HACCP, with performance standards verified by pathogen testing, at every step of food production

- A national food safety plan that sets priorities, adopts strategies, ensures accountability, and monitors progress

- Recall authority, access to records, and penalties for lapses in safety procedures

- Uniform food safety standards for states, consistent with federal policies

- Standards for imported foods equivalent to those for domestic foods

- Food safety to take precedence over commercial considerations in trade disputes

- Universal food safety education for commercial food handlers

- A national system for monitoring cases and outbreaks of foodborne disease and their causes

- Research on methods to control microbial contamination and illness, and on prevention strategies

SOURCE: Some of these suggestions are adapted from Taylor MR. *Food Technology* 2002;56(5):190–194.

CONCLUSION: THE GLOBAL POLITICS OF FOOD SAFETY

At the beginning of the twenty-first century, efforts to prevent microbial contamination of the food supply continue to be held hostage to industries obstructing intervention, agencies competing for scarce resources, inspectors defending obsolete job descriptions, courts defending obsolete laws, and a Congress more anxious to protect the sources of campaign contributions than the health of the public. While many food safety problems have improved since the era of *The Jungle*, the solution to others continues to face formidable political opposition.

Although this chapter has focused on U.S. food safety matters, it begins and ends by recognizing that domestic food safety—like many other political matters—cannot be discussed in isolation from its international dimensions. The safety of the foods we import depends not only on the quality standards set by our trading partners but also on international decisions that might seem only peripherally related to the food supply. Thus, an additional alternative surely should be to insist that the United Nations agencies dealing with trade issues—the Codex Commission and, as discussed in the next part of this book, the World Trade Organization—consider health and safety first in making rules about trade barriers.

As mentioned at the beginning of this chapter, several European countries have reduced outbreaks of foodborne disease by instituting control measures similar to Pathogen Reduction: HACCP. In response to food catastrophes such as mad cow disease in Great Britain and foot-and-mouth disease in cattle throughout Europe, countries such as Canada, Denmark, Ireland, and Great Britain have taken steps to consolidate their food safety activities into single agencies. The European Union has also created a unified Food Safety Authority.[64] The reasons for taking this approach vary from one country to another and may well be designed to promote the interests of food companies and regulators rather than those of the public, as all seem driven primarily by the need for greater efficiency and reduced cost.[65] Although it is too soon to know whether they will also reduce episodes of foodborne illness, these experiments are of great interest. They hold the promise of solving coordination problems as well as providing the strength and flexibility to deal with emerging food safety challenges such as bioterrorism.

International concerns also dominate discussions of food biotechnology, as countries throughout the world grapple with decisions about whether to accept genetically modified food crops produced in the United States. In part 2, we will see that the debates over such foods depend to some extent on safety considerations but relate even more to societal implications. Whether an independent food agency might be more effective in dealing with this broader range of considerations will be taken up in the concluding chapter, as will some thoughts on how the various stakeholders—government, food producers, and consumers—might make food safety issues less political and more focused on health.

PART TWO

SAFETY AS A SURROGATE
THE IRONIC POLITICS OF FOOD BIOTECHNOLOGY

LATE IN THE FALL OF 2001, I ATTENDED A TUFTS UNIVERSITY conference on agricultural biotechnology sponsored by corporations such as Aventis (producer of StarLink corn) and Monsanto (producer of genetically modified cow growth hormone, corn, soybeans, and cotton). Speaker after speaker made the same three points: (1) the number of people in the world is increasing rapidly and food production must increase to keep them from starvation; (2) because the land available for growing food is limited, biotechnology—and only biotechnology—can increase food productivity; and (3) the main barrier to producing genetically modified foods is public doubt about their safety, particularly as expressed by unscientific activist groups such as Greenpeace.[1] Anyone not actively tracking the politics of food biotechnology might be surprised to learn that the chief impediment to eliminating world hunger is a consumer group best known for its opposition to nuclear weapons testing, but this topic is replete with such ironies.

To explain why the ironic politics of food biotechnology deserves attention in a book about food safety, we must begin with some definitions: *biotechnology* and its synonym, *genetic engineering,* are processes by which scientists move genes (DNA) from one organism to another to transfer desired traits. Agricultural biotechnologists move genes from bacteria, viruses, or plants into food plants (the appendix explains how this is done). We call foods containing the new genes by a variety of equivalent terms: *transgenic, bioengineered, genetically engineered (GE), genetically modified (GM), genetically modified organisms (GMO)*, and, occasionally, the pejorative *Franken-foods*.[2] These chapters refer to such foods interchangeably as *genetically modified, genetically engineered,* and *transgenic.*

The speakers at the Tufts conference were intoning the mantra of the food biotechnology industry, the *theoretical* promise that its products will solve world food problems by creating a more abundant, more nutritious, and less expensive food supply. I emphasize theoretical because this promise is not yet realized; the industry is still in its infancy. The speakers were right to be concerned about public acceptance. The commercial products of food biotechnology have caused no end of controversy. In the United States, and particularly in Great Britain, people view the new foods with suspicion, often with dread and outrage. The results: boycotts, destruction of plantings ("ecoterrorism"), legal bans, and trade disputes. Such reactions reflect misgivings about the risks of technological manipulations of food, not only to human health, but also to the environment, to the world economy, and to society as a whole. They also reflect distrust of the motives of the food biotechnology industry and of the ability of government to regulate that industry. This sense of unease—specific for some, vague for others—translates most easily to a simple response: rejection. As people often tell me, "I don't want any GM in my food."

To industry officials and scientists who view risk through a science-based lens, statements like that are antiscientific and irrational. In the early 1990s, they characterized *any* criticism of food biotechnology as ignorant, irresponsible, hysterical, or—my favorite—troglodyte, and as a prominent symptom of a new psychiatric disorder, biotechnophobia.[3] They lamented that well-funded activist groups were deliberately "interweaving political, societal and emotional issues . . . to delay commercialization and increase costs by supporting political, non-science-based regulation, unnecessary testing, and labeling of foods."[4] In that tradition, the Tufts conference speakers complained about the generous funding available to Greenpeace, another irony in light of the disparity between that group's resources and those of the agricultural biotechnology industry.

From its inception, food biotechnology has raised political, societal, and emotional issues: What are the risks of genetically modified foods? What are their benefits? How are risks and benefits distributed? Who makes decisions about them? How will genetically modified foods affect local, national, and international food systems and economies? How should the foods be regulated? Should they be labeled? And: Is it ethical to create such foods in the first place? The questions about risk can be answered scientifically, but the other questions are value-based and *social*. Because questions about ethics and other social matters threaten the very foundation of food biotechnology, the industry and its supporters tend to restrict discussion to questions of safety. From a science-based perspective, if genetically modified foods are safe, there is no sensible reason for regulating, labeling, or opposing them.

The focus on science, safety, and risk obscures the social issues, particularly those having to do with the distribution of economic benefits. Food biotechnology is a huge business, and huge profits are at stake. To survive, the industry must make products that farmers or the public will buy. Politics enters the picture because other stakeholders in the food system have different agendas and hold different values. Scientists want to work on challenging problems that might produce health or economic gains, and, as a necessary benefit, research funding. Government regulators want to ensure that foods are safe, but they also want to avoid congressional intervention and industry lawsuits. As consumers, we all want food that is safe (or safe enough), but many of us also are concerned about social issues. Food biotechnology is political because basic questions—Who benefits? Who decides? Who controls?—require societal resolution and cannot be decided solely by the methods of science.

The debates about food biotechnology are especially complicated because the science itself is so complicated. That most people cannot understand the science behind genetically modified foods is a given. But anyone, trained in science or not, can grasp whether democratic political processes are at work in making decisions about these foods. We will see how questions of democracy—and the lack of an institutional venue for debating the social implications of food biotechnology—underlie much of the distrust of the industry and its government regulators. The desire for democratic processes and the trust they inspire explain why the lack of labeling of genetically modified foods is such a critical point of debate. Labeling places the power to make decisions in the hands of consumers, not the industry.

Although the safety of genetically modified foods is an important issue, it is not the only one of interest. But because safety appears to be the only *legitimate* ground for criticism, it acts as a surrogate for concerns about democratic processes and social implications. The Star-Link corn affair is an example of the use of safety as a surrogate; the arguments focused on allergenicity (science), but the real issues had to do with the company's control over the food supply and evasion of democratic processes of government oversight (social values). The politics of food biotechnology matter because the disputes shift attention away from the underlying issues. If, for example, the roots of world hunger lie in poverty, we should be debating options for redressing economic imbalances. If we want to meet the food needs of the twenty-first century, we ought to be considering a broad range of alternatives, among which biotechnology may or may not be the best. Social problems are manifestly difficult to address, as their causes are multiple and complex. It is understandable that we might find simple, "reductionist" approaches to such problems—like genetically engineering vitamins into rice—preferable to the messy business of political action to address world poverty.

This part of the book deals with how and why the safety of genetically modified foods became a surrogate for concerns about larger social issues.[5] In telling this story, these chapters continue many of the themes noted earlier: industry promotion of economic self-interest at the expense of health and safety, the industry's political efforts to prevent imposition of regulatory controls and labeling requirements, the fragmentation and consequent weakness of government oversight, the imbalance in power between corporate and public interests, and the use of science as a rationale for self-interested actions.

The discussion of these themes begins in chapter 5 with an introduction to the food biotechnology industry—its methods, promises, and realities. Much of the chapter is devoted to a discussion of the "poster child" for the benefits of genetically modified foods, Golden Rice, a rice bioengineered to contain beta-carotene, a precursor of vitamin A. Chapter 6 evaluates the benefits claimed for genetically modified foods, as well as their safety risks: allergenicity, antibiotic resistance, and environmental impact. In chapter 7, I discuss the politics of government oversight of genetically modified foods and describe how the industry convinced federal regulatory agencies to use a strictly science-based approach to risk evaluation, thereby allowing companies to plant first, *then* deal with problems (rather than requiring premarket testing). Chapter 8 focuses on the important societal issues that spark protests against genetically modified foods: consumer choice at the marketplace (labeling), inequities in ownership of plant resources (intellectual property rights or "biopiracy"), the accidental movement of transgenes into conventional crops ("genetic pollution"), and corporate control of the food supply (globalization). Overall, these chapters provide an analysis of where the issues raised by food biotechnology stand today, and how industry, scientists, government, and the public might deal with the ongoing disputes about genetically modified foods.

CHAPTER 5

PEDDLING DREAMS

PROMISES VERSUS REALITY

BIOTECHNOLOGY COMPANIES HAD BEEN WORKING ON AGRICUL-tural projects for 10 years or more when, in 1992, I received a last-minute invitation to talk about the labeling of genetically modified foods at a conference organized by Public Voice, a consumer advocacy group for food and health policy in Washington, DC. As a trained molecular biologist—though a long lapsed one—I was intrigued by the possibilities of the technology. I had not been following the field very closely and was puzzled about why an advocacy group might be concerned about labeling products that were still hypothetical. As it happened, I was not unprepared to address the question. For teaching purposes, I routinely collect scientific articles and newspaper clippings on nutrition topics, and I had accumulated a thick file on food biotechnology. The invitation provided an excuse to see what was in it.

The file surprised me. It immediately revealed that the industry's exciting promise to solve world food problems had little to do with the reality of its research and development efforts. Instead, companies were working on crop products most likely to generate returns on investment. Furthermore, industry leaders seemed to view the public not as an enthusiastic partner in enhancing the food supply but rather as a hostile force threatening their economic viability. The industry and its supporters in science, government, and business framed public questions about the safety or other consequences of food biotechnology as irrational challenges by scientifically illiterate consumers. I could not evaluate their science-based contentions that the techniques were inherently safe and the foods no different from those produced by conventional genetic crosses, however, as none had yet come to market.

Since then, the situation has changed in some ways but not in others. Once the Food and Drug Administration (FDA) approved the marketing of genetically modified foods in 1994, the production of these foods grew rapidly. By 2001, genetically modified varieties accounted for 26% of the corn and 68% of the soybeans planted in the United States as well as 69% of the cotton (the source of cottonseed oil for animal feed). Manufacturers were using ingredients made from transgenic corn and soybeans in 60% or more of processed foods on supermarket shelves—baby formulas, drink mixes, muffin mixes, fast foods, and, as we have seen, taco shells. Early in the twenty-first century, it is not possible to keep genetically modified foods *out* of the food supply.[1]

What should we, as citizens and consumers, make of this situation? This chapter establishes a basis for answering that question by examining the promises of the food biotechnology industry—what it *could* do—in comparison to the reality of its products and actions.

THE THEORETICAL PROMISES

In theory, if not yet in practice, food biotechnology holds much promise for addressing world food problems, most notably the overall shortfall in food production expected early in the twenty-first century. By some estimates, the global demand for rice, wheat, and maize will increase by 40% above current levels as early as 2020.[2] To feed an increasing population on a constant area of arable land, the land must produce much more food—and do so without irreversibly damaging the environment. No technical barriers—again, in theory—prevent the use of genetic manipulations to improve the quantity and quality of the food supply, increase its safety, reduce the use of harmful pesticides and agricultural chemicals, and reduce food costs. Table 11 lists examples of the stunning range of potentially beneficial applications of food biotechnology that are now available or under investigation. Figure 11 illustrates a cartoonist's somewhat ironic view of such possibilities.

These applications could increase world food production, especially given the conditions of poor climate and environmental degradation characteristic of many developing countries, and they also could improve the nutritional quality of indigenous food plants on which so many populations depend. The potential for such improvements explains why industry leaders refer to food biotechnology as "the most important sci-

TABLE 11. Theoretical and current applications of food biotechnology

---

Food Plants (for human use)
Improve flavor, texture, or freshness.
Increase levels of vitamins, protein, and other nutrients.
Increase production of chemicals such as sugars, waxes, or nutritionally
  important components.
Decrease levels of caffeine or other undesirable chemical substances.
Reduce saturated fatty acids in plant seed oils.
Produce drugs such as antibiotics, vaccines, or contraceptives.

Crop Plants (mainly for animal feed)
Introduce herbicide resistance to improve weed control.
Permit growth with minimal use of fertilizers, pesticides, or water.
Increase resistance to damage by insect, fungal, viral, or other microbial pests.
Increase resistance to "stress" by frost, heat, salt, or heavy metals.
Permit fixation of atmospheric nitrogen.
Increase grain content of scarce amino acids.

Food Animals (for human use)
Increase the efficiency of growth and reproduction.
Strengthen disease resistance.
Develop veterinary vaccines and diagnostic tests.
Increase milk production.
Produce milk containing pharmaceuticals.

---

entific tool to affect the food economy in the history of mankind," "the single most promising approach to feeding a growing world population while reducing damage to the environment," and an innovation that will "create miracles to help us feed a hungry world efficiently and economically."[3] Such statements promise that food biotechnology will improve the food supply more effectively than conventional genetic techniques— those that involve selecting plants with desired traits, cross-pollinating them with related stock, and selecting and growing the progeny for many generations under field conditions. As this chapter explains, food biotechnologists consider such methods to be slow and imprecise and far inferior to their own.

The promise that food biotechnology will provide food for a hungry world, however, has yet to be fulfilled and is unlikely to be realized in the immediate future. Many of the applications listed in table 11 pose technical problems of formidable complexity. It is not easy to identify genes for

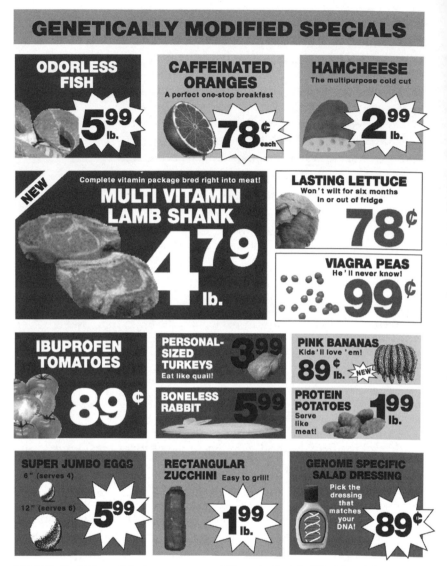

FIGURE 11. This political commentary, "Genetically Modified Specials," appeared as an "op-art" opposite the editorial page of the *New York Times*, July 15, 2000. (© 2000 Jesse Gordon and Knickerbocker Design. Reprinted with permission.)

desired traits, isolate them, insert them into plants, and provide the additional molecular components needed to make them function properly. The slow progress of biotechnology in addressing world hunger does not imply that this problem cannot be solved; given sufficient time, commitment, and funding support, the technical barriers could well be overcome.[4]

Technical problems, therefore, are a temporary barrier and are not the most important one. Instead, the main barrier to producing more food for the developing world is economic. Food biotechnology is a business, and businesses must generate returns on investment. In the food biotechnology business, economic aims (the reality) compete with humanitarian aims (the promises). These purposes conflict: one goal is to produce more and better food for an increasing population, but another is to produce foods with a competitive advantage in today's global marketplace—particularly "value-added" foods processed in ways that generate benefits for consumers and higher profits for manufacturers.[5] Although genetically modified foods might well be expected to meet both goals, they often do not. Like all industries, this one serves investors who demand rapid returns, and financial considerations inevitably influence decisions related to product development. The business imperatives explain why the industry continues to view legitimate public questions about the use, safety, or social consequences of particular products as threats to the entire biotechnology enterprise. Without substantial changes to the economic realities of food biotechnology, its feed-the-world potential remains an unfulfilled promise.

THE ECONOMIC REALITIES

If food biotechnology companies are primarily businesses, then their primary concern is to recover the costs of research and development and to maximize returns on investment. Research costs can be high; it takes years and hundreds of millions of dollars to bring a genetically engineered food to market. Nevertheless, even before the FDA approved the first such food for production, business analysts viewed the industry as one with a huge market potential. In 1992, they predicted that the value of the industry would increase to at least $50 billion by the year 2000. As late as 1998, some were predicting that worldwide sales could exceed $300 billion by 2010. These predictions were overly optimistic, but food biotechnology is still big business. Worldwide sales of genetically modified crops rose from $1.6 billion in 1998 to about $2.2 billion in 1999, and are now expected to rise to $25 billion by 2010.[6]

Regardless of the accuracy of such estimates, the rapid expansion of the food biotechnology industry is impressive. By 1998, about 1,400 companies had invested more than $110 billion in agricultural biotechnology, and the FDA had approved about 50 food products for marketing. By 2001, genetically engineered crops were growing on at least 109 million acres throughout the world, a 25-fold expansion just since 1996. Although 80% of the acres were in North America, Argentina, and China, 10 other countries also had substantial plantings and more than 40 countries permitted field trials of one crop or another, most intended for animal feed.[7] Despite the recent decline in planting of genetically engineered corn that occurred as a result of European opposition (discussed in chapter 8), some segments of the industry are doing very well.

One especially successful agricultural biotechnology company is Monsanto, which has played an unusually active—some might say aggressive—role in the industry. Monsanto is a multinational company based in St. Louis, Missouri, whose corporate motto used to be *Food, Health, Hope*.[8] After the company merged with Pharmacia & Upjohn in 2000 to form an agricultural unit of Pharmacia, it changed the slogan to *A Single Focus: Agriculture/A Renewed Purpose: Value*. Monsanto employed about 14,000 people worldwide in 2002. Its agricultural biotechnology products exceed financial expectations. Its stock price rose by 75% in 1995 and by another 70% in 1996; at that time, company officials estimated that their products would earn $2 billion by the year 2000, $6–7 billion by 2005, and $20 billion by 2010. By 2000, sales exceeded $5 billion, well ahead of projections.[9]

Not all companies are this fortunate or skilled. In 1998, for example, just 8 out of 350 publicly traded food biotechnology companies were profitable.[10] Business analysts attribute the typically poor performance to uneven management, corporate shortsightedness, and product failures. Most companies were slow to invest sufficient funds in research, as was the U.S. government. Investors are leery of regulatory hurdles and consumer opposition. Financial imperatives require food biotechnology companies to work on projects that are technically feasible and likely to repay the costs of investment in short order. Thus, they focus research efforts on "input traits" that will make crops easier and less expensive to grow through control of weeds, plant diseases, ripening, insects, or herbicide-resistance, or will make foods last longer on the shelf and cost less to process. If these characteristics benefit the public, they do so invisibly. Most of the financial rewards go to the companies that produce the seeds and chemicals. In some situations, farmers also benefit.[11]

Monsanto applies its research budget for agricultural biotechnology, which exceeds the combined total of all the publicly funded tropical research institutes in the world, almost exclusively to temperate-zone agricultural problems. The company brilliantly designs its principal agricultural products to establish control of the entire industry. Its flagship product is the herbicide Roundup. Monsanto scientists genetically engineer soybeans and corn to be "Roundup Ready," so their crops grow happily when doused with that herbicide while the competing weeds are killed. Farmers who buy Monsanto's seeds also buy Monsanto's herbicide. The company began selling Roundup Ready soybeans in 1996; just two years later, farmers planted them on one-third of U.S. soybean farmland, covering 25 million acres. The company's research "pipeline" mainly emphasizes Roundup Ready crops designed for animal feed. Monsanto's emphasis on these crops is understandable; annual sales of Roundup exceed those of the next six leading herbicides combined. The company also produces a variety of crops genetically engineered to contain a toxin derived from *Bacillus thuringiensis* (*Bt*). As we saw in the introductory chapter, the *Bt* toxin inhibits the growth of insect pests and has been used for years as a spray on organic farms. Monsanto's patent-protected innovation was to genetically engineer the *Bt* toxin into the plant itself so that insect resistance would not wash off in the rain.

Monsanto's crops grow mainly in the United States and other industrialized countries. Because developing countries lack a viable market for such products, few agricultural biotechnology companies can afford to invest in solutions to the food problems of the developing world. The agricultural needs of developing countries are well defined, and numerous private and public agencies support useful projects, but these funding sources are not coordinated and often tend to favor the priorities of donors more than recipients.[12] For years, Dr. Roger Beachy, the director of a U.S. biotechnology research institute devoted to improving crops in developing countries, complained that he could get little support from industry beyond permission to use patent-protected techniques "for specific crops under certain circumstances."[13]

As complaints about the disparity between the promises and the realities of food biotechnology became more strident, companies began to put more resources into projects that might benefit the developing world. Monsanto's scientists, for example, are genetically engineering oilseeds to contain beta-carotene, a precursor of vitamin A. This vitamin is especially lacking in undernourished populations, and its addition to the diet produces an almost miraculous range of health improvements.[14] Development of such products is time-consuming and expensive, and success is uncertain. Companies introduced genetically engineered papaya in Hawaii, for example, to replenish an entire industry ravaged by viral disease. The fruit grew well in the first seasons, but its developers remain cautious about its long-term viability: "We'd all be nuts to say that this is the final solution. . . . Biological systems evolve."[15] This comment reflects yet another reality; it is one thing to develop a food in a laboratory but quite another to grow it successfully under field conditions. A 1994 statement by one business analyst still applies: "Nearly 20 years into the gene-splicing revolution . . . no one has cured cancer or produced a bioengineered miracle of loaves and fishes for a hungry third world. The industry is still peddling dreams."[16]

Such doubts enrage industry supporters in the United States and, sometimes, in developing countries. Florence Wambugu, for example, is a plant pathologist from Kenya who has worked with Monsanto since 1992 to develop a genetically modified sweet potato that can survive infection from a virus that otherwise would greatly reduce crop yields. At the Tufts University conference I attended in 2001, she predicted that the bioengineered potato would increase worldwide sweet potato production by at least 15%, increase the income of farmers by $41 million, and improve the food security of 1 million people—without any increase in the costs of production. Ms. Wambugu is an eloquent and forceful promoter of biotechnology as the solution to worldwide food shortages, and she does not mince words about the harm caused by "antibiotech lobbies":

> Antibiotechnology protesters . . . deny developing countries like my home, Kenya, the resources to develop a technology that can help alleviate hunger, malnutrition and poverty. . . . As an African, I know that biotech is not a panacea. It cannot solve problems of inept or corrupt governments, underfunded research, unsound agricultural policy, or a lack of capital . . . but as a scientist, I also know that biotech is a powerful new tool that can help address some of the agricultural problems that plague Africa. The protesters have fanned the flames of mistrust of genetically modified foods through a campaign of misinformation. These people and organizations have become adept at playing on the media's appetite for controversy to draw attention to their cause. But the real victim in this controversy is the truth. . . . I know of what I speak, because I grew up barefoot and hungry.[17]

In 2001, her sweet potato was in field trials, and the level of its productivity or acceptance would not be known for some time. Nevertheless, Monsanto has used the potato in its public relations campaigns since 1996 ("the sweet potato project will ultimately be a major contribution to food security for some of the poorest farmers in the world"), and the Biotechnology Information Council, which runs an industry-sponsored public relations campaign, also uses her work: "Florence Wambugu helped develop sweet potato varieties that are resistant to a complex set of viruses that can wipe out three-fourths of Kenyan farmers' harvest. . . . Similar techniques are being used to improve other staple crops of the developing world, including cassava, banana, and potato."[18] These statements are promises. The crops are not yet in production, but the public relations materials do not emphasize that point.

The most highly publicized example of the gap between promises and reality is "Golden Rice," genetically engineered to contain beta-carotene, a precursor of vitamin A. Although this rice also is not yet in production, it has been the industry's primary advertising tool to promote the humanitarian benefits of food biotechnology (see figure 12). This rice raises a variety of issues that illustrate some further points about the interweaving of science and politics in food biotechnology, as we will now see

MAKING RICE "GOLDEN"

Much of the promise of food biotechnology depends on its science, but the realities depend on social as well as scientific factors. Nowhere is this distinction better illustrated than in the case of Golden Rice. To understand why the interplay between the scientific and societal issues makes genetically modified foods so *political*, we need to begin with an explanation of the extraordinary scientific achievement involved in creating Golden Rice.

Biotechnology versus Traditional Plant Genetics

Scientists who are puzzled by public distrust of food biotechnology tend to see its techniques as extensions of those of traditional plant genetics but superior because they are more efficient and precise. Traditional plant breeding can be tedious. Suppose, for example, that you would like to create a tomato with a thicker skin so it can be transported without getting crushed. Using the typical genetic methods, you would grow many kinds of tomatoes and look for a rare plant that produces tomatoes with thicker skins. You might also treat tomato embryos with chemicals or radiation to induce mutations; if you are lucky, a mutation will lead to fruit with a thicker skin. You then grow seeds from these tomatoes into plants, select progeny plants with thicker skins, cross them (through pollination)

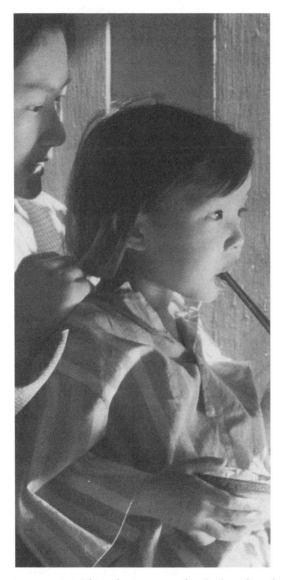

FIGURE 12. This advertisement for the benefits of Golden Rice is part of an industry public relations campaign to promote public acceptance of genetically modified foods; it appeared frequently in 2001 in publications such as the *New Yorker, Scientific American,* and the *New York Times.* The text fails to emphasize that the rice, which "could help alleviate more suffering and illness than any single medicine," is not yet available.

with tomato plants with other desirable traits, and, eventually, end up with thick-skinned tomatoes that breed true. A process like this involves luck as well as skill, takes an average of six to eight years of growing cycles, and can (and often does) result in a tasteless supermarket tomato. Other such manipulations created the full array of fruits, vegetables, and crops that make our food supply so abundant. It is safe to say that virtually all plants that constitute part of today's food supply were genetically manipulated in one way or another. Traditional genetic manipulations permit the transfer of genes only between members of the same species or those that are closely related—apples and pears, for example. In contrast, agricultural biotechnology extends these techniques to address problems of efficiency, time, and species limits on transferable traits.

Because both traditional plant genetics and biotechnology involve similar manipulations and because they both achieve the same result—insertion of new segments of DNA into a plant's existing DNA—biotechnologists maintain that the plants they develop are no different from those produced in old-fashioned ways, and should not be viewed or treated differently by regulatory agencies or the public. As we will see (and as the appendix explains in further detail), the steps involved in creating a transgenic plant are numerous and complex, and they introduce DNA segments that may come from unrelated organisms. Do these differences matter? The response is *no* if one focuses on the similarities: DNA is DNA no matter where it comes from. The response is *yes* if one focuses on differences or the societal implications of the technology. Points of view govern such responses and lead to political controversy.

Golden Rice: The Science

Plant bioengineering is accomplished through *recombinant* DNA technology, through which the DNA segments that comprise a desirable gene from bacteria, for example, are inserted (recombined) permanently into the DNA of an entirely different organism—in this case, a plant. Scientists using recombinant techniques have created insect- and herbicide-resistant crops by taking genes from bacteria and transferring them to corn and soybeans. To develop Golden Rice, they recombined genes and DNA regulatory segments from daffodils, peas, viruses, and bacteria to induce rice to make beta-carotene in its endosperm—the white, starchy part of the grain. Rice, like all grains, consists of three principal parts: a surrounding sheath of nutrient-rich bran, an inner endosperm containing starch and a little protein, and an embryo, which draws on the energy

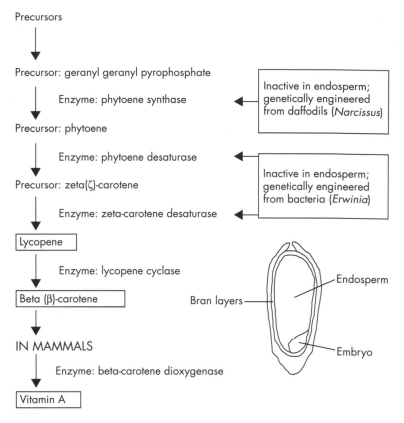

IN RICE

Precursors

↓

Precursor: geranyl geranyl pyrophosphate

↓   Enzyme: phytoene synthase

Precursor: phytoene

> Inactive in endosperm; genetically engineered from daffodils (*Narcissus*)

↓   Enzyme: phytoene desaturase

Precursor: zeta(ζ)-carotene

> Inactive in endosperm; genetically engineered from bacteria (*Erwinia*)

↓   Enzyme: zeta-carotene desaturase

Lycopene

↓   Enzyme: lycopene cyclase

Beta (β)-carotene   Bran layers —   Endosperm

↓

IN MAMMALS

↓   Enzyme: beta-carotene dioxygenase   Embryo

Vitamin A

FIGURE 13. The metabolic steps through which plants make beta-carotene from precursor molecules, and animals convert beta-carotene to vitamin A. An enzyme carries out each step. Rice bran contains information for the complete set of enzymes to make beta-carotene, but some enzymes are inactive in the endosperm. To create Golden Rice, scientists obtain genes (DNA) for the missing enzymes from other plants and bacteria and insert them into the DNA of rice (see tables 12 and 16, pages 158 and 280).

and nutrients in the grain when it begins to grow into a plant (see figure 13). Rice makes small amounts of beta-carotene in its bran layers, but not in the endosperm. Most people just eat the endosperm, however, because millers remove the bran layers when they convert brown rice to white rice (which is why white rice in the United States is enriched with several vitamins and iron).

Rice bran and highly pigmented fruits and vegetables (such as melons or carrots) make beta-carotene in a series of steps in which precursor molecules are converted to beta-carotene by specific enzymes (which are proteins), one for each step. Rice endosperm lacks three of the required enzymes. To insert beta-carotene, researchers Ingo Potrykus and Peter Beyer and their colleagues in Switzerland and Germany obtained genes for the missing enzymes from daffodils and bacteria. They also isolated genes or regulatory DNA segments from peas, viruses, and other bacteria to help the recombinant enzymes function in rice endosperm. After a decade of effort during the 1990s, the techniques worked. The scientists made rice that contained beta-carotene and identified it immediately by its yellow color (hence: Golden Rice). They published this work in 2000. Figure 13 illustrates the pathway of biosynthesis of beta-carotene and the enzymes replaced by genetic engineering. The pathway illustrates an important distinction: beta-carotene is not the same as vitamin A but is a *precursor* of the actual vitamin. We (and other mammals) have enzymes that convert beta-carotene to vitamin A in our bodies.[19]

The technical challenges involved in moving genes from one organism to another—daffodils and bacteria to rice, for example—are daunting, even to experts. Scientists must find the genes for the missing enzymes, reproduce them, and make them function. The "make function" part is particularly challenging. Genes do not work independently. They have to be *regulated,* which means in this case that the rice needs to be "told" when, where, and for how long the genes for making beta-carotene should do so. Scientists must also find, duplicate, and transfer the genes or DNA segments for these regulatory functions into the rice along with the genes for the missing enzymes. Accomplishing these tasks is a technical *tour de force*—an art as well as a science—not least because of the extraordinary number of genes and factors required, each requiring its own separate bioengineering step carried out in just the right order. As an illustration of the complexity of this work, table 17 in the appendix (page 302) summarizes the *less* complicated of the two approaches used to insert beta-carotene genes into rice.

Complicated as they are, the genetic engineering steps are only the *first* part of realizing the humanitarian benefits of Golden Rice. The inserted genes must be transmitted to seeds; the rice must continue to make beta-carotene when taken out of the laboratory and grown in fields; people must accept, buy, and eat the rice; and the beta-carotene must be absorbed, split into vitamin A, and function in the human body. Table 12 lists these requirements in greater detail. These additional tasks also can

TABLE 12. Research steps required to genetically engineer and to produce and use Golden Rice containing beta-carotene, a precursor of vitamin A

Basic Research (see table 17 in appendix for further details)

Isolate the desired genes and regulatory DNA segments from daffodils, bacteria, peas, and viruses.

Transfer the genes and segments to rice embryos.

Grow the embryos; select the rare embryos that accept the desired genes and segments.

Grow the transgenic embryos into plants.

Harvest seeds from the plants.

Test the seeds for beta-carotene.

Repeat the procedures in rice strains able to grow in tropical climates.

Production Research

Grow the transgenic rice for several generations to ensure the stability of the beta-carotene trait.

Evaluate the plants for environmental effects, presence of allergens, changes in nutrient composition, or unwanted effects on yield.

Obtain regulatory approval to grow the rice commercially.

Obtain regulatory approval to market the rice.

Produce the rice in sufficient quantities for distribution and marketing.

Consumer Research

Conduct studies to determine the degree of consumer acceptance of the rice.

Conduct dietary studies to evaluate patterns of consumption of the rice among vitamin A–deficient individuals and population groups.

Clinical Research

Conduct biochemical studies to determine how much beta-carotene is absorbed from the rice, and whether consuming the rice increases levels of vitamin A in the body.

Conduct clinical studies to determine whether consuming the rice is associated with a reduction in symptoms of vitamin A deficiency and improvements in health and survival among individuals and population groups.

---

be difficult to accomplish. One production problem, for example, is the relative instability of transgenic plants with multiple inserted genes; such plants tend to lose the transgenic traits over several generations. Another is that the scientists engineered beta-carotene into a variety of rice that grows best in temperate zones. To succeed in developing countries, the technology must be transferred to locally grown varieties.

The degree of acceptance by consumers is also a matter of concern.

Preliminary surveys suggested that some people found the yellow color unattractive; they thought someone might have urinated on the rice. Scientists can remove the undesirable color by inserting the genes for the additional enzymes in the pathway to vitamin A (which is colorless), but these steps only add to the technical difficulties. Table 12 explains why promotion of Golden Rice as a means to prevent vitamin A deficiency is premature. At best several more years of work will be needed to bring it to market.

Golden Rice: The Politics

White rice is the principal source of energy (calories) for one-third or more of the world's population, but it is not a source of vitamin A. Only animals make vitamin A; plants make beta-carotene, its precursor. The lack of vitamin A is the single most important cause of blindness among children in developing countries and a major contributor to deaths among malnourished children and adults. Children who are even mildly deficient in vitamin A are at increased risk for early death, but health authorities can prevent an astonishing proportion of such deaths—more than half—with supplements of vitamin A (*not* beta-carotene). Supplements are relatively inexpensive and need to be taken once every six months or so, but because they cannot always be obtained by the people who need them most, fortification of a commonly consumed food might be another way to solve a serious world health problem.[20]

Since 1984, the Rockefeller Foundation has dispensed about $4 million annually to fund genetics projects to improve one characteristic or another of rice plants, and it considers Golden Rice to be the greatest achievement of this program. Moving Golden Rice beyond the research stage, however, unexpectedly encountered political problems. Ironically, one of the difficulties was a confrontation with patent rights, as a "thicket of intellectual property claims" governed use of the technology. The companies most likely to benefit from the public relations generated by Golden Rice, among them Monsanto and AstraZeneca, hold proprietary patent rights to as many as 70 of the materials or DNA segments needed for its construction. To solve the legal problems connected with using the technology, Dr. Potrykus and his colleagues contracted with AstraZeneca to market the rice in the United States and other industrial markets. In return, AstraZeneca agreed to help make the technology available to the developing world. It gave the technology to the International Rice Research Institute in the Philippines where scientists are crossing Golden Rice with locally grown varieties. AstraZeneca also said it would give the Golden Rice seeds to farmers earning less than $10,000 a year (a figure that includes most farmers in developing countries) and allow farmers to save the seeds to plant in future years. Monsanto also agreed to give up its intellectual property rights for this rice.[21]

These concessions appear exceedingly generous, but Golden Rice is unlikely to have much commercial potential in developing countries. Its public relations value, however, is enormous. In July 2000, the cover of *Time* displayed a photograph of Dr. Potrykus with the headline "This rice could save a million kids a year . . . but protesters believe such genetically modified foods are bad for us and our planet. Here's why." The story noted that it was "no wonder the biotech industry sees Golden Rice as a powerful ally in its struggle to win public acceptance. No wonder its critics see it as a cynical ploy."[22] Cynics might indeed raise eyebrows at the advertisement shown in figure 14, a component of the biotechnology industry's public relations campaign in 2001. The advertisement features a photograph of a child of indeterminate ethnicity eating a "vitamin-enriched" breakfast cereal presumably made from Golden Rice. It says, "Thanks to biotechnology, researchers are developing a new kind of rice with beta-carotene. . . . In the future it could help prevent serious illnesses, such as blindness or anemia, for many people in developing parts of the world."

Dr. Potrykus—frustrated by the encumbrances of industry patent rights on the one hand and objections by antibiotechnology advocates on the other—emphasizes the humanitarian benefits of his research. He told the Tufts University conference that the 40,000 people dying from malnutrition every day need the technology just to survive. Malnutrition, he said,

> pose[s] immense medical problems for developing countries. Traditional interventions are helpful, but require additional and complementary actions. . . . Applied in "humanitarian projects" they could substantially and sustainably improve the health and life of the poor. Whether the poor will benefit, does neither depend upon scientific, patent right, or economic problems, nor upon socioeconomic, consumer health, or environmental risks. It depends mainly upon the political "success" of radical anti-GMO organizations. Those who try to prevent careful exploitation in humanitarian projects must be taken responsible for their damage.[23]

By "those," Dr. Potrykus meant Greenpeace: "Is there any problem left that could interfere with the exploitation of 'Golden Rice' to the benefit of the poor and disadvantaged in developing countries? It is

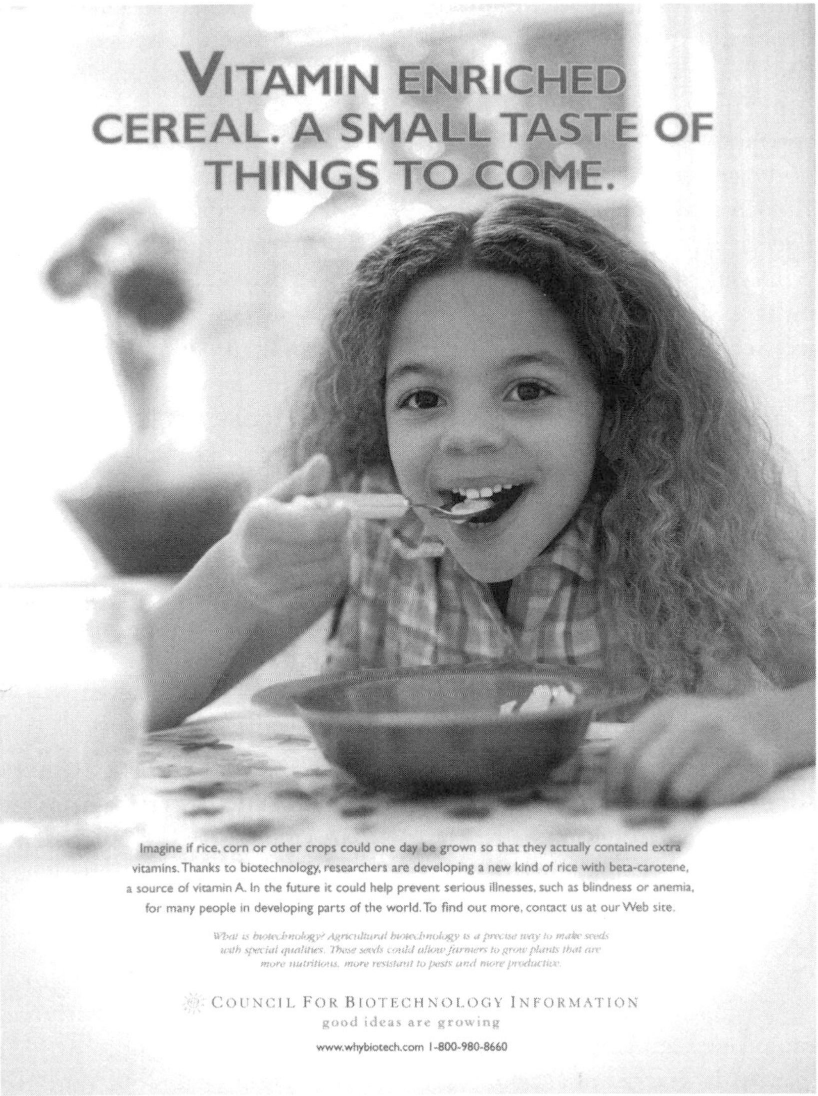

VITAMIN ENRICHED
CEREAL. A SMALL TASTE OF
THINGS TO COME.

Imagine if rice, corn or other crops could one day be grown so that they actually contained extra vitamins. Thanks to biotechnology, researchers are developing a new kind of rice with beta-carotene, a source of vitamin A. In the future it could help prevent serious illnesses, such as blindness or anemia, for many people in developing parts of the world. To find out more, contact us at our Web site.

What is biotechnology? Agricultural biotechnology is a precise way to make seeds with special qualities. These seeds could allow farmers to grow plants that are more nutritious, more resistant to pests and more productive.

COUNCIL FOR BIOTECHNOLOGY INFORMATION
good ideas are growing

www.whybiotech.com 1-800-980-8660

FIGURE 14. This biotechnology industry advertisement appeared late in 2001 inside the front cover of *Food Safety*, a publication of the National Restaurant Association's Educational Foundation. The text suggests that Golden Rice could help prevent nutritional deficiencies among people in the developing world, presumably by replacing the current vitamin-enriched breakfast cereals.

unfortunate that the answer is yes: Greenpeace . . . and associated GMO opponents regard 'Golden Rice' as a 'Trojan Horse.'. . . By their singular logic, the success of 'Golden Rice' has to be prevented under all circumstances, irrespective of the damage to those for whose interest Greenpeace pretends to act."[24] Dr. Potrykus is correct in his assessment of the motivations of Greenpeace. From that organization's standpoint, Golden Rice obscures fundamental issues of societal values—in this case, poverty and control over resources—and is a techno-fix imposed by corporations and scientists without consulting recipients about whether they want it or not. Greenpeace says that the true purpose of Golden Rice is to convince people to accept genetically modified foods.

If Greenpeace frustrates scientists and biotechnology industry officials, it is in part because its tactics are so effective. For one thing, Greenpeace fights science with science. In February 2001, the group challenged the fundamental premise (and promise) of Golden Rice. Greenpeace calculated that adults would have to eat at least 20 *pounds* (9 kilograms) of Golden Rice to meet daily vitamin A recommendations. Greenpeace called Golden Rice nothing but "fool's gold" and said, "It is shameful that the biotech industry is using starving children to promote a dubious product. . . . This isn't about solving childhood blindness, it's about solving biotech's public relations problem."[25]

Greenpeace did its homework. It took at face value the scientists' own estimate that a daily intake of 300 grams (nearly 11 ounces) of Golden Rice should provide the *equivalent* of 100 units of vitamin A. As noted earlier, beta-carotene must be converted to vitamin A in the body. This process is usually incomplete, however, and the amount that is converted into vitamin A is a matter of sharp debate. The scientists who developed Golden Rice assumed that 6 molecules of beta-carotene would yield 1 of vitamin A, whereas U.S. estimates suggest a conversion ratio of 12 to 1.

Greenpeace took the scientists' figures and compared them to recommended levels of vitamin A intake for the U.S. population. By U.S. standards, 300 grams (11 ounces) of Golden Rice provides one-third the recommended level of daily intake of vitamin A for a child aged one to three years, one-seventh the level recommended for an adult woman, and one-ninth the level for an adult man. By such standards, young children would need to eat nearly 33 ounces of raw rice per day, which, when cooked, would amount to 99 ounces, or about 6 pounds—an absurdly large amount. If the Golden Rice scientists had used the higher U.S. conversion ratio, that quantity doubles to an even more absurd 12 pounds.[26]

It must be understood that the U.S. standard is deliberately set high to meet the nutritional needs of about 98% of the population; people with average requirements can prevent vitamin A deficiency at much lower levels of intake.[27] Nevertheless, to meet just 10% of the U.S. standard, young children would still need to eat more than a pound of cooked rice a day. The Greenpeace analysis made it clear that on quantitative grounds alone, Golden Rice would constitute—at best—a partial solution to health problems caused by vitamin A deficiency.

As might be anticipated, the Greenpeace estimations elicited outraged arguments from scientists and the industry. As a nutritionist, I particularly appreciated the arguments because they raged around the kinds of basic questions my colleagues and I like to discuss in nutrition science courses: What standards are appropriate for the intake of nutrients by individuals and populations? How much beta-carotene is converted to vitamin A in the body? How much vitamin A is required to prevent or alleviate the symptoms or consequences of deficiency? The arguments also dealt with an important question in *applied* nutrition: Should nutritional standards for developing countries be the same as or lower than those for industrialized countries? This question is political rather than scientific because of its implications: lower nutrient standards make populations appear to be better nourished. They also make Golden Rice appear to be more effective.

Dr. Potrykus acknowledged: "Greenpeace has identified a weak point in the strategy of using Golden Rice for reducing vitamin A deficiency." He then countered with new calculations based on standards less "luxurious" than those of the United States—those of India, for example. He said, "Golden Rice is not supposed to provide 100% of the vitamin A–supply, but to . . . [be] complementing other dietary components." On this basis, he estimated that 50% of the standard for a child in India could be met by about 100 grams of Golden Rice per day (a quite reasonable 9 ounces, cooked), and that this amount could be reduced even further if his group could bioengineer the rice to contain higher levels of beta-carotene. Although he still viewed the Greenpeace objections as morally irresponsible, he said he shared "Greenpeace's disgrace about the heavy PR campaign of some agbiotech [agricultural biotechnology] companies using results from our experiments. . . . I stressed, however, also, that I am grateful to all those companies, which donated free licenses . . . to allow for the humanitarian use of Golden Rice in developing countries."[28]

The president of the Rockefeller Foundation, Gordon Conway, also agreed that the industry was overselling the promise of Golden Rice:

> The food industry . . . has featured the golden grains as part of a $50 [million] campaign to promote GM foods. The message is that GM is not just about profits, it can save children's lives. All of this hype is premature and dangerous. The science that led us to Golden Rice is at a very early stage. Until the product is fully developed and tested, no one can be sure how well it will work. . . . But some anti-GM activists would like the work to be stopped before we know its real value.[29]

In this statement, Mr. Conway also expressed a common theme: Golden Rice holds so much promise that no questioning of its value is justified.

As it turns out, if Greenpeace activists had known a bit more about basic and applied nutrition, they could have provided even further cause for skepticism about the promise of Golden Rice. To begin with, the "bioavailability" of beta-carotene, the amount that is absorbed and converted to vitamin A, is quite low—10% or less by some estimates—which explains why conversion ratios to vitamin A may be as high as 12 to 1. Also, an enzyme (from the intestine or liver) splits beta-carotene into two molecules of vitamin A (see figure 13). Like all enzymes, this one is a protein that must be synthesized in the body. Beta-carotene, like vitamin A, is fat-soluble, meaning that it requires some fat in the diet to aid its absorption and transport. People whose diets are adequate in fat and protein are able to use beta-carotene more efficiently than those who are malnourished. Furthermore, vitamin A deficiency is often the most visible manifestation of generalized protein-energy malnutrition, in part caused by intestinal or parasitic infections that interfere with the absorption of beta-carotene and its conversion to vitamin A.[30] We do not yet know the extent to which malnourished children—those most at risk of vitamin A deficiency—can absorb and use the beta-carotene in Golden Rice. In addition to such doubts, Golden Rice may prove costly. The companies may be donating the *technology* to create the rice, but farmers will still have to sell it, and people will still have to pay for it. Moreover, in many countries where vitamin A deficiency is common, food sources of beta-carotene are plentiful, but people believe the foods inappropriate for young children, do not cook them enough to make them digestible, or do not consume enough fat to permit much in the way of absorption. It remains to be seen whether the beta-carotene in Golden Rice will fare better under such circumstances. Overall, vitamin A deficiency is a complicated health problem affected by cultural and societal factors as well as dietary factors. In this situation, the genetic engineering of a single nutrient or two into a food, while attractive in theory, raises many questions about its benefits in practice.

In 2001, I sent a brief letter outlining these nutritional points to the *Journal of the American Dietetic Association.*[31] An electronic copy appeared on the Internet and drew responses from colleagues around the world. A British scientist (who identified himself as a Fellow of the Royal Society) wrote, "It would seem to me that the simplest way to find out if vitamin A rice [*sic*] works as a vitamin supplement is to try it out. If it doesn't then what has been lost except a lot of hot air and propaganda; on the other hand if it does work and your letter has delayed its introduction, could you face the children who remain blind for life as a consequence?"

The writer seems to suggest that even if beta-carotene contributes just a little to alleviating vitamin A deficiency, no questioning of the theoretical premise of Golden Rice—and, by implication, food biotechnology—is acceptable. Anyone who raises questions about the potential value of Golden Rice bears moral responsibility for 500,000 cases of childhood blindness and millions of deaths from vitamin A deficiency each year. What I find most striking about such views is their implication that complex societal problems in this case, malnutrition are more easily solved by private-sector, commercially driven science than by societal decisions and political actions.

We already know that questions about the ability of Golden Rice to help people overcome deficiencies of vitamin A will not be answerable for several years. While waiting for the results of future research, it is worth considering more immediate ways to solve problems of vitamin A deficiency. Taken together, the many nutritional, physiological, and cultural factors that affect vitamin A status suggest that the addition of a single nutrient to food will have limited effectiveness. Instead, a combination of supplementation, fortification, and dietary approaches is likely to be needed—approaches such as promoting the production and consumption of fruits and vegetables rich in beta-carotene, educating people about how to use such foods, and improving the quantity and variety of foods in the diet (so beta-carotene can be better absorbed). Perhaps most helpful would be basic public health measures such as providing adequate supplies of clean water (to prevent transmission of diarrheal and parasitic diseases). Long-term solutions to the problem of vitamin A deficiency in particular, and malnutrition in general, continue to depend on societal interventions such as education, housing, health care, employment, and income—all more difficult and complicated, but ultimately more likely to be effective, than genetic engineering. Can genetic engineering usefully contribute to such efforts? Possibly, but that question cannot yet be answered.[32] In the meantime, the industry's public relations campaign continues.

One notable feature of the debates about Golden Rice is that its safety did not emerge as a major point of contention. Greenpeace found much to criticize without emphasizing safety issues but did raise one such issue—environmental effects: "GE rice, like other genetically modified organisms (GMOs) released into the environment, is a form of living pollution and its environmental impact is not only unpredictable and uncontrollable but also irreversible."[24] Dr. Potrykus responded to this charge by explaining that Golden Rice is no different from ordinary rice: "As the pathway [of beta-carotene synthesis] is already in rice (and in every green plant), and the difference is only in its activity in the endosperm, it is very hard to construct any selective advantage for Golden Rice in any environment, and therefore, any environmental hazard." What most concerned Dr. Potrykus was the threat that Greenpeace might engage in ecoterrorism and interfere with test plantings. He warned Greenpeace, "If you plan to destroy test fields to prevent responsible testing and development of Golden Rice for the humanitarian purpose, you will be accused of contributing to a crime against humanity."[33]

In the next chapter, we will examine environmental and other potential risks of genetically modified foods as a basis for evaluating the industry's contention: if genetically modified foods are safe, no opposition to them is justified. We will also examine how Greenpeace and other groups concerned about broader societal issues use questions about safety to raise dread and outrage and rally public support for their goals.

CHAPTER 6

RISKS AND BENEFITS

WHO DECIDES?

IN JUNE 2001, THE PEW CHARITABLE TRUST'S INITIATIVE ON
Food and Biotechnology, a project devoted to establishing an "independent and objective source of credible information on agricultural
biotechnology," conducted a survey of public attitudes toward transgenic
foods in the United States. In answer to the question "How concerned
are you about the safety of eating genetically modified foods in general?"
two-thirds (65%) of respondents expressed some level of concern, and
the rest expressed little.[1] These results seemed to indicate a fairly high
level of anxiety about genetically modified foods. But do they? The answers to questions about food biotechnology sometimes depend on who
is asking them. A few months later, in September 2001, the industry-sponsored International Food Information Council (IFIC) asked the question
in a different way: "What, if anything, are you concerned about when it
comes to food safety?" Only 2% of respondents thought to mention genetically modified foods (as compared to the 30% who mentioned microbial pathogens and the 25% who mentioned food packaging).[2] Regardless of the degree of concern expressed, the surveys suggest that
relatively few people are likely to reject genetically engineered foods entirely on principle (but see figure 15).

Like most else about food biotechnology, surveys of consumer attitudes are political. Industry leaders worry deeply about public acceptance and want to reassure consumers that transgenic foods are safe. It
is very much in their interest to demonstrate that the public is unconcerned, and very much in the interest of antibiotechnology advocates to
demonstrate the opposite. Surveys matter, and those devoted to food

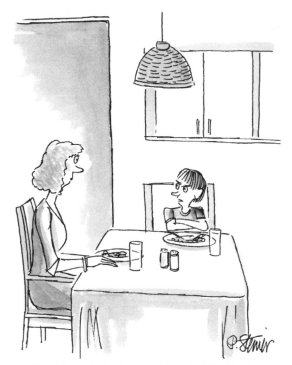

"I say it's genetically altered, and I say the hell with it."

FIGURE 15. Peter Steiner's drawing appeared in the *New Yorker*, July 24, 2000. The boy's comment is a modern version of a dinner conversation depicted by Carl Rose in that magazine in 1928: "It's broccoli, dear." "I say it's spinach, and I say the hell with it." (© The *New Yorker* Collection 2000 Peter Steiner from cartoonbank.com. All rights reserved.)

biotechnology constitute their own growth industry. Researchers have developed careers based on asking people what they think about genetically modified foods.

My personal collection of consumer surveys dates back to 1987, when the now defunct congressional Office of Technology Assessment (OTA) commissioned the Harris organization to convene focus groups and conduct telephone interviews on the topic. Since then, government agencies, university groups, industry groups, professional groups, national magazines, Internet sites, survey organizations, and individual researchers have all tried their hand at figuring out what consumers

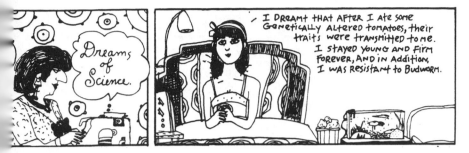

FIGURE 16. Sylvia's dreams of science are based on some of the earliest and most attractive promises of agricultural biotechnology. (© 1990 Nicole Hollander. Used with permission.)

think about genetically modified foods. Groups like the Pew Initiative and IFIC conduct frequent surveys to try to capture changes in attitudes over time.[3]

Despite substantial differences in the surveys—when they were conducted, who asked the questions, how the questions were worded, what they probed, and who answered them—the results are remarkable for their overall *consistency*. I think the following statements constitute a fair summary: Most people do not know very much about the scientific basis of food biotechnology but are intrigued by its promises. They expect the foods to produce benefits for society and, perhaps, for themselves. Although they are uneasy about the safety of the foods (a dread factor), they think the benefits likely to outweigh any risks. They are more likely to favor some genetically engineered foods over others, particularly those that seem to improve health or the environment, or that might save money or time. The cartoon in figure 16 nicely captures these views. On the other hand, the surveys also reveal considerable doubt about the government's ability to ensure the safety of the new foods and even greater doubt about the industry's willingness to make decisions in the public interest—particularly because genetically engineered foods are not labeled (an important outrage factor). As we will see in the next chapter, people in other countries share these attitudes but are more explicitly outraged by the ways biotechnology companies exercise control of the food supply.[4]

The results of these surveys come as no surprise. They are fully consistent with the research on risk communication discussed in the introduction, and they have considerable predictive value. Most people are vaguely or somewhat uneasy about eating the foods, mainly because they are not convinced that the industry and government are doing much to ensure safety or act in the interest of consumers. The lack of labeling is a critical factor: "What are they trying to hide from us?" Food biotechnology leaders, however, behave as if safety is a sufficient reason for trust: if the foods are safe, there is no reason to reject them. The surveys reveal that other concerns—those summarized in table 2 (page 17)—are just as important as safety and are often more important. Such concerns derive from personal values, perceptions, and beliefs that view biotechnology in general, and food biotechnology in particular, as morally, ethically, philosophically, or economically questionable.[5] As I discuss in chapter 8, many antibiotechnology advocates raise fundamental questions about protection of democratic institutions when they point out the ways in which the industry uses science and politics to achieve commercial goals.

Others raise more personal issues of values. In 1998, at the peak of the furor over genetically modified foods in Great Britain, for example, none other than His Royal Highness, Prince Charles, wrote of food biotechnology: "I happen to believe that this kind of genetic modification takes mankind into realms that belong to God, and to God alone. . . . We simply do not know the long-term consequences for human health and the wider environment of releasing plants bred in this way. . . . It is the *unforeseen* consequences which present the greatest cause for concern. . . . I personally have no wish to eat anything produced by genetic modification, nor do I knowingly offer this sort of produce to my family or guests."[6]

One might hardly think it productive to argue with such beliefs, but biotechnology stimulates theological as well as secular debate. Derek Burke, the former chairman of the British government's scientific committee on novel foods, took the secular route: "He [the prince] is raising one more food scare. As far as we can see, the risks of genetically engineering crops are very, very low. You can't walk away from changing the world."[7] A Vatican official also weighed in: "We are increasingly encouraged that the advantages of genetic engineering of plants and animals are greater than the risks. . . . We cannot agree with the position of some groups that say it is against the will of God to meddle with the genetic make-up of plants and animals." Pope John Paul II disagreed; at an outdoor mass attended by 50,000 farmers, he said that using biotechnology to increase production was contrary to God's will and that when farmers "forget this basic principle and become tyrants of the earth rather than its custodians . . . sooner or later the earth rebels."[8] Officials thought it necessary to counter religious arguments, because such values *matter*. Prince Charles's statements contributed to a sharp increase in public opposition to transgenic foods in Great Britain.[9]

British attitudes toward food biotechnology are more extreme than those found in the United States, but what most strongly emerges from surveys on both sides of the Atlantic is the importance of trust. If people do not trust the industry, they must rely on their governments for assurance that food is safe and worth eating. If they do not trust government, they worry more about safety. When, as discussed in chapter 7, U.S. government agencies made industry-friendly decisions to approve transgenic foods exclusively on the basis of science-based perceptions of risk—completely discounting all other considerations—they created a trust vacuum. Without an opportunity to consider the commercial, societal, and political implications of science-based approaches, advocacy groups focused on the one issue open for debate—safety. This chapter examines the health and environmental safety issues raised by genetically modified foods. In looking at these issues, we will see that despite protestations of industry and government to the contrary, it is impossible to separate science from politics in matters related to the safety of these foods.

HEALTH CONCERNS

When scientists first discovered how to move genes from one organism to another, they wondered whether such manipulations could be harmful to health or to the environment. In 1975, researchers met in Asilomar, California, to review the potential hazards of genetic manipulations. To prevent unanticipated problems that might emerge from the new recombinant DNA techniques, they proposed stringent research guidelines. The National Institutes of Health (NIH) soon required recipients of its research grants to follow such guidelines. In an extreme example of caution, residents of Cambridge, Massachusetts, debated whether such experiments should be allowed within the city limits. Later, when time and experience reassured people about the safety of the techniques, the guidelines became less restrictive. In retrospect, the intense anxiety—dread and outrage—about early genetic engineering experiments strikes many scientists as inappropriate to the low level of risk.[10] They view objections to food biotechnology as equally inappropriate.

Industry scientists working on early food biotechnology projects considered their work fundamentally similar to conventional genetics. If the foods did pose risks, these would be small and outweighed by benefits. Indeed, industry leaders believe that the projects are so interesting and potentially beneficial (and, of course, economically viable) that they raise no safety issues whatsoever. Critics disagree. In particular, they question the safety of genetic engineering manipulations that use (1) genes from bacteria responsible for diseases in plants, (2) genes for antibiotic resistance as "selection markers" (see page 176), and (3) regulatory DNA sequences transferred from one organism to another. They wonder whether "in the transgenic plant the harmonious interdependence of the alien gene and the new host's protein-mediated systems is likely to be disrupted in unspecified, imprecise, and inherently unpredictable ways."[11]

Critics ask whether the new proteins made by genetically modified plants might cause allergic reactions. They question the wisdom of planting vast areas of land with crops modified to resist herbicides or insects: will such plants transfer herbicide resistance to unwanted weeds, or toxin resistance to harmful insects? Government regulations do not require agricultural biotechnology companies either to answer such questions in much detail or to do very much to identify the potential consequences of releasing transgenic foods into the environment (consequences such as those that occurred with StarLink corn). The government not only fails to require labeling of genetically modified foods but actively opposes attempts to label such foods. All of this means that companies can decide for themselves what foods to produce and market, and consumers have little choice in the matter. Questions of safety, therefore, cannot be addressed without dealing with issues of regulation, oversight, trust, and control—politics. With politics in mind, we can now examine the principal safety issues: allergenicity, antibiotic resistance, and harm to the environment.

Allergens

It makes sense to think that introducing the DNA for a new gene into a food would also cause that food to make a new protein. That, after all, is the function of genes and the very purpose of food biotechnology. It also makes sense that some people might develop allergic reactions to the new protein; some proteins are allergens. In theory, any food protein can be allergenic. In practice, however, just eight foods cause 90% of food allergies: milk, eggs, soy, and wheat in children, and peanuts, tree nuts, shellfish, and fish in adults. When susceptible people eat these foods, most react with mild symptoms (itching, for example), but for others the result can be deadly. True food allergies—those that involve components of the immune system and threaten life—are relatively rare. Doctors diagnose them in less than 8% of children and 2% of adults in the United States.[12]

Whether the new transgenic proteins in foods might cause allergies is not easy to answer, mainly because many of the transgenes come from microbes never used as food. Furthermore, food allergies are a highly neglected area of medical research, and depressingly little is known about the structural features of proteins that induce immune reactions. Because exceptions are frequent, the few generalizations are highly tentative: allergenic proteins appear to occur in high concentrations in foods, to share some structural similarities, to be less easily digested to their constituent amino acids than are nonallergenic proteins, and to require multiple exposures to induce reactions.

Surveillance of food allergies also is limited. The widespread use of soy proteins—transgenic or not—in foods such as infant formulas, meat extenders, baked goods, and dairy replacements might be expected to increase the prevalence of soy allergies, but the increase would be difficult to detect unless it affected large numbers of people. Worse, because methods to diagnose food allergies are unavailable or imprecise, the allergenic potential of most genetically modified foods is uncertain, unpredictable, and not easily tested.[13]

These research limitations make genetically engineered foods especially vulnerable to charges that newly introduced genes will cause plants to produce allergenic proteins. Industry-friendly scientists recognize that such charges are based on "reasoned concern" but complain that they also are based on "fear through ignorance, and political motivation."[14] Antibiotechnology advocates raise the issue of allergenicity not only because it is scientifically justifiable but also because the industry is unable—or rarely tries—to prove that a newly introduced protein is *not* an allergen (witness StarLink). The government does not require biotechnology companies to test for allergens, and they rarely do. For one thing, testing is difficult. For another, testing is hardly in a company's best interest. Monsanto scientists, for example, wondered whether making soybeans "Roundup Ready" would make them more allergenic. They voluntarily tested and found the proteins in their soybeans to be similar in structure and quantity to those in conventional soybeans. On this basis, they assumed that no new allergens had been introduced but were not required to test for that possibility.[15] Like testing for microbial pathogens, testing for allergens is risky: you might find one.

Indeed, finding an allergen in a new transgenic food is a disheartening experience, and not only for its maker: it is a "shadow . . . cast over
the agricultural biotechnology industry."[16] One such shadow emerged in
the mid-1990s when scientists working for the venerable agricultural company Pioneer Hi-Bred created a transgenic soybean to solve a nutritional
problem—the need for sulfur—in poultry feed. Chicken feathers are
strong because their proteins are linked tightly with sulfur. The sulfur
comes from sulfur-containing amino acids, particularly one called methionine. Soybean proteins are relatively low in methionine, and soy-
based chicken feed must be supplemented with this amino acid—a troublesome expense. Proteins enriched with methionine might solve this
problem. As it happens, Brazil nuts contain a particular protein with two
unusual characteristics: it is exceptionally rich in methionine; it also is
present in large amounts (it accounts for 18% of all the proteins in Brazil
nuts). Pioneer Hi-Bred scientists isolated the gene for the Brazil nut protein and transferred it into soybeans. They recognized, however, that a
protein present in such high concentration might be the very one responsible for allergies to Brazil nuts.

Thus, they thought it prudent to find out if their transgenic soybeans
caused problems for people allergic to Brazil nuts. Ordinarily, this study
would be impossible because few laboratories have the biological materials needed to test for food allergens. By coincidence, Nebraska researchers had collected blood samples from people known to be allergic
to Brazil nuts, and they happened to have on hand all the components
necessary to do the tests. To the company's dismay, the experiments "succeeded." People allergic to Brazil nuts exhibited the same kinds of blood
and skin reactions when exposed to proteins extracted from the transgenic soybeans. Despite a substantial investment in development of the
soybean feed, Pioneer Hi-Bred discontinued the project.[17]

It must be understood that the Food and Drug Administration (FDA)
did not require the company to do such studies, nor do most companies
conduct them. As discussed in chapter 8, allergenicity and other safety
concerns about transgenic foods raise complex regulatory issues. Under
a policy developed by the FDA in 1992, the company was encouraged—
but not required—to consult FDA staff about the need to test products
before marketing them.[18] Pioneer Hi-Bred, a company with a long tradition of ethical practice dating back to the days of its founder, Henry
Wallace, did so voluntarily. Once testing revealed the allergenicity of the
transgenic protein, FDA policy required the company to label its soybeans as genetically modified. Although the soybeans were intended for

chicken feed, the company could not imagine how the beans could be kept separate from the human food supply, and it withdrew them.

In this unique instance, the company recognized that the gene donor came from a food known to be allergenic, was able to obtain blood samples from people allergic to Brazil nuts, and ended the project. Supporters of the FDA policy interpreted these events as a demonstration of its effectiveness; the soybeans never entered the food supply. Others, however, thought that this case proved that the FDA policy favored industry and could not protect consumers against less well studied transgenic proteins. The next case might not be so ideal, and the public less fortunate. Transgenic foods do not have to be labeled (see chapter 7), and avoidance is often the *only* effective way to prevent food allergies. Without labels, people with food allergies have no choice.

In 1993, the FDA asked for public comment on whether and how to label food allergens in transgenic foods and held a conference the next year to consider developing rules on this issue. The agency never released such rules, however, almost certainly because of industry pressure. The initial FDA proposals required "premarket notification"—informing the agency in advance about development of transgenic foods—but the biotechnology industry objected. Industry leaders wanted limits on *any* rules governing the safety of transgenic allergens and demanded that they "sunset" (be withdrawn and disappear) after three years.[19] Since then, international groups have had problems reaching consensus on the level of risk posed by transgenic allergens but do agree about how to minimize risk: developers should gradually introduce products into test markets and then monitor their effects.[13] This approach, no matter how sensible, will not be easy to implement. The unresolved status of FDA policy on transgenic allergenicity means that the industry retains *voluntary* responsibility for protecting the public against uncommon or unidentified allergens in genetically modified foods.

One especially ironic aspect of this situation is that the food biotechnology industry, in achieving an unregulated marketplace, made itself vulnerable to charges of producing allergens (through lack of testing) and covering up the hazards of transgenic foods (through lack of labeling). The StarLink corn episode illustrates this irony. Pioneer Hi-Bred knew in 1996 that soybeans intended for chicken feed could not possibly be kept separate from those intended for human consumption. As described in the introductory chapter, both Aventis and the Environmental Protection Agency (EPA) ignored this lesson at great cost. With their success in finding evidence of StarLink corn in common food products and revealing gaps in the regulatory system for genetically modified foods, advocates could use allergenicity—a safety issue—as a means to oppose the industry's economic and political goals. StarLink's owner could not demonstrate the safety of the corn to the satisfaction of EPA advisory committees and was forced to withdraw it from the market, albeit too late.[20] Supposedly scientific arguments about the degree to which transgenic foods might be allergenic reflect underlying concerns—less easily debated—about who is entitled to decide what people eat.

Antibiotic Resistance

A second legitimate safety issue is antibiotic resistance. In chapter 1, we saw how the routine use of antibiotics as growth promoters in cows and chickens favored the emergence of resistant microbial pathogens, rendering the antibiotics useless against human infections. Plant biotechnology raises similar concerns. In creating new plant varieties, agricultural biotechnologists link genes for antibiotic resistance to the genes they want to transfer into plants; these genes act as selection markers to identify the rare plants that actually accept the new genes. This selection system works because the plants that take up the antibiotic-resistance marker genes are the only ones to survive when grown in a broth containing the antibiotics (see appendix). Given the importance of antibiotic resistance as a public health problem, it makes sense to ask whether genetically engineered foods contribute to that problem. Answering that question requires a brief discussion of how antibiotics work.

Molds and bacteria naturally produce chemicals—antibiotics—that interfere with the growth or reproduction of *other* bacteria but are not nearly so toxic to animals or humans. Antibiotics act by blocking specific steps in the synthesis of structures or in metabolic processes unique to bacteria: cell walls (penicillin), cell membranes (polymyxin B), proteins (streptomycin, chloramphenicol, tetracycline), nucleic acids (rifampin), or folic acid vitamins (sulfonamide, trimethoprim). When animals or humans take antibiotics appropriately—in the right dose for the right length of time—the drugs suppress the growth of all sensitive bacteria. Bacteria, however, are exceedingly small, and the normal digestive tract contains hundreds of billions of them. Among this multitude, some are likely to lack the target structure; these grow in the presence of the antibiotic. Penicillin, for example, has no effect on bacteria that lack cell walls. Bacteria can acquire antibiotic resistance by mutations that change the structure of DNA and favor survival or produce enzymes that destroy the antibiotics or pump them out. The use of low-dose antibiotics "selects" for such bacteria; the drugs kill off most competing bacteria and allow the resistant ones to proliferate.[21]

The use of marker genes for antibiotic resistance in plant biotechnology raises additional concerns. Perhaps the genes for such characteristics will jump to other bacteria, and the bacteria will become resistant to *multiple* antibiotics. Scientists transfer new genes into plants by using special pieces of bacterial DNA called plasmids. Plasmids often contain three kinds of genes relevant to this discussion: (1) genes that enable them to "infect" and transfer selected genes into plants, (2) genes for antibiotic resistance, and (3) genes that enable them to infect many different kinds of bacteria (see appendix). Plasmid-containing bacteria in the intestines of animals or people could transmit antibiotic resistance to other bacteria, some of which might be pathogenic. This possibility is not just theoretical. Some pathogenic bacteria once easily controlled by penicillin are now thoroughly resistant to that drug, and others in ground meat have been found to resist treatment by as many as 12 antibiotics.[22]

Such findings explain why the continued use of low-dose antibiotics in farm animals elicits so much concern. They also explain why health officials want food biotechnologists to stop using clinically important antibiotics as selection markers. They want to avoid any chance—no matter how improbable—that transgenic plants might "lose" their recombinant antibiotic-resistance markers and transmit them to soil bacteria, to animals, or to people. In the worst-case scenario, a plant gene might recombine with the DNA of bacteria living in the intestines of animals or people and pass the trait for antibiotic resistance along to disease-causing bacteria. The antibiotic used in the selection process would then be ineffective as a treatment option. Alternatively, the antibiotic might be useless if people taking it were eating foods containing genes for resistance to that drug.

Perhaps because most scientists believe that such possibilities are exceedingly remote, the question of antibiotic-resistance markers also exists in a regulatory vacuum. Attempts to regulate transgenic antibiotic resistance began in 1990, when Calgene, an agricultural biotechnology company, asked the FDA for an opinion about whether it could use a gene for resistance to the antibiotic kanamycin (neomycin) as a selection marker for constructing transgenic tomatoes and canola oilseeds. This particular resistance gene specifies production of an enzyme able to inactivate kanamycin and related antibiotics. By the time the FDA issued its 1992 policy on genetically engineered plants, kanamycin *already* was in use as a selectable marker for development of more than 30 transgenic crops. In that policy, the FDA made no particular recommendation about antibiotic-resistant marker genes but said that its scientists were evaluating the issue.[18] In 1993, hoping to elicit a decisive response, Calgene petitioned the FDA to permit use of the kanamycin-inactivating enzyme as a "food additive" in genetically modified foods and cotton. In 1994, the FDA convened a meeting of its Food Advisory Committee to consider the Calgene petition.

I was one of four consumer representatives to that committee at the time, all of us united in what turned out to be the minority opinion. We were troubled by the lack of satisfactory answers to our questions about the probability of transferring antibiotic resistance. We urged caution but were heavily outvoted. After the meeting, FDA officials correctly reported that committee members "generally" approved the agency's regulatory approach and agreed that Calgene had addressed the relevant scientific questions. Thus, the FDA ruled that Calgene's evidence met the legal definition of safety for food additives: reasonable certainty that no harm would result from use.

Calgene contended that the kanamycin-inactivating enzyme (like all enzymes, a protein) would be destroyed by cooking or normal digestive processes and was unlikely to function in the intestine. But could the *gene* for antibiotic resistance jump from food or soil to bacteria in the intestines of animals or people? The FDA considered this suggestion too highly improbable to be worth discussion. In approving the kanamycin-inactivating enzyme as a food additive, the FDA explained that its policy is not to regulate genes or DNA: "DNA is present in the cells of all living organisms, including every plant and animal used for food by humans or animals, and is efficiently digested. . . . The DNA that makes up the [kanamycin-resistance] gene does not differ from any other DNA and does not itself pose a safety concern."[23]

In its decision, the FDA emphasized that safety "does not—and cannot—require proof beyond any possible doubt that no harm will result under any conceivable circumstance." Nevertheless, the agency agreed to consider further requests for use of selection markers for resistance to other antibiotics on a case-by-case basis. Subsequently, various groups challenged the FDA about the safety and regulatory status of antibiotic-resistance marker genes and, in late 1996 and early 1997, the agency consulted with outside experts about whether the use of such genes might cause problems. On the basis of those discussions, the FDA drafted a guidance statement for industry. This reassuring document said that antibiotic-resistance genes in food were "not of great concern," as the chance that they might be transferred from plants to bacteria in the intestine or environment was "remote."[24]

It is difficult to know how to interpret the FDA's decisions or guidance suggestions. Either transgenic transfer of antibiotic resistance is a problem or it is not. The FDA's use of the word "remote" suggests that marker genes require no special attention, but its nonbinding guidance document advises developers to evaluate the use of these genes quite carefully. Developers of new plant varieties, according to the FDA, should find out whether their marker genes involve clinically important antibiotics and whether they could transfer resistance to bacteria. If so, developers should use something else. Furthermore, if an antibiotic is the *only* one available to treat a particular infection in animals or people, it should not be used at all.

The inherent ambiguity of the agency's position seemed certain to—and did—elicit contentious comments, but the FDA did not respond to them. In the meantime, countries throughout Europe used concerns about antibiotic resistance as a basis for bans on the development and growth of transgenic food plants, and U.S. groups also used the issue to raise objections about food biotechnology. In 2001, when the Department of Health and Human Services (DHHS), the FDA's parent agency, released the *Action Plan to Combat Antimicrobial Resistance*, its principal recommendation to prevent such problems was a public education campaign to reduce the clinical use of antibiotics—not to reduce antibiotic use in animals.[25]

Overall, the relaxed regulatory environment demanded by the food biotechnology industry raises many of the outrage issues listed in table 2. No matter how remote the health hazards might be, the industry's antiregulatory stance does little to inspire trust. If anything, the stance invites criticism on safety and other grounds. As we will now see, similar considerations affect issues related to the environmental effects—risks and benefits—of genetically modified foods.

ENVIRONMENTAL ISSUES: RISKS AND BENEFITS

The mandate of the FDA is to assure the safety of drugs, medical devices, and foods, and the agency's policy for food biotechnology focuses on consequences that might present direct risks to *human* health. In approving transgenic foods, the FDA does not consider whether they might pose *ecological* risks. They might, for example, displace existing plants and animals, create new plant pathogens, disrupt ecosystems, transfer genes to weeds or wild relatives, reduce crop diversity, or "contaminate" native plants or organically grown foods. Widespread planting of *Bt* crops, for example, might encourage the proliferation of insects resistant to the *Bt* toxin. Similarly, widespread use of herbicide-resistant crops might transfer that resistance to undesirable weeds or encourage further reliance on chemicals—such as Monsanto's Roundup—as pest-management strategies.[26] Despite such concerns, plantings of transgenic crops increased from negligible acreage in 1995 to hundreds of millions of acres within just a few years. Agricultural producers quickly adopted transgenic soybeans, corn, and cotton, largely because they simplify the control of weeds and insect pests by requiring fewer applications of the more toxic chemicals. Farmers, apparently, perceive significant benefits from growing transgenic crops, but how are we, as citizens and consumers, to reconcile the risks and benefits? Let's begin by looking at the risks.

Environmental Risks

When researchers began to examine questions of environmental risk, their early results provided plenty of justification—albeit highly preliminary—for concern. In 1996, for example, farmers planted 2 million acres with Monsanto's *Bt* cotton, but lost thousands of acres when the toxin failed to protect against a bollworm infestation. This event raised the uncomfortable possibility that such huge plantings might promote *Bt* resistance.[27] According to investigative accounts, EPA officials asked Monsanto to evaluate whether the surviving bollworms were indeed *Bt*-resistant, but the agency could not force the company to cooperate: "Further evaluation of the crop is entirely dependent on Monsanto's own reporting."[28] Also in 1996, researchers reported that transgenic oilseed (canola) plants readily transmitted herbicide resistance to related weeds. Because weeds reproduce rapidly and compete for nutrients with crop plants, this finding raised fears that cross-pollination might create herbicide-resistant "superweeds" that could overrun cropland and cause an ecological catastrophe. EPA officials revealed the consequences of the regulatory gap, however, when they explained that monitoring of herbicide resistance is not a federal responsibility: "It is the developer of the product that has the interest in assuring that resistance does not build up."[29]

These early reports on environmental risks were based on single studies and needed further confirmation, but others soon followed. For example, preliminary studies showed that bees and other beneficial insects die when exposed to the *Bt* toxin, but certain harmful moths and tobacco budworms resist it. The *Bt* toxin remains stable in soil for many months, meaning that it exerts continuous pressure to encourage the growth of resistant insects. Herbicide-resistant plants transfer resistance to related weeds, sometimes over great distances through pollen drift.[30] Many such problems can be unintended consequences of large-scale plantings of transgenic crops, and they greatly trouble environmentalists. As I will soon explain, effects on monarch butterflies are the most political of such consequences, but let's look first at the environmental *benefits* claimed for transgenic crops.

Environmental Benefits

As evidence for the benefits produced by genetically engineered crops, the industry notes how quickly growers have adopted them. In theory, the crops should help growers. At the time farmers first began to plant transgenic crops, they were using more than 80 million pounds of conventional pesticides (a term that includes both insecticides and herbicides). Reducing the use of these chemicals should produce economic as well as health benefits, and a major argument for the value of transgenic crops is that they eliminate the need for hazardous pesticides—except Roundup, of course—by millions of pounds annually. This idea is central to the biotechnology industry's public relations efforts. The advertisement shown in figure 17, for example, promotes the ecological advantages of transgenic crops. This advertisement, which much resembles those for the cigarette-selling Marlboro Man, is clearly meant to suggest that genetically engineered crops will save family farms.

As with all issues related to food biotechnology, its benefit to farmers is subject to debate. Also like the other issues, this one is complicated and lacks a firm research base on which to resolve outstanding questions. By 2001, most observers agreed that transgenic cotton required less use of pesticides than conventional cotton, but only in certain areas. In Arizona, for example, the use of transgenic cotton led to a breathtaking decline in the need for pesticides against budworms and bollworms: from 400,000 pounds in 1995 to just 2,000 pounds in 2000. In other states growing such cotton, however, the overall use of pesticides *increased*.[31] When it comes to corn and soybeans, however, the evidence is wide open to interpretation. Here are just a few observations: U.S. farmers who planted *Bt* corn in 1997 did much better economically than farmers who planted conventional corn, but in 1998 they did worse, largely because so much

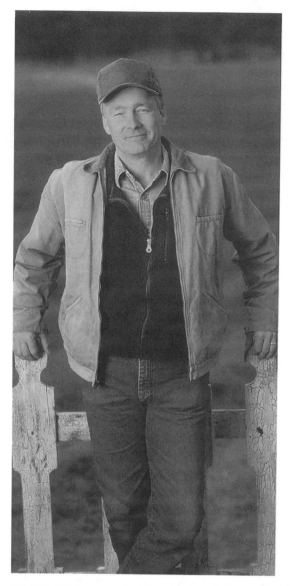

Biotechnology
is helping him
protect the land
and preserve his
family's heritage.

"I'm raising a better soybean crop that helps me conserve the topsoil, keep my land productive and help this farm support future generations of my family."
—Rod Gangwish, farmer

Biotechnology is helping Rod Gangwish to grow a type of soybean that requires less tilling of the soil. That helps him preserve precious topsoil and produce a crop with less impact on the land. Preserving topsoil today means a thriving farm for generations to come.

Biotechnology allows farmers to choose the best combination of ways to help grow their crops. It helps cotton farmers use fewer chemicals to protect their crops against certain pests. And, it's helping provide ways for developing countries to better feed a growing population. And, in the future, it can help farmers grow better quality, more nutritious food.

Biotechnology is also enhancing lives in other ways, helping to create more effective treatments for diseases such as leukemia and diabetes.

Biotechnology is helping create solutions that are improving lives today, and solutions that could improve our world tomorrow. If you're interested in learning more, visit our Web site or call the number below for a free brochure about biotechnology and agriculture.

COUNCIL FOR
BIOTECHNOLOGY
INFORMATION

good ideas are growing

1-800-980-8660
www.whybiotech.com

FIGURE 17. In 2001, the biotechnology industry's public relations campaign featured the equivalent of the Marlboro Man. Rather than cigarettes, however, this advertisement promotes the industry's view of the ecological advantages of transgenic crops (reduced pesticide use, soil conservation), and consequent benefits to society (farm preservation). In 2002, a series of elegant photographs promoted the benefits of genetically modified corn, soybeans, cotton, and papaya.

corn was produced that prices fell and the costs of seeds and pesticides increased. Transgenic crops—cotton as well as corn and soybeans—contributed to an overall decline in pesticide use of 2.5 million pounds from 1997, or just 1% of total pesticide use. Infestations with the European corn borer were relatively low that year, suggesting that fewer pesticides would have been applied anyway.[32] In contrast, an analysis of data from 1999 found that Roundup Ready soybeans alone saved $216 million in the costs of controlling weeds and required 19 million fewer applications of herbicides. The contradictions in these results are due to the large number of variables that have to be considered in such analyses, many of them constantly changing, and some easier to measure than others.[33] What seems most evident from attempts to evaluate benefits is that it is still too early to do so. We do not yet know the overall effects of transgenic crops on cost, productivity, and use of pesticides.

Indeed, one of the chief complaints of environmentalists is that transgenic crops will *increase* the use of agricultural chemicals, especially of Monsanto's Roundup. Farmers planted Roundup Ready soybeans on just 1 million acres in 1996 but on 48 million acres in 2001; they applied Roundup to 20% of farm acres in 1995 but to 62% in 1999.[34] Roundup generates billions of dollars in annual sales, and Monsanto benefits twice; it sells the herbicide *and* the seeds for the crops that resist it. The company's studies show that Roundup Ready soybeans survive when doused with the chemical, and are as nutritious when fed to rats as conventional soybeans.[35] Whether the use of Roundup is environmentally beneficial is, of course, a debatable issue. Monsanto points out that it registered Roundup as an herbicide in 1974 with minimal subsequent evidence of hazard: "Consumers benefit from Roundup Ready soybeans because farmers can control weeds better . . . with less herbicide while using a herbicide with the best environmental profile." To bolster that argument, the company cites two lines of research: Roundup binds so tightly to soil particles that the chemical does not harm nearby vegetation (and, therefore, is unlikely to move to groundwater), and it decomposes naturally to benign substances.[36]

Critics, however, raise alarms about the heavy use of this product: Roundup may induce weeds to develop resistance; it may poison fish, earthworms, or other beneficial creatures; and it may disrupt soil ecology. From a biochemical standpoint, resistance to Roundup is not difficult to achieve. Its active chemical, glyphosate, inhibits the action of an enzyme that helps make three amino acids needed to construct plant proteins. Plants cannot make proteins when this enzyme is blocked. Bacteria, however, are well known to produce a mutant variant of this enzyme that is completely unaffected by glyphosate; they do so through "point" mutations (mutations that alter just one amino acid) or mutations that cause the enzyme to be produced in such large amounts that glyphosate becomes ineffective. Such mutations could occur in plants as well as in bacteria. The transfer of Roundup resistance to weeds through pollination also is probable, and has already occurred. The idea of widespread resistance to Roundup is not improbable, and it alarms the industry as well as environmentalists.[37]

The most highly critical statements about the use, toxicity, and persistence in soil of Roundup can be traced to an exhaustive scientific review published in 1995. The review identifies toxic effects from the chemical itself as well as from ingredients used in its formulation. It describes studies on experimental animals in which Roundup caused eye and skin irritation, cardiac depression, gastrointestinal distress, reduced weight gain, increased frequency of tumors, and reduced sperm counts. In people, Roundup appears as the most common cause of pesticide-related illness among landscape workers and the third most common cause of such illness among agricultural workers. Roundup residues persist in vegetables a year after treatment and in soil for more than a year. Researchers report that Roundup produces toxic effects on beneficial insects, fish, birds, and earthworms; eliminates vegetation used as food and shelter for animals and birds; and reduces the activity of bacteria that fix nitrogen and perform other "friendly" tasks.[38] Whether these effects are worse than those produced by the pesticides replaced by Roundup is a question that demands further research. In the absence of convincing studies, such decisions are a matter of opinion.

Underlying questions about the potential risks of transgenic plantings are more general concerns about what Roundup Ready and *Bt* crops might do to biodiversity. The huge amount of U.S. farmland devoted to transgenic crops borders on *monoculture*—the planting of one variety of a crop to the exclusion of all others. The lack of biological diversity means that any point of vulnerability leaves monocultured crops open to overwhelming attack by insects, weeds, or diseases—and to catastrophic losses. Such vulnerability is illustrated by the splitting of stems of Roundup Ready soybeans when grown in hot climates. When this happened, observers guessed that crop losses could reach 40%. They wondered if the biochemical changes that induce resistance to glyphosate might also cause plants to produce a form of cellulose (lignin) that becomes brittle in hot temperatures typical of southern states and tropical countries.[39]

From such examples, it should be evident that questions about the relative risks and relative benefits of genetically modified foods cannot be answered without further research and experience. As I explain in chapter 7, the industry and its sympathetic government regulators decided in advance—using a strictly science-based approach to risk assessment—that the foods were safe and that few precautions were necessary, and they assumed that any unanticipated consequences of transgenic foods could be handled appropriately by existing regulations. As it turned out, unexpected consequences revealed the inadequacies of this approach. Some examples follow.

THE POLITICS OF UNEXPECTED CONSEQUENCES

Critics of food biotechnology insist that without prior experience, transgenic foods raise safety issues that are difficult to define, predict, or quantify but that nevertheless should be taken seriously and evaluated in advance—*before* the foods are grown extensively and enter the food supply. They invoke the precautionary principle (discussed in the introduction). As support for the need for precaution, they cite the examples to which we now turn. These examples explain why safety issues—especially those that cannot easily be resolved by scientific studies—become matters of politics. A precautionary approach threatens the economics of the entire agricultural biotechnology enterprise.

Toxic Contaminants: Tryptophan Supplements

The classic case of the unanticipated consequences of nutritional—if not food—biotechnology concerns supplements of the amino acid tryptophan. Like all amino acids, tryptophan is a component of proteins in all organisms. Supplements of tryptophan have been used for years as self-medication for insomnia and neurological conditions. In the 1980s, companies began to genetically engineer bacteria to produce larger amounts of tryptophan so that this amino acid would be easier to collect and purify. In 1989, tryptophan supplements produced by a Japanese petrochemical company, Showa Denko, caused eosinophilia-myalgia syndrome (EMS), an unusual constellation of symptoms of muscle pain, weakness, and increased blood levels of white cells (eosinophils). Eventually, more than 1,500 people who had taken the supplements became ill, and about 40 died. The FDA prevented further marketing of the supplement, and the company stopped making it.[40]

This example might just indicate that genetic techniques sometimes lead to unexpected problems, but this particular situation had additional implications. Because tryptophan is a normal component of body proteins, investigators did not think that the genetic engineering processes were at fault. Instead, they suspected that a toxic substance emerged during the manufacturing process, and they attempted to identify it. Victims, however, sued Showa Denko for about $2 billion, thereby introducing liability as an intervening factor. The company not only refused to cooperate with FDA investigations but also tried to discredit the scientists who had linked the syndrome to its product. Showa Denko demanded prepublication copies of the studies under the Freedom of Information Act (most scientists would find this intimidating as well as a nuisance) and used a carefully selected advisory committee to argue that the studies were done poorly and could not be reproduced.

Furthermore, the company sponsored its own research studies, organized a conference to announce the results, and paid for publication of the conference papers as a supplement to the *Journal of Rheumatology*. Not unexpectedly, the sponsored researchers raised questions and produced data that appeared to exonerate Showa Denko. In contrast, the one independent paper ("prepared by US Government employees and entirely funded by the US Government") concluded that the Showa Denko tryptophan supplement caused the EMS epidemic. The government scientists charged that the studies sponsored by Showa Denko were

> based on supposition, surmise, and conjecture. [They] direct attention toward potential biases or confounding events with a low probability of having occurred and a still lower probability of having had a substantial effect on the studies reviewed. In so doing, they direct the reader's attention away from the combined weight of evidence of the studies, which strongly supports a causal association of Showa Denko LT [tryptophan] and epidemic EMS.[41]

To date, the toxic component remains "incompletely characterized," making it difficult to institute preventive measures. In this case, the company's self-interested stance not only interfered with finding the cause of the disease but also failed to resolve lingering uncertainties about the safety of the genetic engineering processes used in manufacturing the supplements.

Toxic Proteins: The Pusztai Affair

Next we turn to the possibility that genetic engineering might cause *foods* to produce toxic substances, in this case, lectins. Lectins are proteins in plants that are naturally toxic to insects and nematode worms. They do not bother us because we cook lectin-rich foods—kidney beans, for example—long enough to unravel the structure of the proteins and destroy their function. In 1998, an investigator in Scotland announced that rats became ill when they ate transgenic lectins, thereby initiating a political furor of quite astonishing proportions.

This story begins soon after the peak of the mad cow disease epidemic in Great Britain, a crisis that resulted not only in the downfall of the British beef industry but also in the loss of public confidence in scientists and government (see concluding chapter). In this context, Dr. Arpad Pusztai, a long-time researcher at the Rowett Research Institute in Aberdeen, applied for and won a competitive contract to see how rats might react to consuming transgenic potatoes containing lectins. Dr. Pusztai isolated genes for lectins from snowdrop plants and transferred them into potatoes. For comparison, he physically inserted purified lectins into other potatoes. He fed the transgenic potatoes to one group of rats and the lectin-added conventional potatoes to another group. All of the rats reacted badly to lectins, but the ones fed the transgenic potatoes fared worse.[42] On August 10, 1998, Dr. Pusztai—bravely or foolishly, depending on one's point of view—appeared on television to announce that the rats fed transgenic potatoes showed signs of growth retardation and some immune system dysfunctions. He said: "If you gave me the choice now, I wouldn't eat it," and it would be "very, very unfair to use our fellow citizens as guinea pigs."[43]

Dr. Pusztai based these comments on studies not yet published or subjected to peer review. Industry officials charged that because of his remarks, "the whole of the biotechnology industry had gone up in smoke," and they would now be faced with consumer opposition that would take years to undo.[44] The head of the Rowett Institute defended the work at first, but quickly changed his mind. After reviewing the data and judging it flawed, he sealed Dr. Pusztai's laboratories, forced him to retire, barred him from speaking to the press, and ordered a formal audit of his data—actions that received front-page press attention and did nothing to calm public alarm about food biotechnology in Great Britain or Europe.

As might be expected from a review of provisional results, the audit committee decided that the data did not support Dr. Pusztai's conclusions. Dr. Pusztai again reviewed his own data and said that they did. Furthermore, he conducted his own peer review; he sent copies of his research reports and the television transcript to scientists who requested these documents, and asked *them* to evaluate the materials. In February

1999, more than 20 scientists from at least 13 countries called a press conference to announce that the findings were just as Dr. Pusztai had claimed.[45] Public calls for a moratorium on food biotechnology research followed immediately. Most scientists (other than the 20 supporters) strongly doubted that genetically modified lectins could have harmed the rats, although they thought the potatoes might have been induced to express higher levels of *other* toxic substances. When the British government rejected demands for a moratorium, critics charged that government officials were "in the pocket of the biotech industry" and had offered huge sums to biotechnology companies to induce them to work in Britain. They also noted that Monsanto had bought off the Rowett Institute in advance with a £140,000 grant.[46]

In May, the British Royal Society weighed in with an anonymous review that judged Dr. Pusztai's studies flawed and inconclusive. Dr. Pusztai called this clandestine peer review "deprecable because many influential committees are redolent with advisors linked to biotechnology companies."[47] The *Lancet*, a leading medical journal, agreed, calling the Royal Society's review "a gesture of breathtaking impertinence."[43] The Prince of Wales expressed sympathy for Dr. Pusztai's plight. Industry commentators, however, said Dr. Pusztai was "largely responsible for the British public's mistrust of genetically modified food" as well as for subsequent governmental actions to regulate, label, or ban genetically modified foods.[48]

In October 1999, in an act that itself generated a huge outcry, the *Lancet* published Dr. Pusztai's data as a short research letter. The journal fueled the controversy by including another report in the same issue suggesting that snowdrop lectins interact with human white blood cells in some peculiar way that demands further investigation. An editorial in the same issue, however, stated that such experiments were incomplete, insignificant, inadequately controlled, and uninterpretable.[49] Justifying the journal's decision to publish evidently flawed research, the *Lancet*'s editor chided critics for their "failure to understand the new, and apparently unwelcome, dialogue of accountability that needs to be forged between scientists and the public." He quite sensibly pointed out, "Risks are not simply questions of abstract probabilities or theoretical reassurances. What matters is what people believe about these risks and why they hold those beliefs. [The] data are preliminary and non-generalisable, but at least they are now out in the open for debate."[50]

By one report, a member of the Royal Society with ties to biotechnology companies accused the editor of acting immorally by publishing research known to be "untrue" and implied that doing so would "have implications for his personal position." With or without such threats, the editor's argument did not convince scientists skeptical of the quality of the research, and they heavily criticized the journal for publishing it.[51] Whatever the scientific merits of Dr. Pusztai's work, his treatment reinforced public suspicions that no group with a vested interest in food biotechnology would act in the public interest. If a problem with transgenic foods did emerge, the government and much of the scientific establishment would support the industry above all other considerations.

Killing Monarch Butterflies

We now turn to the most widely publicized—and most fiercely debated—example of unintended consequences—the effects of Bt crops on *friendly* insects, in this case, monarch butterflies. Monarch butterflies lay their eggs on milkweed plants that grow throughout fields of corn. Of course the Bt toxin kills monarch larvae that hatch from the eggs; the toxin is *supposed* to kill insect larvae. When Cornell University investigators dusted laboratory milkweed leaves with pollen from Bt corn, the results were only to be expected: the test larvae grew more slowly and died more quickly than those fed leaves dusted with pollen from conventional corn or with no pollen at all.[52] This research note, taking up less than a page in a scientific journal (albeit the prestigious *Nature*), elicited an immediate response: "Will the conjectured absence of butterflies flapping their wings on Iowa farms provoke political firestorms among Washington policymakers?" Indeed, yes. Farmers did not want to be termed "butterfly-killers," and neither did Congress. Legislators proposed an appropriation of $200,000 to study the effect of transgenic foods on monarch butterflies and also introduced legislation to require labeling.[53] Monarch butterflies became the symbol of antibiotechnology protests, as illustrated in figure 18.

From the industry standpoint, killing butterflies and other friendly insects is normal collateral damage, no worse than the effects of conventional pesticides. Using this argument to deflect appeals for preservation of an already endangered species, however, would be unlikely to succeed. Thus, the industry employed different strategies. The first was to discredit the science by pointing out, correctly, that one small laboratory study should not be taken too seriously until it is confirmed. Second, the industry funded new studies, reportedly at $100,000 each, to repeat the

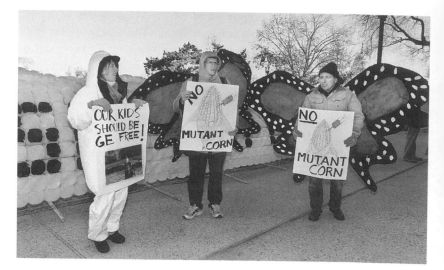

FIGURE 18. The FDA's Washington, DC, hearings on genetically modified foods in November 1999, drew demonstrators dressed as monarch butterflies. This photograph appeared in the *New York Times Magazine*, December 12, 1999. (© 1999 AP/Wide World Photos by J. Scott Applewhite. Reprinted with permission.)

work in field trials. Third, it organized a scientific symposium to publicize the results of those trials.[54] The industry-funded studies produced the expected conclusion: transgenic crops pose no risk to monarch butterflies. This outcome was so certain that the industry sponsors distributed a news release *prior* to the conference: "Scientific symposium to show no harm to monarch butterfly."[55] The conference itself, however, proved rather contentious. Some participants complained about manipulation by the industry: "It was dirty pool and the fox was guarding the chicken coop. . . . It was not conclusive."[56] Independent scientists were appalled by the industry's heavy-handed control of a meeting at which researchers—many with only preliminary results to report—were supposed to be presenting and discussing them in a careful and deliberate manner.

Further studies attempted to resolve the issue. One reported that pollen from *Bt* corn did not harm black swallowtail butterflies. The authors concluded, "at least some potential nontarget effects of the use of transgenic plants may be manageable," but "the plain fact of the matter is that growing food has nontarget effects. . . . Our challenge is to minimize them."[57]

Another found just the opposite, but came to the same conclusion: *Bt* pollen on milkweeds in corn fields caused "significant mortality" of monarch butterfly larvae: "This is telling us that with naturally deposited pollen there's a good probability you'll get some mortality."[58]

Although it might seem self-evident that *Bt* pollen kills "nontarget" insects as well as those it is intended to control, the industry and its federal regulators have taken heroic—and expensive—steps to prove the trivial nature of such collateral damage. In December 1999, the EPA "called in" (translation: asked for) comments from researchers on the toxicity of *Bt* corn pollen. In February 2000, the U.S. Department of Agriculture (USDA) held a conference to respond to that call-in and to set research priorities for determining the safety of *Bt* pollen for monarch butterflies. Its own in-house researchers spent two years investigating this question (conclusion: "negligible" risk).[59] In September 2000, the EPA issued a preliminary report concluding that the butterfly population was not at risk from *Bt* pollen. In the meantime, agricultural biotechnology companies had pooled resources in partnership with those agencies to fund extensive field trials. The results of these trials appeared as a collection of six papers in the *Proceedings of the National Academy of Sciences* in September 2001. The final paper concluded, "The impact of *Bt* corn pollen from current commercial hybrids on monarch butterfly populations is negligible." Its lead author said, "I don't think there's a need to consider monarchs at risk due to this technology." The *New York Times* headline repeated the conclusion: "Reports say threat to monarch butterflies is 'negligible.'"[60]

My reading of this extraordinary scientific effort to prove the obvious comes to a slightly different interpretation: negligible under some circumstances, but not others. The papers provide substantial evidence that certain types of *Bt* corn produce more lethal pollen than others. They find that monarch butterflies are more likely to survive in fields planted with lower amounts of genetically modified corn, treated with lower levels of insecticides, and weeded less vigorously (unweeded fields contain more milkweed plants). The butterflies survive better when they are not near the center of the fields where pollen counts are higher, and when rain washes the pollen off the milkweed plants.

Such results may be debatable, but no such debate took place—for reasons of politics. The papers were to appear just at the time the EPA was about to decide whether to renew the licenses (registrations) for planting *Bt* corn and cotton. The EPA asked the journal to release the papers on the Internet prior to publication so the agency would appear to have considered the results in coming to the decision—one it had already made.[60] In announcing the decision, the EPA said: "Adhering to a process that emphasized up-to-date scientific data and methodologies, numerous opportunities for public involvement, and balanced decision-making, EPA maintained a transparent review process to ensure that the decision was based on sound science."[61] Critics did not find the process so transparent, not only because they had no chance to review the studies beforehand, but also because some of the data had been classified as "confidential business information" in an unusual concession to the industry. When the EPA did make the confidential information available, it required readers to agree not to copy or discuss it. In this instance, as in so many others, science alone cannot settle social questions of transparency or trust.

THE POLITICS OF RISKS AND BENEFITS

When dealing with questions about the risks of genetically modified foods, industry leaders are fond of saying that nobody has died yet from eating them. This may be a correct assessment, but it misses the point. In a situation in which the risks of genetically modified foods are questionable but so are the benefits, point of view becomes the critical factor in interpretation. Regardless of the remoteness of safety concerns, the intensity of criticism—and the vulnerability of the industry—have prompted government agencies to take safety issues seriously. In 2002 alone, the General Accounting Office (GAO) chided the FDA for not doing a better job of validating information provided by food biotechnology companies, disclosing its evaluation methods, and developing new testing methods to ensure the safety of genetically modified foods. The White House Office of Science and Technology Policy asked the FDA, EPA, and USDA to strengthen restrictions on field testing to prevent escape of transgenes, and scientific panels of the National Academies urged more careful safety evaluation of genetically modified plants and animals.[62]

Regardless of the outcome of such actions, the safety questions discussed here—whether genetically modified foods cause allergies, antibiotic resistance, higher production of lectins, or the death of monarch butterflies, and whether they decrease or increase the use of pesticides— are not necessarily the primary issues. Genetically modified foods *already* pervade the food supply. The experiment is in progress; its results will emerge in due course. Whether such an experiment is in the public interest—or for that matter is in the interest of the industry—will also be revealed in time. If food biotechnology is political, it is because the public has no choice but to participate in this experiment. Thus, the important question is *who gets to decide*. In the next chapter, we will consider how agricultural biotechnology companies—particularly Monsanto—convinced regulatory agencies that questions about societal risks and benefits do not need to be addressed before planting transgenic foods, that the foods require no special labels, and that the public has no choice about whether to consume them.

CHAPTER 7

THE POLITICS OF
GOVERNMENT OVERSIGHT

AMONG THE LESSONS OF THE STARLINK CORN EPISODE IS THIS: genetically modified ingredients pervade the U.S. food supply, but consumers cannot identify them because the foods are not labeled. This situation was not inevitable. Federal agencies made "science-based" decisions that transgenic foods are equivalent to conventional foods (DNA is DNA no matter where it comes from) and require no special regulatory oversight. In this chapter, we will see how the biotechnology industry lobbied successfully for this approach, using the now familiar mantra: the techniques are inherently safe, the products are no different than those produced through traditional genetics, and labeling is not only unnecessary but misleading.

In choosing this approach, federal regulators permitted companies to develop genetically modified foods without having to alert regulatory agencies (premarket notification), evaluate the safety of the products in advance (premarket testing), or label them once they were ready to market. In approving transgenic foods, they restricted the debate to science-based issues of safety. If the foods appeared safe for human health they could be marketed: plant first, then deal with problems. As discussed earlier, this approach differs from the method required by the precautionary principle: demonstrate safety *before* planting. The science-based approach also excluded debate about the societal issues summarized in table 2 (page 17). The regulatory agencies interpreted their mandates to mean that they could not consider dread-and-outrage factors when making decisions about genetically modified foods.

This chapter examines how food biotechnology companies achieved a "plant first" regulatory environment. To understand the politics of the current system, we must recall that Congress wrote the principal laws affecting food safety in 1906, long before anyone knew anything about DNA, let alone transgenic foods. As noted earlier, the discovery of recombinant DNA techniques in the 1970s stimulated discussion about how to assure their safety. At hearings in 1983, Congress reviewed arguments for federal regulation of biotechnology. The following year, under pressure from the pharmaceutical industry, the White House Office of Science and Technology Policy (OSTP) proposed a "Coordinated Framework" for the regulation of biotechnology and issued a final version in 1986. The pharmaceutical industry argued that because DNA is DNA, drugs produced through recombinant techniques require no special considerations, laws, or agencies. The OSTP agreed and established four principles: (1) existing laws are sufficient for regulation, (2) regulation applies to the products, not the processes by which they were developed, (3) safety should be assessed on a case-by-case basis, and (4) agencies should coordinate their regulatory efforts.[1]

This last principle would prove especially challenging because the Coordinated Framework distributed regulatory responsibilities among a large number of federal entities: three offices reporting directly to the president; three cabinet-level federal agencies; two major subagencies within one cabinet-level agency; eight centers, services, offices, or programs within major agencies; and five federal committees—all operating under the authority of 10 distinct acts of Congress. Any regulatory plan of that complexity suggests that coordination will be difficult—impossible is more like it—and that oversight will be plagued from the start by gaps, duplication of effort, and overlapping responsibilities. Like the oversight scheme for food safety, the Coordinated Framework reveals the need for a single food agency.

The Coordinated Framework applies to foods as well as drugs and assigns three agencies to their regulation, two at the cabinet level—the U.S. Department of Agriculture (USDA) and the Environmental Protection Agency (EPA)—and a subagency of a third (the Department of Health and Human Services), the Food and Drug Administration (FDA). Genetically modified foods, however, do not easily fit into the existing regulatory categories of these agencies, leaving much room for interpretation. Moreover, the three agencies operate under different laws. The Plant Pest Act allows the USDA to regulate transgenic crops as *plant pests* when they contain genes or regulatory DNA segments from potentially harmful organisms: insects, nematodes, slugs, and snails, but also bacteria, fungi, and viruses. Because just about all gene donors are on this list, most transgenic plants require USDA permits to allow them to be field-tested, transported through interstate commerce, or imported. Over time, the USDA has modified its regulations to make it easier for companies to plant genetically engineered crops without having to obtain permits.[2]

In contrast, the Federal Insecticide, Fungicide and Rodenticide Act (FIFRA) requires the EPA to "register" transgenic foods as *plant-pesticides* (or, as they are now called, *plant-incorporated protectants*). If a crop is bioengineered to contain the toxin from *Bacillus thuringiensis (Bt)*, for example, the EPA considers it to contain a pesticide and regulates the plant as it would any pesticidal chemical. Ordinarily, makers of *Bt* crops must submit voluminous information about the toxin's effects on health and the environment, but the EPA can and does grant exceptions.

To further complicate matters, the FDA regulates transgenic foods as *food additives* under the provisions of the Food, Drug, and Cosmetic Act. Unless food additives are generally recognized as safe (GRAS), meaning that they have a history of safe use, they require premarket approval; manufacturers must submit evidence demonstrating "reasonable certainty" that an additive will not be harmful if used appropriately. In practice, the FDA has jurisdiction over all genetically modified foods, although it shares regulatory authority over plants that have to be field-tested or transported across state lines with USDA, and those containing the *Bt* toxin with EPA. Dealing separately with two—let alone three—agencies is guaranteed to be a lengthy, complicated, and expensive process, and food biotechnology companies complain that the regulations are cumbersome and restrictive. They also complain that the regulations are contrary to the intention of the Coordinated Framework because they hold genetically modified foods to *higher* safety standards than conventional foods.[3] To evaluate such contentions, let's begin by examining the FDA's role in regulating transgenic foods and the ways in which the biotechnology industry has influenced that role.

THE FDA'S "SCIENCE-BASED" APPROACH

The FDA's main function is to regulate drugs, and its food activities are decidedly secondary. By the early 1990s, the FDA had approved at least 15 recombinant drugs for medical use, with recombinant insulin among the earliest in 1982. The benefits of many of these drugs seem evident. Recombinant insulin, unlike that obtained from pigs, has an amino acid structure identical to that of human insulin and can be produced in unlimited quantities. So can recombinant enzymes used in food manufacture such as chymosin, an enzyme used to coagulate milk in the early steps of cheese making. In the past, cheese makers obtained chymosin as part of a mixture called rennet, which had to be extracted from the stomachs of calves and was expensive and of inconsistent composition. Scientists bioengineered the gene for chymosin into bacteria, and the FDA approved the recombinant enzyme in 1990. Such drugs and enzymes elicited few objections from critics of biotechnology, mainly because of the obvious advantages. Transgenic chymosin, for example, does not require the slaughter of baby calves. Also, manufacturers did not publicize its origin, as they saw "little to gain from waving the biotech flag."[4] Transgenic drugs did not become controversial until they affected food more directly, as was the case with the cow growth hormone, recombinant bovine somatotropin (rbST)—a drug that affects *milk*. Because the approval process for this drug was so evidently political—interweaving considerations of science, safety, commercial objectives, and societal issues—and because it paved the way for subsequent FDA approval of transgenic foods, the case of bovine growth hormone is worth close examination.

The Politics of Bovine Growth Hormone (BGH): More Milk

The politics of this animal drug begin with its very name. Proponents of the drug use the scientific term *bovine somatotropin* (bST), whereas critics tend to use the more recognizable *bovine growth hormone* (BGH). Both put an *r* in front to distinguish the genetically engineered drug from the natural hormone in cows. For simplicity, this chapter uses rBGH. Whatever it is called, the recombinant hormone increases milk production in cows by 10–20%. It proved controversial from the start, and questions about its safety continue to be debated, especially in Canada and Europe. Monsanto developed the bioengineering capacity to create rBGH in the early 1980s, and the company quickly promoted it as a means to increase the efficiency of dairy farming. Although this use might appear to be of great benefit to consumers as well as to farmers, critics soon raised questions about the possibility of adverse effects of the drug on human health, animal welfare, and the economic viability of small dairy farms. Furthermore, consumers would have no choice about whether to buy products resulting from use of the hormone, as milk from cows treated with rBGH (shorthand: rBGH milk) would not be labeled as genetically engineered.[5]

When the FDA approved rBGH as a new animal drug in 1993, available analytical methods could not easily distinguish milk from treated and untreated cows.[6] Because the naturally occurring BGH in cow's milk was indistinguishable from rBGH, the agency ruled that labeling would be misleading because the milks are the same. Monsanto and other biotechnology companies viewed disclosure as a threat to the future of agricultural biotechnology. If rBGH failed in the marketplace, the entire industry might be in jeopardy. The industry extolled rBGH and the equivalent hormone in pigs as "biotechnological miracles that would give consumers more for their money at less cost to the environment," but worried that "ignorance, nostalgia and a Luddite view of technology" would prevent the drugs—but also transgenic foods in general—from reaching the marketplace.[7]

Industry leaders had grounds for concern. By 1989, when Monsanto was testing rBGH on commercial farms in nearly every important dairy state, the drug was already under attack by groups concerned about family farms as well as by those suspicious of any kind of genetic engineering. Several supermarket chains refused to carry milk from rBGH-treated cows, and the owners of Ben & Jerry's announced that they would label ice cream packages with a statement opposing use of the hormone. Before the drug had even been approved for commercial use, the state legislatures of Wisconsin and Minnesota temporarily banned sales of rBGH. By 1992, four major supermarket chains, two large manufacturers of dairy products, and the nation's largest dairy cooperative joined the boycott, as did many small farmers, dairy cooperatives, and grocery chains.[8]

The Safety Issues. Bovine somatotropin stimulates milk production. The hormone, a protein, is always present in cow's milk at low concentrations. Milk from rBGH-treated cows contains both the natural and recombinant hormones. Neither the natural nor the recombinant hormone is likely to affect human health; the cow hormones differ in structure from the human hormone, are not biologically active in humans, and do not promote human growth. Furthermore, like all proteins, cow hormones are largely digested to their constituent amino acids and, therefore, inactivated in the human digestive tract.

In 1990, Monsanto said that its studies had satisfied any doubts about whether rBGH milk is safe for human consumption. That year, FDA scientists reviewed more than 130 studies of the effects of rBGH on cows, rats, and humans and also concluded that the hormone does not affect human health. Critics called this conclusion an unprecedented display

of conflict of interest: FDA scientists had produced a favorable evaluation of evidence in support of a drug not yet approved by their agency.
Others accused the FDA of colluding with Monsanto because agency scientists could not have conducted the review unless the company had disclosed confidential studies that were not available for evaluation by the
general scientific community. A panel of experts recruited by the National
Institutes of Health (NIH), however, concluded that milk from rBGH-
treated cows was essentially the same—and therefore as safe—as milk
from untreated cows. According to one rBGH supporter, the hormone
had been tested on 21,000 cows and described in more than 900 research
papers by 1992 with no indication of harm to human health.[9]

Nevertheless, critics continued to raise doubts about the safety of
rBGH-milk on two grounds: antibiotics and a substance called *insulin-
like growth factor-1* (IGF-1). The concern about antibiotics derives from
observations that cows given rBGH develop more frequent infections of
their udders (mastitis). The more milk cows produce, the more likely they
are to develop mastitis, and rBGH increases milk production. Because
farmers treat the infections with antibiotics that can linger in milk and
meat, eating foods from treated animals might contribute to selection for
antibiotic-resistant bacteria. On this basis, the General Accounting Office (GAO) urged the FDA not to approve rBGH until issues related to
mastitis could be resolved. Federal regulations require the FDA to test for
antibiotic residues in milk, but the agency is able to test for just a small
fraction of animal drugs in common use—just 4 out of 82 in one study—
suggesting a lack of ability to monitor such substances. Because of this
regulatory gap, another federal committee recommended that the FDA
ban rBGH until the antibiotic risks could be evaluated. The Republican
administration in power in 1992, however, was committed to a policy of
industry deregulation, and it ignored the recommendations.[10]

IGF-1 concerns critics for three reasons: (1) rBGH increases levels of
this factor in cow's milk, (2) IGF-1 in cows is chemically identical to human IGF-1, and (3) higher levels of IGF-1 in cow's milk might stimulate
premature growth in human infants or cancer in adults. It is difficult to
evaluate this last contention given the current state of research. Population studies associate high levels of IGF-1 in blood with a higher risk of
prostate cancer in men and breast cancer in premenopausal (but not post-
menopausal) women and, perhaps, with a greater risk of high blood pressure, but these findings do not necessarily have anything to do with drinking milk; high IGF-1 levels could be due to genetic or other dietary causes.[11]
The factor ought to be inactivated during processing and digestion, but

some seems to be absorbed intact. The research gaps have encouraged lingering doubts, demands for reassessment of the safety of rBGH, and lawsuits against the FDA. They also encouraged one anti-rBGH activist, Robert Cohen, to go on a hunger strike in 1999—one of the more extreme forms of protest against foods made with transgenic ingredients.[12]

The Social Issues. Protests about the safety of rBGH obscure an underlying issue—its economic impact. The production of milk in the United States has long exceeded demand, and the government has long subsidized the dairy industry through purchases of surplus milk. Monsanto contends that costs to farmers will decline because fewer cows will produce more milk, and the savings will be passed on to consumers. This last benefit seems doubtful, mainly because dairy prices are tightly linked to federal support programs. If prices fall, levels of taxpayer-supported federal spending would increase to protect farm incomes. Critics also raise concerns about the effects of rBGH on the cows themselves; higher milk production stresses cows and leads to more frequent mastitis and sores at injection sites (an issue of animal rights). Although Monsanto asserts that appropriate veterinary and herd-management practices minimize such problems, farmers report them regularly. The FDA, however, views these complaints as raising no new concerns about animal health.[13]

Use of rBGH also raises questions about effects on rural life. If people drink less milk to avoid rBGH, or if it increases veterinary costs, the drug might contribute to the ongoing attrition of small dairy farms. Jerry Cohen, then an owner of Ben & Jerry's, told the FDA Food Advisory Committee in 1993: "We do know that the use of BGH will increase the supply of milk at a time when we already have a tremendous surplus. It does not make any sense to exacerbate this problem with a product about which there are so many legitimate doubts, a product whose principal beneficiaries will be chemical companies and corporate agribusiness."[14] That the product affects milk itself raises issues. As ethicist Arthur Caplan explained, "Is there any product in the world that has tried harder to sell itself as wholesome and pure than milk? . . . It is a food for innocent, trusting children, culturally laden with symbolism. Any adulteration of milk . . . is seen as taboo."[15] Despite this range of concerns, Monsanto only needed to overcome doubts about the safety of the drug for human health to obtain FDA approval.

Monsanto's Campaign for Approval. Monsanto's efforts to obtain FDA approval for rBGH began as soon as it produced the drug. At the company's request, the FDA permitted distribution of rBGH for limited use on an experimental basis in 1985, and subsequently affirmed the safety of rBGH milk and meat in 1988, 1989, and again in 1990, as did the NIH in 1990 and the Office of Technology Assessment (OTA) in 1991. When the FDA's approval of rBGH as a new animal drug appeared imminent in August 1993, Congress imposed a 90-day moratorium on sales. The U.S. Senate, concerned about the fate of small dairy farms, asked for a moratorium lasting an entire year, but House opposition forced a compromise resulting in the shorter time limit.[16] After lengthy deliberations, advisory committee consultations, and public hearings, the FDA approved rBGH as a new animal drug in November 1993 and ruled that milk produced by cows treated with the hormone would not need to be labeled. In announcing this decision, FDA commissioner Dr. David Kessler stated: "There is virtually no difference in milk from treated and untreated cows. . . . In fact, it's not possible using current scientific techniques to tell them apart. We have looked carefully at every single question raised, and we are confident this product is safe for consumers, for cows and for the environment."[17] The FDA approval applied only to Monsanto's rBGH, although approvals for similar products from other companies seemed sure to follow. Industry representatives hailed the decision as a victory for Monsanto, an indication of reduced regulatory barriers, and a precedent for approving forthcoming products of agricultural biotechnology.

This resounding success was no accident. As early as 1987, business analysts expected rBGH to generate millions of dollars in annual sales. The potential for large returns on investment explains Monsanto's unusually aggressive sales tactics and political actions to promote this otherwise problematic product. Public relations firms working for Monsanto engaged in the usual sorts of lobbying activities in support of rBGH approval but also sent "secret agents and spies" to infiltrate citizen's groups opposed to use of the hormone.[18] As a member of the FDA Food Advisory Committee, I attended hearings on rBGH prior to its approval. The FDA had invited interested companies to provide one witness each. Monsanto sent *nine*, some of them supposedly "independent" witnesses (one was a pregnant dairy farmer from upstate New York) whose connections to the company emerged only when FDA officials required them to declare who paid for their travel to the meeting. The company took full advantage of its connections in government, enlisting an influential former Congressman—to whom the secretary of agriculture owed his appointment—to discourage federal studies of the economic effects of rBGH.[19]

Monsanto wielded other kinds of influence. It withheld consent to publish a peer-reviewed article by independent researchers who used the company's data to measure amounts of white blood cells—an indicator of mastitis—in rBGH milk. Monsanto reserved the right to publish its own data first but delayed doing so for several years; this delay effectively prevented the FDA from considering the independent analysis during the rBGH approval process. Monsanto researchers argued that mastitis white cell counts depend on how much milk is produced, whether or not the cow is treated with rBGH. In contrast, the independent investigators found milk from rBGH-treated cows to contain more white cells, although they could not say whether the higher counts were due to the drug itself or to the higher milk yield. Eventually, they published the results and revealed the dispute.[20]

In another incident, Monsanto lawyers pressured Fox Television to refuse a four-part series on rBGH commissioned by one of its Florida stations from two staff investigative reporters. The station suspended the reporters and did not air the series. The reporters documented sales of rBGH-milk by Florida grocers who had pledged not to sell it, and inadequacies in state screening methods for antibiotics in the treated milk. They also said that Monsanto had offered as much as $2 million to Canadian regulators who were considering approval of rBGH, and had made large gifts to universities whose researchers provided data in support of FDA approval. They established a Web site to describe their side of the story and filed a whistle-blower lawsuit against the television station. The case went to trial in mid-2000; it resulted in a clear win for the reporters. The jury agreed that Fox "acted intentionally and deliberately to falsify or distort the plaintiffs' news reporting on BGH," and awarded a judgment of $425,000 in damages.[21] These incidents were only the most public—and documented—of Monsanto's actions, most of which took place behind closed doors in Congress, at the FDA, and (as rumored) at newspapers planning to run stories on the possible hazards of rBGH.

Monsanto's Campaign against Labeling. Monsanto steadfastly resisted demands for labeling of rBGH milk and recruited dairy industry executives to persuade the FDA to establish favorable labeling guidelines. The company hired two Washington law firms to monitor dairies for advertising and labeling violations and to instigate legal action against milk processors who had "inappropriately" misled customers through labeling practices.[22] The FDA asked the Food Advisory Committee to hear testimony on the labeling issue. A Monsanto official explained the company's position. Because its surveys indicated that 60% of consumers thought that rBGH labeling implied a safety or contamination risk, mandatory labeling would violate the spirit and intent of the labeling laws and would also "diminish the credibility of the food label and would represent a clear step backward from the wonderful progress that has been achieved."[23] Because the FDA seemed already to have decided the issue and the Advisory Committee's role was just that—to advise—critics viewed the hearings as a "public relations smokescreen" and "a regulatory charade."[24]

Some dairy companies, concerned that consumers might not want to buy milk from hormone-treated cows, began labeling their products "BGH-free." Monsanto and its industry supporters objected and asked the FDA to establish guidance "rules" on the labeling of dairy products derived from cows *not* treated with rBGH. In February 1994, the FDA stated that it could not require such labeling, but companies could voluntarily say they were not using rBGH, provided "that any statements made are truthful and not misleading." Although this ruling might sound permissive, the FDA considers "misleading" to apply to any suggestion that untreated milk is superior. Thus, the agency views *BGH-free* as misleading because all milk contains some natural BGH. The term *rBGH-free* also is misleading because the recombinant and natural cow hormones cannot be distinguished. Dairy companies may use such terms only if they provide an explanation of the context: "No significant difference has been shown between milk derived from rBGH-treated and non-rBGH-treated cows."[25]

Vermont, which boasts of its quality dairy products, defied the FDA ruling and passed legislation requiring rBGH milk to be labeled: "Vermonters have the right to know what is in the food they eat. . . . In particular, there is a strong public interest in knowing whether or not rBST has been used in the production of milk and milk products."[26] Industry groups acting on behalf of Monsanto quickly and successfully challenged this law in the courts. When several major milk marketers launched new brands certified as coming from cows that had not been treated with the hormone, Monsanto warned them that their labels "might create the impression that something is wrong with milk from treated cows."[27] By May 1994, Monsanto had sued at least two dairy companies on this basis, a situation that made it appear as if "everyone is terrified of Monsanto. . . . It is quite ominous."[28] In Vermont, only a small fraction of farmers continued to use rBGH. Companies like Ben & Jerry's used their rBGH-free status as a marketing tool, as shown in figure 19: "We oppose recombi-

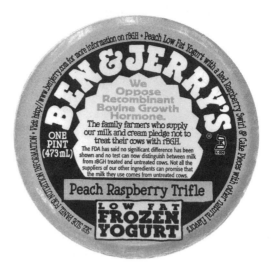

FIGURE 19. Soon after the FDA's approval of
recombinant bovine growth hormone (rBGH),
Ben & Jerry's used product labels to display the
company's policy on this drug. These statements
conform to the FDA's 1994 guidelines on voluntary labeling of milk products derived from
cows that had not been treated with rBGH.

nant bovine growth hormone. The family farmers who supply our milk
and cream pledge not to treat their cows with rBGH."

Monsanto's Revolving Door to the FDA. A nagging concern throughout the deliberations over rBGH was the revolving door through which
employees of Monsanto and FDA exchanged positions. In Washington,
DC, the law firm King & Spalding filed a brief with the FDA on behalf
of Monsanto arguing that the agency could not legally justify a labeling
requirement for rBGH milk. The primary author of the document was
a former FDA chief counsel.[29] Furthermore, three FDA staff members
involved in rBGH regulatory decisions had previously worked for Monsanto, either directly or indirectly. This connection led several members
of Congress to question whether the FDA had colluded with Monsanto
in approving the drug, and they demanded a GAO investigation.[30] The
GAO reviewed more than 40,000 pages of documents, interviewed 54
people, and evaluated the financial disclosures and conflict-of-interest
statements of all FDA employees involved in the rBGH approval. Al-

though the GAO concluded "there were no conflicting financial interests," its report raised discomfiting questions. One FDA employee, Dr. Margaret Miller, worked for Monsanto from 1985 to 1989 as a laboratory supervisor responsible for evaluating tests that measured rBGH and IGF-1 levels in cow blood, tissues, and milk. Within a year or so of leaving Monsanto, she was helping draft FDA responses to citizens' petitions seeking to halt sales of rBGH milk and to congressional queries about rBGH. She also contributed advice on matters directly related to rBGH approval. GAO investigators said she had followed the letter of federal ethics regulations, but expressed some concerns about her adherence to their spirit. They said the FDA commissioner was so "visibly surprised" in 1993 to learn of Dr. Miller's employment with Monsanto that he ordered an internal review of her activities. Although the internal review also concluded that she had not violated ethical standards, it said her participation in rBGH matters "does raise questions."

GAO investigators were even more troubled by issues related to the role of Michael Taylor. Mr. Taylor, whom we encountered in chapter 2 as the courageous USDA official responsible for instituting Pathogen Reduction: HACCP, began his career as a lawyer with the FDA. He left the agency to work for King & Spalding, the firm representing Monsanto, but returned to the FDA in 1991 as deputy commissioner for policy, and he held that position during the time the agency conducted its rBGH safety review. At the time, Mr. Taylor had been with the FDA for more than two years, but newly passed ethical guidelines applied only to the first year of employment, so his activities were "not covered by the appearance of loss of impartiality provisions."[31]

Mr. Taylor is a coauthor of the FDA's 1992 policy statement on genetically engineered plant foods (discussed below), and he signed the *Federal Register* notice on labeling of rBGH milk. Although other FDA officials responsible for those policies shared his views, court documents later released as a result of a 1999 lawsuit revealed considerable disagreement about the policies within the agency. FDA officials told the GAO that Mr. Taylor had recused himself from matters related to rBGH and "never sought to influence the thrust or content" of the agency's policies. Nevertheless, Congressman Bernard Sanders (Ind-VT) viewed Mr. Taylor's involvement as casting doubt about the impartiality of the rBGH review process. Mr. Sanders said the ethics rules in this situation "were often stretched to the breaking point and were broken on a number of occasions. The FDA allowed corporate influence to run rampant in its approval of BGH. . . . This is exactly the kind of thing that sends consumers the message that federal bureaucrats care more about corporate profits than they do about consumer health and safety. . . . The bottom line is that Monsanto's product received favorable treatment when it probably should not have."[32]

Monsanto's Political Success. Monsanto succeeded in obtaining FDA approval of rBGH without a labeling requirement. In March 1995, the company claimed that it had sold 14.5 million doses of rBGH during the previous year and that 13,000 dairy farmers, representing 11% of the potential market, were using the hormone. Sales were especially strong in New York (where 10% of dairy farmers used the drug) and Wisconsin (15%), but were especially weak in Vermont. Although early sales fell short of expectations, Monsanto says that rBGH broke even in 1996, increased sales by 30% in 1997, and has been profitable ever since. As one sympathetic observer explained, "a profit-oriented company like Monsanto wouldn't make that kind of investment for a product that's not successful . . . rBST is saving dairy farming."[33]

USDA economists maintain that the controversy over use of rBGH has had little effect on consumer demand for milk, principally because of lack of evidence of harm.[34] Consumer attitudes toward rBGH milk in the United States are difficult to evaluate, however, not least because of the lack of labeling. Surveys that deliberately probe outrage factors tend to identify substantial concern about the safety of rBGH, especially among people who do not trust the FDA or perceive little benefit from the product. In contrast, industry-sponsored surveys reveal lukewarm opinions on the matter. For example, respondents to a 1994 survey reacted positively, but only slightly so (scoring 6.18 on a scale where 10 is strongly positive), to this reassuring statement: "The National Institutes of Health, the American Medical Association, and several other independent medical groups have found milk from cows that receive BST is unchanged, safe, and nutritionally the same as milk currently on grocery store shelves. Given this information, how acceptable do you find the use of BST?"[35]

Despite such attempts to guide public opinion, surveys demonstrate consistent support for labeling rBGH and all transgenic products. Although the industry demands that the marketplace decide the commercial fate of the hormone, consumers cannot easily make their opinions known if the products are not labeled. One index of underlying public opinion is the spectacular growth in sales of organic ("rBGH-free") milk from $16 million in 1996 to almost $31 million in 1997, a rate of increase substantially higher than that of nearly any other food product.[36] I have heard Monsanto officials say that company scientists developed rBGH because it was technically possible to do so and that they had given no thought to its societal implications. In 1996 I visited the company offices in St. Louis and met Monsanto scientists who had worked on the project. They told me that they believed rBGH would help produce more milk, and more milk would help to alleviate world food shortages. Whatever the motives, once the company committed research funding to rBGH, it needed to recoup the investment, and it appears to have done so. Furthermore, Monsanto's determined effort to achieve approval of rBGH succeeded in a more important respect. Because rBGH raised more safety issues than the transgenic foods that followed, its approval smoothed the way for subsequent FDA actions on herbicide- and Bt-resistant crops. During the time the FDA was responding to pressures to approve rBGH, its staff was also working on policies for approval of transgenic foods.

The Politics of Transgenic Food Plants

Until now, this chapter has examined the politics of a genetically engineered drug, albeit one involved in food production. We now turn to genetically engineered foods themselves. In mid-1992, the FDA issued a policy statement on the regulation of plant foods produced through biotechnology. Figure 20 outlines this policy. As explained by FDA commissioner Dr. David Kessler, the agency developed the policy to be "scientifically and legally sound and . . . adequate to fully protect public health while not inhibiting innovation."[37] He said the policy reflected the prevailing view among senior FDA officials that foods produced through recombinant DNA techniques raised no new safety concerns and therefore could be overseen by applying the agency's existing rules for food additives. In FDA-speak: "In most cases, the substances expected to become components of food as a result of genetic modification of a plant will be the same as or *substantially similar* to substances commonly found in food" (emphasis added). The FDA would only require pre-market review for foods that contained known allergens or toxins or were substantially altered in nutrient content.[38]

The doctrine of *substantial similarity*, or *substantial equivalence* as it later came to be called, meant that the FDA would be taking after-the-fact action to recall products if they caused problems. The agency's safety evaluation would focus on changes in the "objective" characteristics of

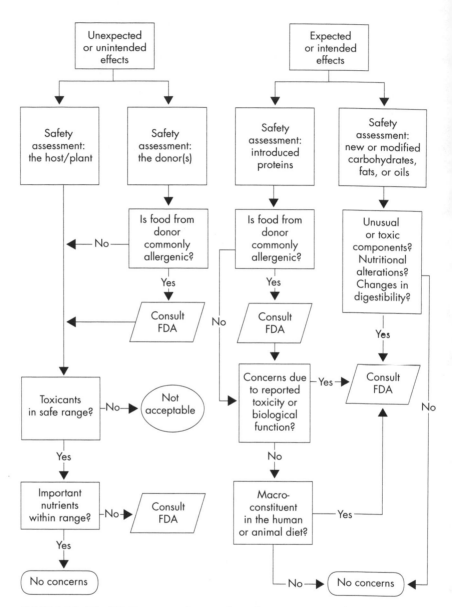

FIGURE 20. The FDA's 1992 policy on the safety assessment of genetically modified plants. Companies did not need to consult FDA unless the transgenic plants contained allergens, toxins, or unusual components, or exhibited significant alterations in nutrient content. (Source: FDA. *Federal Register* 57:22984–23005, May 29, 1992.)

foods—new substances, toxins, allergens, or nutrients—not on the techniques used to produce them. To determine whether transgenic foods raised safety concerns, the FDA would hold private "consultations" with industry. These would be *voluntary*. The agency would require them only when the objective characteristics raised safety questions; otherwise, companies would not need to obtain approval in advance, conduct premarket safety evaluations, or label the foods in any special way. These policies remained in place until 2001, when the FDA required premarket notification.[39]

The food biotechnology industry welcomed these 1992 "efforts by the White House to provide . . . as much regulatory relief as possible," and viewed the policy as "a very strong incentive for investment in the agricultural/food biotechnology area."[40] One investment analyst summarized the FDA's announcement as an "assurance that after all a company's planning for a picnic, the government won't rain on it."[41] Consumer groups, however, criticized the policy as inadequate to protect public safety and threatened mail campaigns and legal challenges. A 1999 lawsuit, for example, obtained 44,000 pages of documents related to the FDA policy. The documents revealed that some FDA scientists had been concerned about the lack of data on safety risks and thought the policy too favorable to the industry. Overall, the (ultimately unsuccessful) lawsuit concluded, "There is more than enough evidence to convince a reasonable man or woman that current FDA policy is unscientific, unwise, irresponsible, and illegal."[42] Other critics attacked the idea of substantial equivalence as a basis for policy. "Substantial equivalence," they said, "is a pseudoscientific concept because it is a commercial and political judgment masquerading as if it were scientific. It is, moreover, inherently antiscientific because it was created primarily to provide an excuse for not requiring biochemical or toxicological tests. It therefore serves to discourage and inhibit potentially informative scientific research."[43]

In the meantime, critics seized on the lack of labeling as a cause for action. Celebrity chefs in New York City called for a boycott of genetically engineered foods. The chef leading the boycott, Rick Moonen (then at Oceana, New York City), explained to the press: "As a chef, I am responsible for every plate of food in my restaurant. . . . The consumers put their dietetic, religious and allergic confidences in my hands, and with no requirements for safety testing, I am not permitted to fulfill my obligations. But what is most disturbing to me is the idea of selling the food without a label."[44]

Some commentators understood that the no-labeling policy of "least

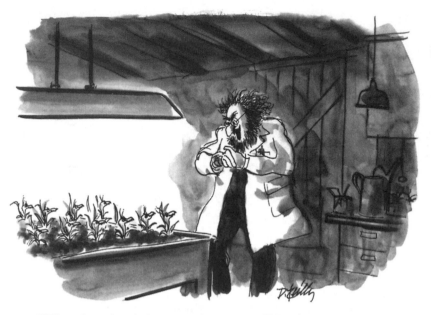

"There's splendid news from the F.D.A., my pretties!"

FIGURE 21. The FDA's relaxed regulatory stance on genetically modified foods elicited this response from *New Yorker* cartoonist Donald Reilly. (© The New Yorker Collection 1992 Donald Reilly from cartoonbank.com. All rights reserved.)

regulatory resistance" would increase public suspicion of genetically engineered foods, especially since press accounts had begun referring to them as *Frankenfoods,* and cartoonists were taking full advantage of this satirical opportunity. Figure 21 gives one such example. To allay public fears, a federal study recommended a formal review of the entire federal regulatory framework for food biotechnology in order to establish a more equitable balance between promotion of the industry and protection of the public, but no such review took place. The FDA went forward with the policy and by the end of 1995 had approved the marketing of tomatoes genetically engineered to reach optimal ripening after they were picked; squash resistant to viruses; potatoes and corn resistant to insects; and cotton, corn, and soybeans resistant to herbicides. By mid-2001, the FDA had accomplished 52 consultations on these and other genetically modified food plants, meaning that they could now be marketed.[45] The first of these consultations began in 1991 and concluded in 1994. Because it established the precedent for approval of subsequent foods, we now examine the politics of Calgene's delayed ripening tomato, the "Flavr Savr," and the fate of transgenic tomatoes in the United States and Great Britain.

The Politics of Transgenic Tomatoes, Labeled

To biotechnology companies looking for commercially viable projects, tomatoes are a good investment. Americans expect tomatoes to be readily available, regardless of season. In the early 1990s, American farmers were producing more than 13 pounds (5.9 kilograms) per capita of fresh tomatoes and another 75 pounds (34 kilograms) for processing; the market for fresh tomatoes was worth $3–5 billion annually, and that for processed tomatoes even more. Most supermarket tomatoes are bred for disease resistance, appearance, and durability rather than taste, are picked when green, and are the bane of consumers longing for "backyard" flavor and freshness. Tomatoes taste better when they are picked ripe. They also have a higher content of solids—sugars and starches—that make them more economical to process into tomato paste and sauce.[46] For these reasons, several biotechnology companies were working on tomato projects.

Calgene's Flavr Savr. Beginning in the mid-1980s, Calgene, a California-based biotechnology company, invested $25 million and eight years of effort to alter the gene in tomatoes that causes softening. They constructed the tomato to contain its own gene, but with the DNA in reverse order. This manipulation slowed the gene's action, delayed ripening, and allowed the tomato to be picked at a more mature stage of ripeness and taste. Calgene expected its trademarked "MacGregor's tomatoes, grown from Flavr Savr seeds," to capture at least 15% of the market as soon as they became available. The company's initial marketing strategy differed from Monsanto's approach to rBGH milk; it was utterly transparent. Calgene *labeled* the tomatoes as genetically engineered: "Thank you for buying MacGregor's tomatoes. . . . Since 1982, the MacGregor's team of hard-working professional men and women has successfully applied the latest developments in genetic engineering, tomato plant breeding, and farming to solve an age old problem—how to supply an abundance of great-tasting tomatoes all year round." Figure 22 depicts the tomato-shaped package insert containing these statements.

Calgene's strategy differed from Monsanto's in another respect. In 1989, it *voluntarily* sought FDA guidance on the regulatory status of this first

FIGURE 22. A 1992 press kit for Calgene's genetically modified Flavr Savr tomatoes (neither approved nor marketed at that time) contained this proposed package label. The label not only disclosed the genetic modification but also explained its key elements: a reversed gene for softening and an antibiotic-resistance marker. The FDA approved the tomatoes in 1994, but Calgene never mass-marketed them.

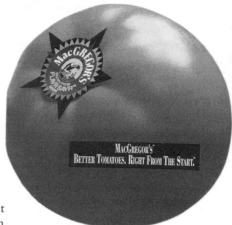

transgenic food, long before it was ready to market. The company's motivation was quite explicit: public relations. If the FDA approved the tomato, consumers would believe it safe to eat. The ensuing ordeal lasted nearly four years. A former Calgene scientist, Dr. Belinda Martineau, recounts these events in her lively 2001 book, *First Fruit*. The FDA, she says, "put Calgene through the wringer" in what turned out to be "a long, hard, even painful process."[47] The wringing began in 1991 with a consultation with FDA about whether the Flavr Savr would be subject to the same regulations as conventional tomatoes. The answer: not exactly. Instead, the FDA asked Calgene to provide extensive information about the tomato's safety and nutrient content. The company published a book in response to this request in 1992. Calgene then asked the FDA for a ruling on whether its scientists could use the gene for resistance to the antibiotic kanamycin (neomycin) as a selection marker, and petitioned for approval of the kanamycin-resistant gene as a food additive. While the FDA was dealing with these requests and asking for more data, the company did some public relations and lobbying. It convinced the Biotechnology Industry Organization, then a trade association of mostly pharmaceutical biotechnology companies, to represent the interests of agricultural biotechnology companies as well. Calgene officials met with high-ranking political leaders at the White House and provided members of Congress with bacon, lettuce, and Flavr Savr sandwiches. They also supplied tomatoes for press tastings and industry-sponsored events.[48] I ate Flavr Savr tomatoes for lunch at a 1994 biotechnology industry meeting in New York City. I thought they tasted like *tomatoes,* better than supermarket varieties but not nearly as good as those available at farmers' markets in August.

The FDA review process went slowly because the science was in its infancy and Calgene researchers had to scramble to respond to the agency's requests. Dr. Martineau's book describes the haste with which Calgene scientists conducted the research. Eventually, the FDA ran out of issues for which it could demand evidence and asked the Food Advisory Committee to review the Calgene materials. I was a member of the committee during that review. We had no obvious reason to think the Flavr Savr unsafe. The tomato contained its own gene and seemed more innocuous than rBGH. The use of the antibiotic-resistance marker gene was the one issue debated. Nevertheless, some of us were troubled by the FDA's insistence that our discussion focus exclusively on safety questions. We were prohibited from raising any other issues—the effect that transgenic tomatoes might have on local tomato growers, for example. The benefit of the tomatoes to consumers seemed to be a taste only marginally better than that of standard supermarket varieties. Furthermore, the Flavr Savr would be expensive—two or three times the price of conventional tomatoes—and the higher cost identified it as a luxury product targeted to an upscale market. Such factors, and whether anyone needed such a tomato, were not open to consideration.

The FDA approved the tomato in May 1994, a decision enthusiastically applauded by the agricultural biotechnology industry. Some consumer groups observed that the FDA's review had been an anomaly because Calgene had volunteered for it and companies were not required to produce safety data. Some antibiotechnology groups such as the Pure Food Campaign led by Jeremy Rifkin, threatened picket lines, tomato dumpings, boycotts, and legal challenges. Mr. Rifkin said, "Calgene has miscalculated in the most profound way. It spent an enormous amount of money and it never asked the simplest question: Do people want this tomato? And I say people don't want this tomato. The bottom line is, who needs it?"[49] Despite such objections, I thought people would buy the tomato if they perceived the improved taste to be worth the increased cost. Within days after the FDA approval, Calgene began test marketing the tomatoes in California and Illinois—priced competitively. By all reports the first Flavr Savr tomatoes flew off the shelves.

It soon became evident that problems other than pricing would determine the Flavr Savr's success. The company developed the tomatoes in California but grew them in Florida, where they did not easily adapt to local climate, pest, or commercial contracting conditions. During transportation, the tomatoes turned to mush. Calgene was unable to solve these problems and gave up on the product. Despite the marketing disaster, the tomato produced commercial benefits. FDA approval of the relatively benign Flavr Savr paved the way for subsequent approvals of Calgene's seed oils, herbicide-resistant cotton, and other transgenic foods. Calgene hoped that these products might prove profitable and help overcome its reported losses of more than $80 million; it continued to report losses through 1994. In 1995, Monsanto bought nearly half the company and owned all of it by 1997.[50] The Flavr Savr gamble made it easier for other companies to obtain FDA approvals for their products, and the entire industry owed Calgene a debt of gratitude. Although the FDA subsequently approved transgenic tomatoes produced by other companies, no such varieties were available fresh in supermarkets late in 2002.

GM Tomato Paste. During the FDA committee review, I was surprised by Calgene's determination to grow fresh tomatoes for sale in supermarkets—no matter how upscale—because processed tomatoes seemed to be a more secure business opportunity. People eat more processed tomatoes than fresh (on pizza, for example), and the higher content of solids in transgenic tomatoes meant that turning them into sauce and paste would be more efficient and less costly. European biotechnology companies that were genetically engineering their own tomatoes understood that such price advantages could be passed along to consumers. In the halcyon preprotest days of 1996, the British company Zeneca, which had obtained FDA approval for transgenic tomatoes the previous year, began to use them in tomato paste. The British grocery chain Sainsbury sold the paste with the prominent label shown in figure 23: MADE WITH GENETICALLY MODIFIED TOMATOES. Sainsbury and other retailers knew their customers. Before putting the labeled paste on its supermarket shelves in January 1998, Safeway, for example, spent 15 months consulting with consumer groups, conducting focus-group research, and preparing advertising materials. Its promotional materials, like those for Calgene's Flavr Savr, reflected the company's certainty that consumers would accept the product.

> Scientists have now identified the gene that makes tomatoes turn soft during ripening, and they've also found a way of switching the gene off. This means that the tomatoes can be left to ripen on the plant until they have their full flavour and colour. . . . [They] remain firm after harvesting . . . with reduced wastage. As less tomatoes go to waste, best use is made of water, a scarce commodity in California where the tomatoes are grown. In

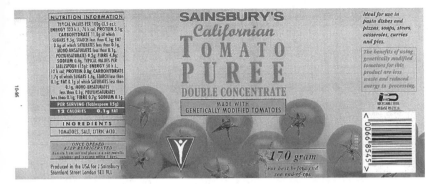

FIGURE 23. British grocery chains sold genetically modified tomato paste labeled as such in 1998. As public opposition to such foods increased, retailers instituted GM-free policies and refused to stock products made with transgenic ingredients.

addition, as the tomatoes contain less water, less energy is used during processing. Together, these improvements mean that Safeway's tomato puree, made from genetically modified tomatoes, is available at a reduced price.[51]

By mid-1998, Sainsbury's had sold about 1 million units of the tomato paste, and a spokesman for Safeway said that it and Sainsbury's "are adamant that their clearly labelled GM tomato purees have consistently out-performed the non-GM alternative." He also said that 99% of people who bought the "GM" puree were aware of its origins.[52] This last figure hardly seems credible, even for the British population, especially because one result of the publicity generated by Dr. Pusztai's potato lectin research (discussed in chapter 6) was to surprise the public with the revelation that supermarkets were full of genetically modified foods.

The furor over that revelation and the subsequent events in the Pusztai affair led to consumer protests and a drop in sales of the transgenic paste. Retailers had plenty of other foods to sell and saw little reason to defend controversial items. Seven supermarket chains, Sainsbury's among them, announced that they no longer intended to sell genetically modified foods, and planned to take "reasonable steps" to ensure that the products did not contain such ingredients.[53] In this instance, the political implications of a safety issue caused a successful and cheaper product to be removed from the market. In the next chapter, we will examine how antibiotechnology advocates accomplished such GM-free policies. In the meantime, let's leave the science-based approach of the

FDA and consider a particularly political aspect of the EPA's regulatory approach: how one of its regulatory targets, *plant-pesticides,* instead came to be called by a euphemism, *plant-incorporated protectants.*

THE EPA'S EUPHEMISM-BASED APPROACH

The FDA is not the only agency that has to deal with questions of labeling; the EPA has its own set of labeling problems related to transgenic foods. The Coordinated Framework makes the USDA and the EPA the primary agencies for deciding whether transgenic plants are safe to grow in fields. Under the framework's curious division of responsibility, the USDA regulates herbicide-resistant *plants* such as those that are Roundup Ready, but the EPA regulates *pesticides* and, therefore, Roundup itself. The laws that govern EPA actions are designed to deal with the safety of such chemical pesticides. Under those laws, the EPA requires pesticide makers to obtain permits—"registrations"—before releasing the chemicals into the environment. Registrations require safety evaluations.

At issue was what to do about the *Bt* toxin. The toxin is a pesticide, but it is genetically engineered into plant tissues. In 1994, as part of its response to the Coordinated Framework, the EPA proposed to apply the laws governing chemical pesticides to transgenic crop plants containing *Bt* and other such toxins and, by analogy, call them *plant-pesticides.* This expanded definition made sense, according to the agency, because the large-scale application of *Bt* crops "could result in new or unique exposures of nontarget organisms, including humans."[54] As we have seen, however, the primary concerns about transgenic crops containing such toxins are about what they might do to the environment: displace existing crops, create resistant weeds, disrupt ecosystems, reduce crop diversity, or, as the most emotionally charged of such problems, kill monarch butterflies. Furthermore, widespread plantings of transgenic *Bt* crops might undermine the use of this toxin in organic agriculture. Organic growers use *Bt* as a temporary spray that washes off in the rain. The permanent integration of the transgenic *Bt* toxin into widely planted crops could spread the *Bt* trait by pollinating related weeds or organically grown crops and promote *Bt*-resistance in insect pests.[55]

To monitor such possibilities, the EPA proposed that developers of transgenic plants register them in the same way as conventional pesticides; evaluate their environmental fate, ecological impact, effects on human health, and potential for inducing resistance; and label them as plant-pesticides. Despite EPA's assurance that the rules would help companies resolve regulatory uncertainties, inspire confidence, and attract investors, most segments of the industry were not pleased. Some industry groups objected that complying with these regulations would cost companies from $60,000 to $1 million per product. Others called the proposals anachronistic, burdensome, and unnecessary, and said such rules would "exert a profoundly negative effect on agricultural research and on the commercialization of biological pest management strategies." In 1996, a coalition of 11 professional societies told Congress that the EPA policy was "scientifically indefensible" because it did not require conventional vegetables to undergo such scrutiny, although many contain naturally occurring chemicals that inhibit pests. Still others called the policy an approach to regulation that "flies in the face of everything science has taught us about risk and the scientific basis of plant genetics." The biotechnology industry's position on the proposed rules was nowhere near unanimous, however, as some of the larger companies *favored* the regulations because they were likely to force smaller competitors out of business. On this basis, a spokeswoman for the Institute of Food Technologists said, "It is not in the public's interest to concentrate all of this research in a few multinational companies. . . . We want to keep the playing field level for all participants." Environmental groups, although "pleased that EPA plans to regulate such crops the way it regulates traditional chemical pesticides," thought the rules inadequately focused on the overuse of chemical herbicides and too generous with exemptions.[56]

While these debates continued, the EPA operated as if the rules were in place but refrained from issuing final regulations. In 1999, the Biotechnology Industry Organization (BIO) challenged the EPA's use of "plant-pesticides" as a designation. This term, it argued, could reduce confidence in the safety of the crops because "pesticide" connotes "kill." Instead, BIO argued, the EPA should encourage consumer acceptance of transgenic crops by labeling them "plant-expressed protectants." Agency officials agreed to consider this demand.[57] Two years later, just prior to renewing the registrations of several varieties of *Bt* corn, the EPA dealt with the question of what to call such crops.

The *Federal Register* notice on this burning question takes up 46 pages of fine print. Parts of it are wonderfully academic and professorial, as respondents to the request for public comment paid close attention to the precise meanings of words. Some, for example, argued that "plant-pesticide" is inappropriate and inaccurate because it means "pest killer," and this meaning is wrong because genetic modifications do not kill pests but, instead, make the plants undesirable to pests or invulnerable to attack. Furthermore, plants labeled as pesticides "might be poorly received by the public, and the public perception of a promising branch of science could be tarnished." Others asked why the agency would attempt to fix something that was not broken; if the EPA changed the name "plant-pesticide" to "a more euphemistic name to satisfy one interest group, other interest groups will soon be urging it to change the names of other types of pesticide products to have better marketing potential." Others suggested alternatives such as "Frankenplants," "Pandora pesticides," or "alien pesticides." Still others contended that use of *plant-expressed protectants* "obscures the legal issues and attempts to mislead the public into believing that these pesticides are not pesticides at all." The EPA's explanation of the reasons for its eventual decision to choose "plant-incorporated protectants" is worthy of an advanced college text in postmodern English:

> EPA believes the adjective "plant-incorporated" more accurately conveys the sense that these pesticides are produced and used in the plant. EPA will therefore utilize this adjective in concert with the term "protectant" to describe this type of pesticide. EPA chose the adjective "plant-incorporated" rather than the adjective "plant-expressed," because the word "expressed" represents a technical term of art, and in this instance it appeared preferable to use the term "incorporated" which also encompasses a meaning found in the common English dictionary . . . i.e., "joined or combined into a single unit or whole." The term "plant-incorporated" may thus be better understood by the general public than the term "plant-expressed.[58]

With this euphemism firmly in place, the EPA could conclude its evaluation of the health and environmental risks of five types of *Bt* corn and renew their registrations for seven years. During these years, companies would have to collect data to demonstrate that these corn varieties did not lead to insect resistance or unexpected health or environmental consequences. The renewed registrations did not include StarLink corn.[59]

This example is not the only time that EPA has altered the use of terms in response to the political goals of industry. EPA registers pesticides in four categories based on their level of toxicity. All carry warning labels—or used to. Late in 2001, the agency agreed that makers of pesticides registered in the least toxic category did not need to place the word *caution* on their labels. The public, said officials, had difficulty understanding the hierarchy of warnings about regulated pesticides, which ranged from "caution" at the low end to "poison" (accompanied by a skull and crossbones) at the high end. The agency was unable to think of a milder word than "caution," so it chose to use nothing at all.[60]

Such examples may seem trivial—humans are not much affected by the *Bt* toxin and the least toxic pesticides are, by definition, not very toxic—but they indicate the degree to which federal agencies respond to the commercial and political concerns of the regulated industries rather than to the health or safety concerns of the public. They also reveal the lack of transparency—the openness of federal processes to public scrutiny and debate—in decision-making processes that affect this industry. Overall, they raise serious questions about inequities in the political process and the effects of such inequities on democratic institutions. The inequitable distribution of political power illustrated here is at the root of public distrust of genetically engineered foods, as we will see in the next chapter.

CHAPTER 8

THE POLITICS OF
CONSUMER CONCERN
DISTRUST, DREAD, AND OUTRAGE

WE HAVE SEEN HOW SCIENTISTS AND FOOD BIOTECHNOLOGY COM-
panies promote transgenic projects by focusing on technical achievements,
safety, and visions of improving the world's food supply, as expressed by
the often repeated phrase "biotechnology—and only biotechnology—can
help the world produce the food necessary to meet the population needs
of the 21st century." This statement, however, immediately raises credibility issues. Can biotechnology really solve world food problems? What
is the industry doing now to address such problems? Are there other methods—perhaps less technical—for solving them?

Food biotechnology first developed bovine growth hormone, *Bt* corn,
and Roundup Ready soybeans, all possessing *agronomic* traits designed
to help food producers. The industry also worked on *processing* traits,
such as insertion of the reversed gene for ripening into tomatoes. More
recently, the industry began developing foods with *quality attributes* (such
as nutrient content) that might benefit consumers directly. Until such
foods become available, the public has little to gain from genetically modified foods—in price, nutritional benefit, or convenience. Evidence for
benefits to the environment or to people in developing countries is also
uncertain. In this situation, any risk—no matter how remote—seems
pointless, especially when food biotechnology raises so many other issues of concern.

This chapter examines the politics of consumer concerns about genetically modified foods, particularly as focused on issues that extend beyond safety and most inspire distrust: labeling, "biopiracy," genetic "pollution," and globalization. These are "outrage" issues. They emerged in

response to the industry's conduct of business in its own interests and the government's collusion in promoting those interests. They are connected to "dread" issues of human and environmental *safety,* but in complicated ways. When people object to food biotechnology by focusing on safety issues, they often do so because they have no other choice. Scientists, federal regulators, and biotechnology companies dismiss outrage considerations out of hand and only permit debate about safety issues. Safety is, as we have seen, a matter of interpretation, highly political, and difficult to separate from the "who decides" factors listed in table 2 (page 17).

In part, the passion that underlies arguments about the safety of genetically modified foods derives from the lack of opportunity to debate their politics and their implications for society. What, for example, does it mean for us as a democratic society that more than half the foods on supermarket shelves contain genetically modified ingredients, but their presence is not labeled? Perhaps it makes no difference whatsoever, but without a formal venue for discussing such questions, people concerned about democratic values will focus on safety questions and use them to generate outrage. This chapter examines the societal issues that underlie public distrust and the reasons why they need to be included in dialogue, if not consensus, about the future of food biotechnology.

THE POLITICS OF DISTRUST

We have seen that the narrowing of debate about food biotechnology to questions of safety has produced two unanticipated effects. The first is to induce outrage. When scientists and companies say, as they often do, "All we have to do to gain public support for food biotechnology is to educate the public that our products are safe," they frustrate anyone who cares about democracy in decision making. Such statements miss a key point: other issues also matter. A second effect, ironically, is to force the debate to focus on a greater range of safety issues, none of them easily resolved. Advocates say: You refuse to hear my concerns about the effects of food biotechnology on rural life, access to seeds, or corporate control of the food supply? Fine, let's talk about *safety.* Let's look at unintended consequences, toxins, allergens, superweeds, *Bt* resistance, antibiotic resistance, and effects on monarch butterflies and (as discussed below) on native corn growing in Mexico. Although most scientists might dismiss such hazards as remote or of little consequence, they cannot prove the concerns insignificant. Just enough evidence exists to fuel ongoing debate and discredit any scientist or regulator who categorically states that genetically modified foods are safe. Safety matters, but so do the other issues to which we now turn.

Labeling: Transparency in Marketing

Labeling continues to be a political issue rather than a simple matter of consumer information, largely because the industry opposes it so strongly and the government supports the industry's position. The public consistently demands disclosure, but the Food and Drug Administration (FDA) insists that labels would be *misleading*. The agency's logic: labels would erroneously imply that genetically modified foods differ from conventional foods and that conventional foods are in some way superior. Although the FDA justifies this position as science based, the policy is clearly political: "Don't ask, don't tell."[1] Whether genetically modified foods differ from conventional foods depends on how one views the construction methods. Based on a review of the steps needed to construct Golden Rice, for example, it is quite possible to make the opposite argument: the foods significantly differ (see tables on pages 158 and 280). Whether labeling implies inferiority also is debatable. If genetically modified foods offer significant advantages, why not flaunt them? Calgene intended to advertise its transgenic tomato as *superior,* and British supermarkets had no problem selling products prominently labeled as genetically modified (pages 212 and 215). Alternatively, if the foods offer no advantages to consumers, the issue boils down to one of choice at the marketplace. Overall, the lack of labeling suggests that something about transgenic foods is best hidden.

The industry tries hard to prove that the public does not really care about disclosure, but independent surveys almost always report substantial support for labeling. Survey results depend on who asks the questions and how they are worded. In May 2001, for example, 62% of respondents said *agree* in response to a question asked this way: Tell me if you agree, disagree, or if you don't know whether information about genetic modification should be required on food labels.[2] In contrast, here is an industry-sponsored question: "The U.S. Food and Drug Administration (FDA) requires special labeling when a food is produced under certain conditions: when biotechnology's use introduces an allergen or when it substantially changes the food's nutritional content, like vitamins or fat, or its composition. Otherwise, special labeling is not required. Would you say you support or oppose this policy of FDA?" Only 27% answered *oppose*.[3]

Regardless of survey results, the makers of transgenic foods are convinced that labeling would have a chilling effect on sales. Unlike vitamin-enriched or organic foods, transgenic foods offer no obvious benefit, and the demise of the British tomato paste reinforced industry fears. Nevertheless, in July 1999 federal officials met with scientific, industry, and advocacy groups to reconsider whether genetically modified foods should be labeled. Commentators interpreted this move as a shift in policy toward regulations based less on science and more on the "dreaded social, political, and economic criteria." Soon after, "a battered Clinton administration" announced hearings for late 1999, suggesting that the FDA might admit its policy failure in this area and develop labeling rules for transgenic foods.[4]

This FDA action also reflected politics: Congress was getting involved in this area. In November 1999, 21 members of Congress, led by Representative Dennis Kucinich (Dem-OH), introduced legislation to require labeling of genetically modified foods. Their rationale for the Genetically Engineered Food Right to Know Act directly contradicted the position taken by the FDA. The bill assumed that because genetic engineering *does* change foods in significant ways (in regulatory terms, produces a *material* change), "federal agencies have failed to uphold Congressional intent by allowing genetically engineered foods to be marketed, sold and otherwise used without labeling that reveals material facts to the public."[5] If passed, the bill would have required all foods containing genetically modified ingredients to be labeled as indicated in figure 24. The label would not apply to drugs; to restaurants, bakeries, or other establishments preparing food for immediate consumption; or to organic crops inadvertently contaminated by nearby transgenic crops. Congressional support, though growing, was insufficient to pass the bill by the end of 2002.

Although the bill's initial supporters included at least three Republicans, the response was predictable: overwhelming opposition from the food industry and its supporters in the Republican-controlled House of Representatives. Food trade groups objected that the warning was unnecessary, unscientific, confusing to the public, and too big to put on labels. A representative of the National Food Processors Association said that the bill placed "Politics ahead of sound science. . . . [Kucinich] apparently believes that Congress—rather than the FDA, the scientific community or the public—is best equipped to address food biotechnology and consumer concerns. . . . Laws and regulations should be based on the best science available, rather than on political pressure from activists opposed to the use of

FIGURE 24. The Genetically Engineered Food Right to Know Act of 1999, introduced by Representative Dennis J. Kucinich (Dem-OH), required this label on packages of foods made from genetically modified ingredients. The bill did not pass.

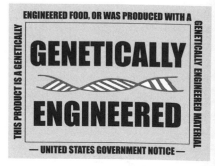

this technology."[6] In contrast, at least 18 consumer and industry groups announced support of the legislation; these included the American Corn Growers Association and the National Farmers Organization, both of which represented producers hurt by the refusal of European countries to buy their commingled conventional and transgenic crops.

In preparing for the 1999 hearings, the FDA was forced to deal with societal questions it had ignored in its 1992 policy. Did the policy best serve the public? Was additional information needed? Who should be responsible for communicating such information, and how should it be made available?[7] As an invited speaker to the first of the hearings, I thought they might indicate a breakthrough in FDA policy. I had heard FDA officials refer to labeling as the "L-word." Labeling caused them no end of trouble, much of it brought on by their resistance to dealing with societal considerations. I thought the FDA needed to approve labeling for three reasons: public demand, the threat of Congressional intervention, and the inability of the industry to overcome public distrust without it. The FDA argued that writing labeling rules would be difficult, as agency staff would have to establish thresholds and deal with foods with multiple ingredients. This objection seems spurious, however, as plenty of FDA officials know how to write *Federal Register* notices. Objections that genetic modification is not *material* also seem weak. The FDA already allowed label statements for production processes: made from concentrate, previously frozen, organically grown, kosher, and irradiated, for example.

In a move that seemed precedent breaking, the FDA conducted focus groups to assess consumer opinions about the labeling issue. To the agency's apparent surprise, practically all of the participants wanted labels to say whether foods were produced through genetic engineering. The FDA report on the focus groups said, "What is striking about participants' initial discussion of their reasons for wanting biotechnology labeling is the widespread perception that the information they want the label to provide is how the food product was produced, rather than the compositional effect of the process on the food product."[8] It is understandable that the FDA found the results "striking"; the agency had already decided otherwise. While the focus groups were in progress in May 2000, the FDA proposed a plan to require premarket notification for transgenic foods but to make labeling *voluntary*. FDA Commissioner Jane Henney said this plan would "show that all bioengineered foods sold here in the United States today are as safe as their non-bioengineered counterparts" and "will provide the public with continued confidence in the safety of these foods."[9] Six months later, after wading through 35,000 public comments on the matter, her agency issued still-interim rules for voluntary labeling. These led the *New York Times* to begin its account with, "Seeking to calm public anxiety . . ." and to quote Commissioner Henney: "What any product doesn't need is for there to be suspicion on the behalf of consumers that something is being slipped by them." Because the revised rules made labeling voluntary and retained restrictions on use of the term *GM-free*, consumer groups called them "purely public relations."[10] The FDA's subsequent warnings to companies to stop using "GM-free" labels or to states seeking to enact GM-label laws, also did not reassure consumer groups that the agency was acting in the public interest.[11]

What seems most surprising is how much the industry's unyielding opposition to labeling damages its own cause. If public trust is the key to successful marketing, biotechnology companies should freely disclose their methods, economic goals, and products. This idea cannot be news to the industry. In 1992, I was not alone in saying, "The labeling issue is really this simple: consumers are more likely to buy the food products of biotechnology if they think the foods are worth the price and if they trust the producer. Trust requires disclosure. . . . All the evidence suggests that consumers will welcome superior products—those that are cheaper, taste better, and have better nutritional value—no matter how they were produced."[12] This advice made sense at the time. Industry leaders ignored it because they chose to blame public resistance on scientific ignorance; if people knew the foods were safe, they would buy them. Labels might suggest that the foods were *not* safe. Later events proved the error of this view. People bought the genetically modified tomatoes because they thought they tasted better or were priced competitively. Public views of biotechnology in the United States then depended on perceived benefits and, as such, were logical, consistent, and predictable.

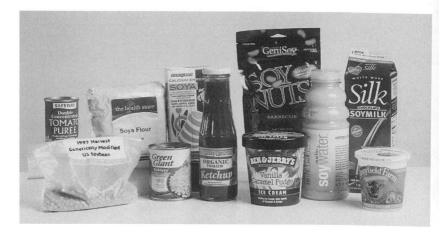

FIGURE 25. These foods bear labels designating their GM status. Those on the left are British or Irish products explicitly labeled either as genetically modified or as "GM-free." The labels of the American products on the right, all purchased in 2000, state that they do not contain genetically modified ingredients. (Photo by Shimon and Tammar Rothstein, 2000.)

An alternative possibility is to decide the risks and benefits of each new food on a case-by-case basis and allow the marketplace to determine success or failure—as it does for other consumer goods. Under this approach, labeling is essential. If the foods are worth buying, labeling should *encourage* purchase (as Calgene thought it might do for the tomato). Whether the industry's unwillingness to subject transgenic foods to marketplace forces was due to fear of rejection, arrogance, or stupidity may never be known, but this position led to results that were hardly in its best interest: public erosion of confidence, questioning of the value of *any* genetic modification of food, demands that government regulations address the societal—as well as safety—implications of the technology, and a steady increase in the labeling of foods as "GM-free." By 2000, as shown in figure 25, many food products in Great Britain and the United States bore labels indicating whether or not they were genetically modified.

Intellectual Property Rights

When biotechnology companies patent the processes for creating transgenic foods, they demonstrate that they are motivated more by interests of economic self-protection than by concerns about feeding the world. Patented transgenic foods cannot be grown without a license and, therefore, require a fee. United States intellectual property laws permit patent owners to exclude anyone else from making, using, or selling protected aspects of transgenic plants for 20 years. The roots of current patent coverage date back to 1930 when the U.S. Patent Office granted limited intellectual property rights to plants propagated through methods that did not involve pollen. In 1970, Congress extended the rights to plants developed through traditional methods of pollination and cross-fertilization. Later, the Supreme Court granted full patent rights to microbes developed through recombinant techniques; the first was patented in 1980. The Patent Office extended full protection to transgenic plants in 1985 and to transgenic animals in 1988.[13] Companies viewed these extensions as an incentive to develop new products. By 1995, the Patent Office had issued 112 patents for genetically engineered plants.

Patents elicit public distrust of the food biotechnology industry for the six distinct reasons discussed next: ownership, enforcement, injustice, "biopiracy," animal rights, and "terminator" technology.

Ownership. Control of the "discoveries" of genetic engineering creates distrust because of the extraordinary breadth of some of the patents. One, for example, grants exclusive rights to all forms of bioengineered cotton; another covers all uses of reverse genes such as those used to create the Calgene tomato; yet another gives Monsanto exclusive rights to methods using certain antibiotic-resistance markers. Competitors of the companies holding such patents find their scope stunning, "as if the inventor of the assembly line had won property rights to all mass-produced goods," or "as if Monsanto had just patented the yellow pages as a method for finding a telephone number."[14] Such concerns are quite justifiable. For example, just four companies control 65% of the patents owned by the top 30 companies working on transgenic seeds: Pharmacia (which, in 2002, owned Monsanto, Calgene, and other agricultural biotechnology companies), DuPont (Pioneer Hi-Bred), Syngenta (Zeneca, Novartis, and others), and Dow Chemical (Mycogen). Monsanto, for example, alone owns more than 100 patents for the processes used to construct transgenic corn and soybeans.

Enforcement. The aggressive tactics used by biotechnology companies to protect their patent rights cannot help but elicit distrust. To pick just one example: Monsanto added a $5 technology fee to each bag of Roundup Ready soybeans when the seeds became available in 1996. The company required farmers to pledge never to harvest the seeds, and to permit its agents to inspect the fields for three years. It used crop consultants and independent investigators as informants, and pursued more than 200 "plant piracy" cases in the courts. A spokeswoman explained, "Monsanto has invested a lot of money . . . and we will protect that investment."[15]

Injustice. Questions of justice cause distrust of genetically engineered foods because of court decisions that consistently favor the patent rights of food biotechnology companies. Biotechnology patents rank second only to software patents in generating lawsuits. In a case considered critical to the continued economic viability of the industry, an Iowa seed company challenged patent protection as monopolistic and contrary to Congressional intent. The company, Farm Advantage, purchased 600 bags of Pioneer Hi-Bred corn seed from a third company for about $54,000 and resold the seeds to customers. In 1999, Pioneer Hi-Bred sued Farm Advantage for violating its exclusive patent rights. The Farm Advantage attorney asked the court to dismiss the case. In 2001, the Supreme Court ruled in favor of Pioneer, a decision seen as a victory for companies holding patents on transgenic processes.[16] A spokeswoman for Monsanto explained that the court "clearly wanted to protect the rights of investors."[17]

Biopiracy. This is the pejorative term applied to the private appropriation of public biological resources, particularly the patenting of indigenous plants for corporate profit at the expense of poor farmers in developing countries.[18] For example, a Texas company obtained a patent for several lines of basmati rice, a staple grain consumed in India for millennia and an important source of income for that country. India requested a reexamination of the patent. Although protests eventually induced the Patent Office to refuse most of the company's claims, the initial approval lent credence to the idea that U.S. companies were stealing native plants from developing countries. When Monsanto's patents on transgenic soybeans raised similar alarms in China, the company said farmers in that country could use the technology without restriction. But why, ask critics, "should someone be entitled to transfer a resource from the public domain to the private domain?"[19] Patenting is unquestionably political; its ostensible purpose is to promote useful inventions that benefit society. If so, according to one academic expert,

It is reasonable to question the extent to which plant and animal patents are likely to benefit society as a whole, particularly in an era when the Western patent system is being imposed internationally against the wishes of numerous countries. . . . If, on the other hand, the protection of the natural rights of inventors is the primary justification for patents, then it is perfectly reasonable to question the extent of those rights. In particular, it makes sense to consider what belongs in the genetic commons as dis-coveries and the natural heritage of humankind rather than industrial or government property.[20]

Animal Rights. The patenting of animals generates distrust for reasons of religion, ethics, and animal rights. Various organizations—animal-rights groups and others—believe that the genetic engineering of farm animals adversely affects family farmers, is cruel to animals, endangers living species, or is flatly unethical. Perhaps in response to such concerns, the Patent Office stopped issuing patents for transgenic animals in 1988. In 1993, it resumed processing of the 180 animal patent applications that had accumulated during the moratorium, but fewer companies were at-tempting to patent farm animals by that time, largely because persistent technical problems and costs had encouraged them to shift to more prof-itable areas of research. Lobbyists against animal patents such as Jeremy Rifkin, a leading critic of biotechnology, continue to object to Patent Office policies for reasons of philosophy and economic inequity: "We believe the gene pool should be maintained as an open commons, and should not be the private preserve of multinational companies. . . . This is the Government giving its imprimatur to the idea that there is no dif-ference between a living thing and any inert object. . . . It's the final as-sault on the sacred meaning of life and life process."[21] Mr. Rifkin helped organize a coalition of church groups representing 80 religious faiths and denominations to oppose patenting on the grounds that animals are cre-ations of God, not of humans. Others also find the idea of patenting an-imals repugnant on moral, ethical, and religious grounds.[22]

"Terminator" Technology. No patent issue elicits greater distrust of the food biotechnology industry—and of its government regulators—than patent protection through "terminator" technology. As yet another irony of the politics of food biotechnology, the terminator was the work of a USDA *government* scientist who recognized that the insertion of cer-tain genes and antibiotic-resistance marker sequences into plants could stop them from reproducing. When treated with a suitable antibiotic, these genes lead to the production of a protein that prevents seed ger-

mination. This trick prevents plants from cross-pollinating bioengineered traits into weeds (a good thing). However, it also acts as a "technology protector system," meaning that farmers cannot collect seeds and grow them. Instead, they must buy seeds protected by a biotechnology company's patents, and must do so every year. Before the USDA researcher had even developed the technology, he won a patent for it in collaboration with a seed company, Delta and Pine Land.

When Monsanto attempted to buy Delta and Pine Land, it appeared as if the true purpose of terminator technology was to protect private property and make farmers even more dependent on seeds and chemicals controlled by corporations. Critics feared that use of this technology would devastate farmers in poor countries who typically save their seeds from one year to the next. On this basis, the Consultative Group on International Agricultural Research recommended in 1998 that its 16 member institutes ban research on terminator genes. The following year, U.S. rural development groups, alarmed about the possible effects of the technology on global food security and biodiversity, organized their constituents to demand that USDA cease sponsorship of terminator research.[23] This research evoked vivid images—and street theater—of corporate science conducted for profit rather than for the good of society (see figure 26).

The already high profile of critics of this research rose even higher in June 1999 when the president of the Rockefeller Foundation, Gordon Conway, challenged Monsanto to stop work on terminator genes. In his view, this work was so controversial that it placed the entire food biotechnology enterprise at risk—including its potential to feed the developing world. The use of this research, he said, "particularly by the poor and excluded, is being threatened by the mounting controversies in Europe and to some extent in the United States. There is a real danger that the research may be set back, particularly if field trials are banned. . . . The agricultural seed industry must disavow the use of terminator technology to produce seed sterility."[24] Mr. Conway also suggested that Monsanto invest more in research to solve food problems in developing countries, and voluntarily label its products. In response, Monsanto officials issued a "terse statement" terming their conversations with Mr. Conway "frank and productive. We will continue to reach out to people like Prof. Conway to discuss the challenges and opportunities of biotechnology applications in agriculture."[25]

Nevertheless, his remarks hit home. In October 1999, Monsanto announced that the company would "make no effort to market" terminator

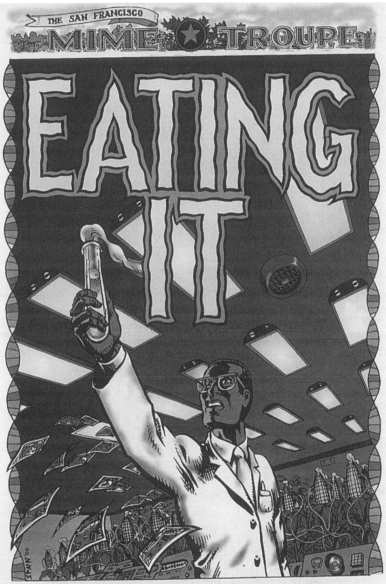

FIGURE 26. This flyer advertises a play produced by the San Francisco Mime Troupe in summer 2000: "In her laboratory, Dr. Synthia Allright-Bloom is hard at work on a bio-genetic engineering discovery that could feed the world." The Mime Troupe presents free plays in public parks.

seeds (even though the possibility of doing so was still years away), thereby averting "a public relations disaster in an industry already under attack on other, more serious fronts."[26] Earlier that year, a Monsanto spokesman said that "seed sterility has become a surrogate for the entire debate on biotech. . . . We are recognizing now though that there is something psychologically offensive about sterile seed in every culture."[27] Other motives, however, may have influenced Monsanto's retreat on this issue. The Justice Department's antitrust division had delayed Monsanto's purchase of Delta and Pine Land. When Monsanto merged with Pharmacia and Upjohn late in 1999, it withdrew the purchase offer (lawsuits ensued). The USDA, citing the many beneficial applications of the ability to turn genes on and off, continues to conduct terminator research, leaving plenty of room for ongoing distrust—and outrage—about how government and industry plan to use this technology.[28]

Genetic "Pollution"

A third major issue of distrust arises from the inadvertent transfer of transgenic pollen to organically grown or native plant species. The high level of public concern about this issue is revealed by the political battle that took place over the USDA's proposed rules for certifying foods as "organic." Scientists and the food biotechnology industry are also concerned about pollen spread, but for a different reason—its political and economic consequences. Such consequences are best illustrated by the discovery of transgenes in native varieties ("landraces") of maize growing in Mexico, and the ensuing uproar over publication of this finding.

Organic Foods. Because practices related to organic farming were inconsistent, organic farmers attempted to set up a voluntary certification program but could not reach consensus on how to do that. They asked Congress to establish mandatory rules for designating food as organic, and legislators did so in 1990 when they passed the Organic Food Production Act and established a National Organic Standards Board to advise the USDA about implementation. The board, realizing that Congress had passed the legislation before bioengineered foods were on the market, recommended "as a policy matter" that genetically modified foods be excluded from those considered organically grown.[29]

In proposing standards, the USDA was especially sensitive to objections that *organic* implied criticism of other agricultural methods. In what appeared to be a compromise forced by mainstream agricultural producers, the agency asked for public comment on whether *organic* could be applied to foods that had been genetically modified, irradiated, or fertilized with reprocessed sewage ("sludge"). Buried in a 120-page and especially impenetrable *Federal Register* notice were a few short paragraphs unlikely to shed light on the department's position on these issues. For example:

> We do not consider non-synthetic substances that have been treated with a synthetic substance, but which have not been chemically altered by a manufacturing process, to be synthetic under the definition given in the Act. . . . We have included toxins derived from genetically engineered bacteria on the proposed National List primarily so that we can receive comment on the proper classification of these substances and on whether they should be allowed, prohibited, or approved on a case-by-case basis.

Translation: the USDA considers genetic engineering and irradiation to be processes that do not alter the fundamental nature of food and, therefore, proposes to include transgenic foods on the Federal List of foods certified as organically grown.

When the USDA invited comments on this idea, the agency got them. By February 1998, just two months after publication of the notice, 4,000 people had filed comments, many of them along the lines of "USDA should not permit corporate agribusiness lobbyists and bureaucrats in Washington to force-feed the rules to organic farmers and their customers." In response to the deluge, the USDA postponed the comment deadline and scheduled public hearings. By March, an extraordinary grassroots campaign based on the Internet, notices on milk cartons, and other low-cost efforts had elicited 15,000 comments, nearly all of them negative. I can attest to the breadth and persistence of this effort; for weeks, I received daily electronic mail instructions about how to file comments on this issue. By the deadline, the USDA organic standards docket contained an astonishing 275,603 letters, with genetic engineering eliciting the most criticism.[30]

Eventually, the USDA responded to public demand and dropped the controversial proposals; it would not permit genetically modified, irradiated, sewage-fertilized foods, or animals fed antibiotics to be labeled as organic. The organic foods industry and its constituents hailed the decision as a decisive victory: "Organic food stores are no longer just little co-ops with tofu and bean sprouts. . . . They alerted their customers, and the customers rejected the proposed rules."[31] Biotechnology industry representatives criticized the decision as "political, not based on any realistic assessment of risks, benefits, or science," and USDA officials reassured them that the organic standards did not "reflect a judgment about the safety or utility of biotechnology. . . . USDA has not drawn official conclusions about biotechnology labeling for conventional agriculture products. In general, USDA is doing a great deal to promote biotechnology as a key part of mainstream US agriculture efforts."

Mexican Native Corn. Plant pollen does not follow USDA rules; it follows air currents. During the FDA's 1999 food labeling hearings, organic farmers testified that genetically altered pollen threatened the ability of their crops to qualify for organic certification. Later, the StarLink episode demonstrated how easy it was to commingle genetically modified seeds with conventional seeds. By 2001, transgenes could be found anywhere anyone looked for them: in fields certified as organic, fields of conventionally grown crops, grain shipments to Japan, food aid to Latin America, fields in countries that had banned transgenic crops, and "GM-free" products. Events the following year confirmed such observations. Monsanto and Aventis CropScience admitted that genetically modified canola seeds, not yet approved by the FDA, "might have found their way" into planted crops, and Australian scientists showed that genes from genetically modified canola readily transfer to conventional canola in neighboring fields.[32]

Such incidents evoke images of accidents: Pandora's box and genies out of bottles. They also evoke a more sinister image—the Trojan horse— the *deliberate* manipulation of the food supply to undermine regulatory controls and consumer choice at the marketplace. As Friends of the Earth explained, "Legal frameworks were supposed to be adequate to ensure that GMOs wouldn't endanger the environment or human health. Biotech companies were supposed to comply with those frameworks. Regulatory bodies were supposed to monitor and oversee GMO releases to ensure they were complying with the legal frameworks. But the reality shows a completely different picture."[33]

Nowhere is the reality more starkly displayed than in the case of transgenic "pollution" of native maize grown in Mexico, where corn originated and where corn biodiversity is treasured. Early in 2000, letters to *Science* warned colleagues that the "introduction of transgenic maize varieties in Mexico may pose a risk to landraces or wild relatives of maize in its ancestral home," and "the direction of gene flow is more likely to occur from [transgenic] cultivars to the wild plants." According to *Sierra* magazine, transgenic corn came to Mexico "courtesy of the North American Free Trade Agreement (NAFTA), which opened the Mexican market to cheap grain from *el norte*"; Mexico now imports three times as much corn from the United States as it did prior to NAFTA. To protect the country's corn heritage, Mexico banned the cultivation of transgenic varieties in 1998 but is unable to completely enforce this ruling.[34]

In 2001, researchers from the University of California, Berkeley, found transgenic corn growing in 15 of 22 remote areas of Oaxaca and Ixtlán and reported these findings in the prestigious British journal *Nature*. Val Giddings of the Biotechnology Industry Organization (BIO) told a reporter from *USA Today* that the report posed no *safety* issues: "If there's any impact at all, it's likely to be positive. There are zero human health implications, zero environmental impact implications."[35] Perhaps so, but the uncontrolled spread of genetically modified traits to plants where they are not supposed to be has 100% implications for public trust in the industry and its government regulators—and for generating outrage.

To head off such reactions, industry supporters launched a remarkably nasty public relations campaign to discredit the Berkeley investigators. The campaign focused on their science and their politics. The researchers made two claims in the *Nature* paper; transgenes existed in native maize, and the transgenes were unstable (meaning that they could spread more easily). The discrediting campaign focused exclusively on the second claim. A public relations firm—one that specializes in using the Internet to lobby—recruited scientists to write letters identifying flaws in the methods used to demonstrate genetic instability. On this basis, the editor of *Nature* did something highly unusual (if not unprecedented) in such scientific disputes. Stopping just short of calling the paper fraudulent, he published some of the critical letters along with an editorial note: "The evidence available is not sufficient to justify the publication of the original paper." The researchers admitted some errors in methods, but reaffirmed their original conclusions.[36]

The public relations campaign also focused on the researchers' politics. The senior author, Dr. Ignacio Chapela, held an untenured faculty appointment in the Berkeley plant biology department that auctioned itself into partnership with Novartis in 1998. Dr. Chapela had led faculty opposition to that partnership. Other faculty had accused his coauthor, a graduate student in that department, of antibiotechnology vandalism of their experimental crops (a charge he denied). Reporters investigating the matter guessed that Monsanto and other proindustry groups were behind the public relations campaign but were hiding that connection. Colleagues sympathetic to Dr. Chapela pointed out that most of the writers of the critical letters to *Nature* received all or part of their research funding from an institute affiliated with Novartis (by this time, Syngenta), but also had not disclosed their competing interests.[37]

In the furor over the paper and its near retraction, one crucial fact is easily overlooked: nobody challenged the observation of transgenes in native corn. Indeed, Mexican scientists soon confirmed traces of transgenes in up to 36% of samples tested.[38] In this sense, the public relations campaign succeeded brilliantly. It focused attention on complicated scientific issues and deflected attention from the crucial social issue—the escape of genetically modified traits into wild plant stocks. Regardless of the scientific merits of the research, the ferocity of the attack made it clear that neither the scientific establishment nor the biotechnology industry have much interest in keeping the new genetic traits under control.

Globalization

Globalization elicits dread and outrage for two principal reasons. The first is the potential loss of national identity and autonomy to multinational corporations bent on maximizing profit. The second is the possibility that international regulatory bodies established to deal with globalization issues might make decisions that favor corporate interests at the expense of public welfare and social justice, especially in the areas of health, environmental protection, and food safety. From a business perspective, globalization is about open markets, low wages, and minimal regulations. Regulations, from this perspective, are costly and complicated barriers to selling products on international markets. If, for example, a country decides to invoke the precautionary principle and require premarket testing and labeling of genetically modified foods, it could refuse to buy U.S. crops that were not segregated and labeled. It is easy to see how international disputes about such matters could become difficult. Such disputes are resolved through three international bodies: the World Trade Organization (WTO), the Biosafety Protocol, and the Codex Alimentarius.

The increasingly powerful WTO is the most important of these bodies. Countries belonging to the United Nations created the WTO to develop, administer, and—most notably—enforce their trade agreements. The purpose of the WTO is to promote free trade, ideally through guarantees of fair and consistent treatment of exports from all member countries. WTO rules require member states to (1) consider all other members as equal trading partners, (2) treat all foreign corporations just as they treat their own, and (3) eliminate all competitive practices that might give them an unfair advantage. In practice, however, richer countries can and do use the rules to their own advantage. The WTO especially raises suspicions because it conducts negotiations in secret.

The WTO replaced the General Agreement on Tariffs and Trade (GATT) in 1995. From 1947 to 1994, GATT nations negotiated reductions in tariffs and other trade barriers through a series of discussion "rounds" identified by their location (the Uruguay Round of 1986–94, for example). By the time WTO succeeded GATT, the principal negotiations no longer concerned tariffs or intellectual property rights as much as they did issues related to environmental protection and food safety. For years, critics have complained that eliminating trade barriers will force countries to adhere to the lowest common denominator in food safety and environmental standards. As evidence, they point to WTO decisions that prevent France from rejecting hormone-fed beef raised in the United States or require the United States to accept Malaysian shrimp caught in nets that trap sea turtles. If WTO decides that genetically modified foods are safe, no member country is permitted to reject them.[39]

One reason why President Bill Clinton invited the WTO to meet in Seattle in 1999 was to resolve the "huge biotech problem" with European countries that were refusing American exports of transgenic corn and soybeans. Although most of the public demonstrations during that meeting were aimed at globalization in general (and labor and biopiracy issues in particular), they also focused on trade issues related to genetically modified foods.[40] By the time of that meeting, international and national government groups were debating whether to allow the production or import of genetically modified foods, to require them to be labeled (and, if so, at what threshold level), or to ban them outright.

International decisions about such issues are difficult to track, as they change constantly in response to political pressures. When the European Union approved sales of transgenic corn in 1996, the biotechnology industry was optimistic that Europeans would readily accept genetically modified foods. In 1997, however, the European Parliament required the foods to be labeled, and in 1999 the European Union also required manufacturers to conduct risk assessments, public consultations, and post-market safety reviews. Some national governments permitted transgenic crops to be grown, but others did not. In mid-2000, *Time* magazine classified countries by their attitude toward genetically modified foods—pro-GM (Argentina, China), cautiously pro (Canada, U.S., India), very cautiously pro (Brazil, Japan), or strongly anti (Britain, France)—but the policies of these countries changed constantly in response to new infor-

TABLE 13. Actions of selected countries and the European Union regarding planting, labeling, or importing of genetically modified foods, 2001

Country	Action Taken
Argentina	Permits planting.
Australia	Permits planting, but also requires posting of locations of planting sites, investigation of violations, and imposition of fines. With New Zealand, issues guidelines for labeling.
Brazil	Permits planting, but requires permits and labeling.
China	Permits planting, but requires certification of production, sale, and import as safe for humans, animals, and environment.
Japan	Establishes labeling threshold of 5% for genetically modified corn or soybeans.
Philippines	Rules that failure to label foods containing genetically modified ingredients is punishable by prison (up to 12 years) and fines (up to $2,000).
Saudi Arabia	Bans import of transgenic animals; requires health certificates for transgenic plants; requires mandatory labeling of processed foods containing genetically modified ingredients.
Sri Lanka	Bans all transgenic foods as of September 1, but later postpones ban indefinitely.
Thailand	Bans new field trials; approves Roundup Ready soybeans.
European Union	Requires member states to ensure the traceability of genetically modified foods at all stages of marketing; restricts new product approvals to 10 years with renewal for another 10 years; establishes public registers for field-testing sites; phases out use of certain antibiotic-resistance markers; establishes labeling threshold of 1%. France, Italy, Luxembourg, Austria, Denmark and Greece declare moratorium on planting until these rules take effect.

SOURCE: *Food Chemical News*, 2001.

mation, ongoing pressures, and decisions of international bodies attempting to deal with issues raised by these foods.[41] To illustrate the complexity of the international picture, table 13 summarizes decisions about transgenic foods made by various countries *just* during the 2001 calendar year.

The inconsistent decisions of international bodies in dealing with genetically modified foods do little to engender trust that the system will operate in the public interest. In 1999, for example, the Biosafety Protocol, an international committee formed as a result of the 1992 biodiversity treaty forged in Rio de Janeiro, proposed to require shipments of transgenic foods to be approved *in advance* by importing countries. The United States refused to sign the treaty, which was also opposed by other large food-exporting nations such as Canada, Australia, Chile, Argentina, and Uruguay. The reason: the requirement could institute "a draconian regime that we have never seen before except for highly toxic and hazardous substances."[42] In January 2000, delegates from 130 nations adopted the treaty, but with compromises; they permitted genetically modified foods to be exported without advance notice but allowed countries to decide for themselves whether transgenic foods, seeds, and microbes posed a threat to the environment. If countries decided to prohibit imports on that basis, they could. Industry leaders considered the compromise as a win and hoped that the treaty would help counter the perception that food biotechnology was not adequately regulated. Some European countries viewed such trade agreements as barely masked attempts to achieve political goals. Many Europeans resented U.S. trade restrictions against countries that conduct business with Iran, Libya, or Cuba, and perceived the aggressive marketing of American transgenic crops as arrogant, controlling, and insensitive. They thought the phrase, "what's good for G.M. is good for America," now meant that genetic modification had replaced General Motors as the symbol of United States corporate power.[43]

Europeans particularly resented the lack of labeling, as it left them little choice at the marketplace. If labels were required, however, U.S. companies would have to take several complicated and expensive actions: segregate conventional crops from transgenic crops in fields as well as during storage, transport, and processing; document the traceability of the crops; and establish thresholds for levels of transgenic contamination. U.S. food producers oppose these measures as impractical and expensive, and international authorities have yet to agree on the lowest level of contaminating transgenes that will permit crops to be labeled "GM-free."

The views of different countries on such issues are "harmonized" by the WTO, but also to a lesser extent by the Codex Alimentarius (food code) Commission of the United Nations. In 1994, an international consumers' group petitioned the Codex to develop standards for mandatory labeling of transgenic foods because "the burden of labeling should fall on those who wish to use and profit from biotechnology and not on those who choose not to use it"; the group renewed such requests through the 1990s. By 1999, public opinion in Europe, especially in Great Britain, overwhelmingly favored labeling and segregation of conventional crops from transgenic crops. When the European Union asked the Codex Commission to require labels for all foods containing identifiable transgenic ingredients, only the United States and Argentina (which also exports transgenic crops) opposed this proposal.[44] U.S. Codex representatives argue that the true purpose of calls for labeling is to protect European trade restrictions: "a mandatory process-based label on genetically engineered food has the potential to be perceived by many consumers as a warning label that the product is unsafe, and therefore could be misleading and, consequently, inappropriate as a mandatory international guideline. Foods derived from biotechnology are not inherently less safe than other foods."[45] Such arguments, along with the other concerns discussed here, convince critics that the goal of the food biotechnology industry is to control the world's food supply for private profit, and that neither the industry nor governing bodies can be trusted to make decisions in the public interest—whether or not the products are safe.

THE POLITICS OF ANTIBIOTECHNOLOGY ADVOCACY

We have seen that objections to genetically engineered foods focus as much on issues of distrust as they do on matters of safety, and are likely to continue to do so unless the industry ceases acting in ways that engender suspicion. Public protests against transgenic foods occurred more swiftly and dramatically in Europe, especially in Great Britain, than in the United States, not least because the British were better informed about the issues. At the peak of the "GM crisis" early in 1999, the seven largest daily newspapers in Great Britain ran hundreds of articles on the subject, nearly all of them negative. Many of the articles focused on the extent to which the Clinton administration pressured the British government to accept American transgenic crops and collaborated in efforts to get those crops approved by the European Union.[46]

Antibiotechnology advocacy—international and domestic—is a constant source of worry to the industry. Such advocacy forms part of a larger trend in organized opposition to other aspects of globalization. During the 1990s, the number of international nongovernmental organizations increased from 6,000 to 26,000, and thousands of such groups exist in the United States alone. These groups are increasingly effective at the corporate, national, and international levels, and business analysts consider them especially difficult to manage because of their skill at using the Internet—an uncontrollable venue—to mobilize support. Yet another irony is the complaint of industry leaders that groups opposed to food biotechnology are so well funded. They point to Greenpeace, for example, which attracts a worldwide income of more than $100 million annually. This amount may seem large, but it is minuscule in comparison to the annual income of the large biotechnology corporations whose officials make that complaint.[47]

Advocacy has been slower to develop in the United States than in Europe, perhaps because Americans generally are less politically active, but also because they tend to have more positive attitudes toward technology, greater trust in regulatory agencies, and less immediate contact with agriculture. Nevertheless, opposition to food biotechnology exists in this country and appears to be growing. Advocacy groups include environmental organizations (such as Environmental Defense, the Union of Concerned Scientists, and the Sierra Club) but also an extraordinary variety of less familiar organizations such as the International Center for Technology Assessment, the Foundation for Deep Ecology, the International Forum on Globalization, and the Rainforest Action Network. Countless local groups like NW Rage (Northwest Resistance against Genetic Engineering) educate members "to resist the intrusion of genetic engineering . . . into our lives."[48] Coalition groups like Genetically Engineered Food Alert demand that food companies refuse to use genetically modified ingredients. Most organizing occurs through dozens of antibiotechnology Internet Web sites and electronic mail services that keep subscribers well informed about the daily actions of companies, government regulators, and critics.[49] Biotechnology companies appear helpless in the face of such tactics and make little attempt to counter them beyond statements on their own Web sites and in the public relations campaigns of the Council for Biotechnology Information (figures 12, 14, and 17).

Away from the Internet, action against food biotechnology takes many forms, nearly all of which mix safety with other issues to evoke distrust, dismay, contempt, or outrage. To begin with, advocates write books—lots of them. My personal collection includes two or three dozen, of which at least ten were written for a popular audience just from 1998 to 2002.[50] Books on the ethics of food biotechnology form an additional publishing genre. I am not the only person who collects such volumes. The geneticist Richard Lewontin reviewed his own collection of books and found that most opposed genetically modified foods for reasons that he judged muddled. He said, "whatever fears [one] might have of possible allergic reactions to food produced from genetically modified organisms, they are not more unsettling than the allergies induced . . . by the quality of the arguments about them. . . . Even the most judicious and seem-

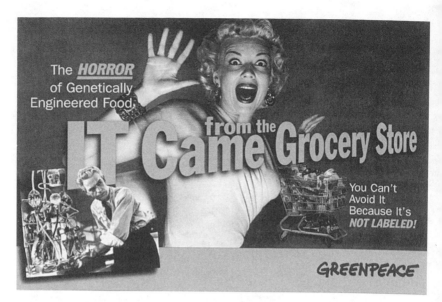

FIGURE 27. Greenpeace uses cards like this one to generate support for campaigns to stop sales of genetically modified foods. Text on the back of the card explains why companies should stop selling genetically engineered food and what consumers can do to encourage that action. (Courtesy of Greenpeace, 2000.)

ingly dispassionate examinations of the scientific questions turn out, in the end, to be manifestoes."[51] By this, he seemed to mean that critics do not clearly distinguish scientific concerns about safety from concerns about social issues.

The books have a political effect, but not always the one intended. Among the most recent, only one favors food biotechnology: *Pandora's Picnic Basket.*[52] Although written by a scientist who claims to be objective, this book also can be viewed as a manifesto. An instructor in my New York University department assigned it to a graduate class on contemporary food issues. He said the class found the science parts useful but also found the book infuriatingly patronizing, biased in coverage, and lacking in coherent social analysis. Informing the public about science is valuable, but that alone is not nearly enough to help people understand how scientific and social issues interact in matters of public policy.

Greenpeace is especially adept at producing materials that use scientific concerns about safety to score points about distrust. Figure 27 gives my favorite example: using the "horror" of transgenic foods to empha-

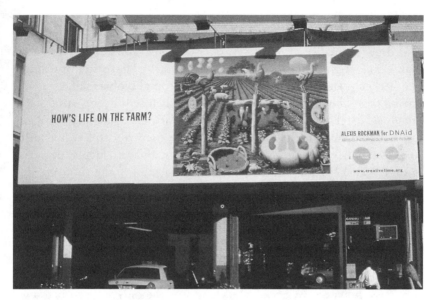

FIGURE 28. In conjunction with an exhibition of artworks on the theme "artists picturing our genetic future," Alexis Rockman's *The Farm* appeared on a lower Manhattan billboard (Lafayette and Houston Streets) in fall 2000. (Courtesy of Alexis Rockman and Creative Time; photograph by Charlie Samuels.)

size the lack of transparency in marketing. Another example: at the time of the 1999 WTO meeting in Seattle, a coalition of more than 60 non-profit groups (The Turning Point Project) placed a series of full-page advertisements on food biotechnology and globalization in the *New York Times*. One, headlined "Unlabeled, Untested . . . and You're Eating It" (October 18, 1999), listed common food products containing genetically modified ingredients and discussed the hazards of toxicity, allergic reactions, and antibiotic resistance. Subsequent advertisements provided lengthy and thought-provoking discussions of various health, environmental, or economic consequences of biotechnology or economic globalization, along with information about how to learn more about such issues. Figure 28 gives yet another example—this one, a painting—of the commingling of safety and social issues as they apply to transgenic foods.

This commingling of safety with other issues is most visible in street demonstrations. The 1999 FDA labeling hearings, for example, attracted protests in all three cities where they were held (figure 18, page 190). The

Oakland, California, hearing attracted 500 antibiotechnology demonstrators and received much attention from the press, largely because it also drew a smaller group of counter-demonstrators. These were researchers and graduate students from the nearby University of California, Berkeley, Department of Plant and Microbial Biology, infamous for having been "bought" by Novartis the year before (the department had auctioned itself to Novartis in an exclusive partnership arrangement giving that company the right to select faculty, review research results prior to publication, negotiate licensing agreements, and veto faculty decisions in some areas).[53] They said they were demonstrating "out of concern that the public was not being informed about the benefits of biotechnology."[54]

Advocates also use the legal system to pursue antibiotechnology goals. In 2001 alone, 36 states considered bills aimed at transgenic foods: restricting plantings or sales; requiring labeling, notification, tracking, or evaluation of environmental impact; banning terminator technology; or prohibiting the use of such foods in school lunch programs. Few such bills pass, however. By 2001, Maryland was the only state to ban a genetically modified food, in this case fish in waterways that connect to other bodies of water.[55] Consumer groups, chefs, and some scientists have filed lawsuits and organized petition campaigns to compel the FDA to institute labeling and safety testing. The Alliance for Bio-Integrity (Iowa City, IA), led by Steven Druker, has filed such suits. Other suits argue that transgenic manipulations make it impossible to observe religious dietary laws; one was cosigned by 113 Christians, 37 Jews, 12 Buddhists, and 122 people who checked, "my faith is not easily categorized." Still others have filed antitrust lawsuits based on the idea that the industry's control over seeds inhibits competition. A petition organized by Mothers for Natural Law collected an astounding number of signatures—nearly 500,000—from people favoring transparency in labeling. Jeremy Rifkin organized a class-action suit against Monsanto arguing that the company is part of an international conspiracy to control the world's corn and soybean supply through intimidation and deceptive business practices. Regardless of the outcome of the bills and lawsuits, they force attention to be paid to societal as well as safety issues.[56]

Such methods may annoy (and sometimes infuriate) biotechnology companies, government regulators, and scientists, but they are traditional ways of taking political action in a pluralistic democracy; they are legal, fair, and—given the many reasons for distrust—thoroughly justifiable. Transgenic sabotage, however, is another matter. When Ingo Potrykus complains about "those who would damage humanitarian projects" (discussed in chapter 5), he worries most that vandals will destroy test plantings of Golden Rice. In Great Britain, Greenpeace and other groups conducted "destruction actions" against test plots of transgenic crops, sometimes dressed in full-body anticontamination suits and goggles. In the United States, numerous incidents of uprooting transgenic crops, trashing laboratories, burning genetic engineering materials, and making personal threats against scientists cross a legal line and enter into the realm of food terrorism.[57] Such actions undermine the legitimacy of the political goals they are designed to accomplish, as do the controlling actions of corporations (see concluding chapter).

TOWARD DIALOGUE, IF NOT CONSENSUS

Protests against genetically modified foods—or the threat of such protests—affect the behavior of retailers who understand that consumers can choose to buy organic products, now labeled as such. Many companies label their products "GM-free" (see figure 25, page 226). In the late 1990s, Gerber's and Heinz announced that they would stop using genetically modified ingredients in their baby foods, and McDonald's "quietly" told farmers to stop growing Monsanto's transgenic potatoes. Frito-Lay told its suppliers not to grow transgenic corn, and Archer Daniels Midland warned its grain suppliers to begin segregating bioengineered crops. Corn growers viewed such developments as a clear sign that "GM organisms have become the albatross around the neck of farmers."[58] The loss of both domestic and foreign sales outlets coupled with more general problems of overproduction caused corn prices to drop to their lowest point in ten years. As a partial remedy, the American Corn Growers Association advised its members to consider planting only conventional seeds. Wall Street analysts were well aware of this problem, seeing current events as very bad news for farmers, seed companies, and seed stocks. They predicted that premium prices would go to conventional rather than transgenic crops because "GMOs are good science but bad politics."[59] Their predictions were correct; corn acres planted in genetically modified seeds fell from 25 million in 1999 to just over 16 million in 2001. By then, more than half of the Midwest grain elevators required segregation of transgenic seeds, and 20% were offering premium prices for conventional corn or soybeans.[60] In part because of objections to transgenic varieties, revenues from U.S. corn exports fell drastically from 1996 to 2000. Exports to Japan fell from $2.4 billion to $1.5 billion (a decline of 38%), to Taiwan from $960 million to $460 million (52%), and to European Union countries from $413 million to $69 million (83%).[61] Despite these reactions, genetically engineered traits are widely dispersed in the environment, and transgenic ingredients pervade the food supply.

Figuring out what to do about this confusing picture preoccupies federal agencies responsible for the regulation of transgenic foods. They worry that food biotechnology will suffer the fate of nuclear power and that its potential benefits will be lost to humanity. Like public protests over early recombinant-DNA experiments, those over food biotechnology may become muted if companies produce genetically modified foods that really do make farming more efficient or benefit consumers. What cannot be predicted is the strength and persistence of public distrust or the willingness of the industry to respond to it and submit the products and marketing methods to greater scrutiny. To help the industry gain public approval, federal agencies recruit advisory organizations to bring together groups of disparate stakeholders to seek points of agreement. As a participant in several such meetings, I can attest that they require people with differing perspectives to listen to one another (itself a step forward) and to attempt to identify issues of consensus. These meetings invariably identify labeling, segregation, traceability, and government oversight as necessary first steps toward achieving public confidence. Although reaching consensus on such steps may never be possible, such meetings permit participants to discuss matters that extend beyond safety and place societal issues of trust firmly on the agenda.

The messy political debates about food biotechnology are not likely to be resolved soon without major changes in the ways the industry conducts business. Genetically engineered foods may be relatively safe by the standards of science-based approaches to risk assessment, but industry decisions have caused them to rank high on the dread-and-outrage scale. To inspire public confidence, the industry must share control of the food supply with consumers. Until people actually have some choice about whether to consume transgenic foods, there is little reason to accept them. Companies need to label the foods and keep them separate from conventional foods. They also need to make more serious efforts to ensure that transgenes do not escape into the wild. They must work with organic farmers to prevent transgenic contamination of organic crops, and they must stop using public relations to "sell" people on the idea that the products are necessary and safe. If biotechnology companies want to convince people that their foods are beneficial, they must make products that *are* beneficial—to consumers and to society. Finally, they must stop acting so aggressively against people who raise questions about the products, stop prosecuting small-scale "violators" of patent rights, and stop insisting that science education—important as it is—will solve the industry's public relations problems. Even some industry supporters understand that biotechnology companies need to become less disingenuous, and set some restraints on "their insatiable appetite for control."[62] If food biotechnology does have benefits for individuals and society— and it is still too early to say whether it does—such benefits can only be achieved when the products are viewed as low in science-based safety risk as well as in value-based dread and outrage.

If companies are going to claim that their work will solve world food problems, they need to put substantial resources into working with scientists in developing countries to help farmers produce more food under local conditions. Such efforts could prove worthwhile if supported by policies designed to support sustainable and organic agriculture, protect against environmental risks, and prevent exploitation of small farmers or of consumers. For some years now, I have suggested that the industry institute a "tithing" program and apply 10% of income to research on projects that address the food needs of developing countries, regardless of their eventual profitability. This approach might indicate that the industry recognizes the difference between its commercial and humanitarian goals. Although I am not aware of any company that has taken on this challenge, I continue to believe that to be perceived as credible, the industry must *be* credible.

If government agencies want to promote food biotechnology, they are going to have to regulate it more effectively. They must insist that companies label, segregate, and ensure the traceability of genetically engineered crops, provide adequate areas of refuge, and keep their transgenes from pollinating out of control. Government regulators should be working with industry to figure out how to label the products and establish workable thresholds for transgenic contaminants. On the international level, they should stop obstructing multinational agreements and cooperate with government policies of other countries. They should grant consumer protection at least the same level of priority as promotion of industry objectives. Federal regulators must recognize as well that science-based decisions also have political dimensions and must find ways to consider societal and environmental implications when approving genetically modified foods.

And what should the public think or do about food biotechnology? As with other aspects of food politics, much depends on point of view. Eating foods containing transgenic ingredients appears unlikely to cause direct harm to human health, but at the moment there also is little evidence for benefit. If a goal is to reduce pesticides in the environment, genetically modifying foods may be an appropriate method for achieving that goal, but so may other methods that also deserve consideration. If the ultimate goal is to ensure food security for the world's population, other means to do so deserve equal time and resources. Overall, the role of genetically modified foods in these larger aspects of the food system is as yet uncertain and unlikely to be known for some time to come.

With that said, we now turn to the concluding chapter in which we will examine some emerging food safety issues. Like food biotechnology, these issues are relatively low in science-based risk but relatively high in dread: mad cow disease, foot-and-mouth disease, anthrax, and other potential weapons of food bioterrorism.

THE FUTURE OF FOOD SAFETY

PUBLIC HEALTH VERSUS BIOTERRORISM

SAFE FOOD IS ONE OF THE GREAT ACHIEVEMENTS OF TWENTIETH-century public health, a result of scientific advances in refrigeration, pasteurization, insecticides, and disease surveillance. This book proposes that food safety also depends on politics. Any doubts about that idea should be thoroughly dispelled by the events of September 2001, when terrorists used airplanes as weapons of destruction and an anonymous correspondent sent letters filled with anthrax spores to civic and media leaders. One consequence of these events was to reveal the vulnerability of food and water supplies to malevolent tampering. Another was to expose the glaring gaps in federal oversight of food safety.[1]

This concluding chapter examines emerging food safety threats in these contexts. Some of the threats are diseases that affect farm animals and only rarely cause disease in humans. Even so, their effects on human welfare can be profound: massive destruction of food animals, loss of livelihoods and community, and restrictions on personal liberty. The outbreaks of mad cow disease and foot-and-mouth disease that occurred in Europe in the 1990s and early 2000s, for example, were destructive, but they occurred as accidental results of production practices. In contrast, bioterrorism is deliberate—the purposeful use of biological or chemical materials to achieve political goals. Bioterrorism introduces a new and especially frightening political dimension to food safety risk: the *intention* to cause harm, regardless of who gets hurt.

In this chapter, we will see how bioterrorism brings up questions of food security and expands the common meaning of that term. In the United States, food security usually refers to the reliability of a family's food supply; people who lack food security qualify for federal or private food assistance. Since the anthrax mailings, food security has also come to mean "food safe from bioterrorism." We begin our discussion of this definitional transition with diseases of farm animals: mad cow disease, foot-and-mouth disease, and anthrax. In recent years, these diseases did not exist or were rare veterinary problems posing relatively little risk to human health. Today, we are concerned about their potential to make us ill, create havoc in the food system, or become tools of bioterrorism. The chapter concludes with a discussion of how we—as a society and as individuals—can take action to address the problems and politics of food safety, now and in the future.

THE POLITICS OF ANIMAL DISEASES

Because one consequence of globalization is the rapid transport of food across national borders and over long distances, a disease that affects the food supply can travel rapidly from one country to another. Animal diseases have trade implications; if a country harbors sick animals, no other country will accept its meat. Trade implications have political consequences.

As we will see, the British epidemics of mad cow disease and foot-and-mouth disease occurred as inadvertent results of meat production practices. In contrast, the U.S. anthrax mailings were a deliberate act. All three risks, however, rank high in dread; they are involuntary, uncontrollable, and cause exotic disease. Just as important, they undermine trust in the food supply and in government and divert resources from more pressing matters of public health.

Mad Cow Disease: Prions and Species Jumps

Mad cow disease emerged as a highly publicized food safety crisis of the mid-1990s, largely confined to Great Britain. The story of this disease is relevant to our discussion for its interweaving of politics and science and its effect on public confidence. The manner in which British officials handled the mad cow crisis, for example, later contributed to public distrust of genetically modified foods. Prior to the early 1980s, hardly anyone had heard of the disease, but by 1999 it had affected at least 175,000 British cows. Its results were catastrophic: destruction of more than 4 million cattle, estimated costs of $7 billion, transmission to at least 18 countries, and worldwide rejection of British beef. By 2001, although "only" about 120 people had died of the human variant of mad cow disease, more deaths—perhaps as many as 100,000—were expected.[2] Because this story reveals many aspects of the modern politics of food safety, it is well worth recounting.

The mad cow epidemic originated in the late 1970s when the political climate in Great Britain favored cost cutting and deregulation—in this case, of the meat-rendering industry. This industry converts the otherwise unusable (offal) parts of dead animals into "meat-and-bone meal" used to supplement the diets of farm animals. In Britain, rendering then involved the use of organic solvents and steam applied under high pressure; this process sterilized the resulting mess and killed anything that might be infectious. The solvents were dangerously flammable, however, and the energy costs high. In the late 1970s, the British industry—but not renderers in other countries—adopted a cheaper method, one that omitted solvents and cooked the offal at lower temperatures. Most rendering plants in Great Britain switched to that system by the early 1980s.[3]

The new method killed most bacteria and viruses. It did not, however, inactivate *prions*, a generic term for the highly unusual infectious agents believed to cause a disease called scrapie in sheep and related diseases in other animals. These invariably fatal diseases affect the brain and nervous system; they are called spongiform encephalopathies because they cause sponge-like holes in the brains of animals and people. Prion diseases present fascinating biological problems. They appear to involve transmission via *proteins* (rather than bacteria, viruses, or DNA), as well as "species jumps" from one kind of animal to another. In the era before mad cow disease, prion diseases seemed to be confined to their particular host animal. Scrapie, for example, affected sheep in Britain for at least three centuries but did not bother people. Instead, people exhibited their own specific and rare form of the disease, as did cows; both appeared spontaneously and were considered "sporadic." At this point, we need to know the names of these diseases: scrapie in sheep, bovine spongiform encephalopathy (BSE) in cows, and Creutzfeldt-Jakob Disease (CJD) in people.[4] Because of the way sick cows behave, BSE soon became known as mad cow disease. In turn, mad cow disease soon emerged as the link between prion diseases in sheep and in people.[5]

BSE first appeared soon after cows ate the inadequately rendered meat-and-bone meal supplements. These supplements almost certainly contained offal from sheep infected with scrapie; Great Britain raises far more sheep than cattle, and scrapie is common in British sheep. Later, they surely also contained offal from cows with as yet unrecognized BSE. Veterinarians observed the first case of BSE in a cow in 1984 and confirmed the disease in 1985. During the next few years, the number of BSE cases in cows increased, signaling a growing epidemic. In 1988, an investigating committee deduced that the sheep disease must have jumped to cows. At this point, the British government banned the use of offal in cow feed and required farmers to report BSE cases and to destroy suspect cattle, all the while repeatedly reassuring the public that British beef posed no health risk.

Despite the new regulations, government officials promised support to the beef industry. The prime minister, John Major, said he was "absolutely determined to reduce the burden of regulation on business."[6] Although the government vehemently denied it, beef producers often ignored the 1988 feed ban and nearly half of all the BSE cases occurred in cows born *after* that year. In 1990, the government appointed yet another BSE review committee, but, according to a later investigation, pressured its members to declare beef safe to eat. Meanwhile, cases of BSE in cows continued to rise, reaching a peak in 1993 and then declining gradually as the use of rendered meat-and-bone meal ceased. During the next few years, scientists became increasingly convinced that mad cow disease might be transmitted to people. Britain banned the use in human food of mechanically recovered meat from cow vertebrae (lest it be contaminated with brain or nervous tissue), but health officials continued to deny any risk from this practice. The European Union, however, banned the sale of British beef for three years, noting that the disease seemed to be a particularly British problem.[7]

These actions came much too late. In 1996, British doctors identified ten young people with a previously unknown variant of Creutzfeldt-Jakob Disease (vCJD). The new disease differed from the slowly progressing CJD that typically occurs in older people. It affected *young* adults, it looked different, and it progressed much more rapidly. Dismayed scientists immediately suspected that the new variant disease represented yet another species jump, this time from cows to people. People who "caught" the new disease must have eaten BSE-contaminated beef before the offal-feeding bans went into effect or during the period of government delays, denials, finger pointings, and failures to enforce rules.[8]

By all accounts, British officials did not handle this new crisis any better and only grudgingly admitted the link between mad cow disease and the human variant. In what appeared to be an act of explicit manipulation, the agriculture minister, John Gummer, appeared on television to show his faith in British meat: he fed a hamburger to his four-year-old daughter. Overall, the government seemed to be acting on behalf of the cattle industry rather than protecting public health. Reinforcing a familiar theme in this book, the *Lancet* blamed the secret ways in which government and expert committees operate—and the lack of public accountability—for the failure of government to do something to stop mad cow disease and prevent its transmission to people. It pointed to "the weaknesses of separating agricultural and medical science, and of allowing one Government department to protect the interests of both the food consumers and the farming industry."[9]

The appearance of the new variant disease in people caused a further crisis, this time in international trade. The European Union banned member countries from buying British beef, and McDonald's and other such companies quickly removed it from sale. To protect the industry, the British government stopped permitting older cows (which are more likely to have developed BSE) to be used as food and began destroying them at a rate of 15,000 per week. By the end of 1998, the crisis subsided, and the European Union ended its ban. When that order took effect the next year, France continued to refuse to accept British beef. British officials threatened legal action: "We have science and the law on our side and it is regrettable that the French had ignored science and defied the law."[10] Soon after, BSE turned up in cows in Germany, Italy, Spain, and Japan, most likely because the animals had been fed meat-and-bone meal exported from Great Britain. Human cases of vCJD also appeared outside of Britain, perhaps because people ate British beef before the offal ban took effect.

In the United States, federal agencies first took action against BSE in 1997, when the USDA banned imports of European cattle and sheep and the FDA banned the use of animal proteins as feed for ruminant animals. In 2000, the agencies banned imports of rendered animal products from 31 countries that had either reported BSE in their cattle or could not demonstrate that cattle were free of the disease. Food safety officials say the absence of mad cow disease and vCJD in the United States is due to such preventive actions. Others, however, are skeptical that the country can remain free of either disease. More than 30 shipments of animal by-products from prohibited countries entered the United States after the ban, but regulatory agencies could not track what happened to at least half of them, perfectly illustrating the need for a system of food traceability. FDA officials said that most of the by-products ended up in pet food, but this fate cannot be confirmed (and would be unlikely to reassure pet owners, regardless). Inspections revealed that 20% of about 2,500 feed mills handling meat-and-bone meal took no precautions to prevent the meal from getting into animal feed. No federal agency tests for prohibited material in feed for cattle. Worse, the bans on use of meat-and-bone meal do not apply to other farm animals such as pigs or chickens because officials assume that feed for these animals never enters the food supply for cows or people. This assumption, as we learned from the Star-Link episode, is overly optimistic.[11]

Because evidence of BSE in U.S. cows would be catastrophic for the industry, the USDA commissioned a three-year study from the Harvard Center for Risk Analysis, a group sponsored in part by industry. This study, based on a "probabilistic simulation model" (translation: assumptions and best guesses), said mad cow disease posed only minimal risk to American cattle or people: "Our analysis finds that the U.S. is highly resistant to any introduction of BSE or a similar disease. . . . Measures taken by the U.S. government and industry make the U.S. robust against the spread of BSE to animals or humans should it be introduced into this country." The report did not say that BSE could never enter the country, just that "The new cases of BSE would come primarily from lack of compliance with the regulations enacted to protect animal feed. . . . Even if they existed, these hypothetical sources of BSE could give rise to only one to two cases per year." Therefore, "the disease is virtually certain to be eliminated from the country within 20 years after its introduction."[12]

These conclusions may reassure or not depending, as usual, on point of view. A spokesman for the National Cattlemen's Beef Association said they gave "consumers and cattle producers the assurance of the safety of the American beef supply," and the president of the American Meat Institute agreed: "The U.S. is free of many animal diseases that plague other nations, testaments to the success of government-industry efforts." British observers, however, thought such groups must be "in denial." Other countries, they said, also claim not to have mad cow disease but find it as soon as they look for it; any failure to test for it in large numbers of cattle is a serious mistake. But, as a BSE researcher in Oregon explained, "let's face it, no country wants to find the disease."[13]

Early in 2002, the General Accounting Office (GAO) criticized the Harvard study as based on flawed assumptions, and identified glaring weaknesses in U.S. inspection, testing, and enforcement policies against animal (and, therefore, human) prion diseases: "While BSE has not been found in the United States, federal actions do not sufficiently ensure that all BSE-infected animals or products are kept out or that if BSE were found, it would be detected promptly and not spread to other cattle through animal feed or enter the human food supply."[14] A meat industry spokesman dismissed the GAO report as a "rehash" and complained that it failed to recognize that "the risk of BSE ever occurring in the United States is extremely low and getting lower every day."[15] As if to admit its unease with the current level of protection, however, the USDA announced that it was considering a variety of more stringent bans on use of brain, nervous tissue, and other offal from older and "downer" cows (those that died before slaughter), and that it had commissioned another report from the Harvard Center to evaluate such options.[16]

All in all, the experience with mad cow disease confirms that the British beef industry, like that in the United States, acts in its own self-interest regardless of consequences for public health. It also confirms that no government agency willingly makes decisions in the public interest if those decisions oppose industry interests. Finally, the mad cow experience reveals the international nature of diseases that affect the food supply. Two examples: in Japan, British meat-and-bone meal caused a case of mad cow disease, which, in turn, induced a scare responsible for a 50% drop in Japanese imports of U.S. beef, and the first case of vCJD in the United States occurred in a young British woman living in Florida. All borders are porous, food problems are global, and international strategies are required to ensure the safety of any country's food supply.[17]

Foot-and-Mouth Disease: A Contagious and Virulent Virus

Such lessons were firmly reinforced in spring 2001 when an epidemic of foot-and-mouth disease devastated cattle not only in Great Britain but also in other European countries. By the time the epidemic ended, officials had destroyed 4 million animals, quarantined entire communities, and witnessed the destruction of British tourism. Foot-and-mouth disease only occasionally infects humans, but it is a severe political threat—to governments, economies, communities, and international relations.[18]

The cause of foot-and-mouth disease is a virus with several particularly dread-inspiring attributes. It spreads rapidly in air and water and over long distances, is highly contagious by inhalation or contact, and can be transmitted through shoes, clothing, automobile tires, pets, and wild animals. It affects cattle, sheep, goats, pigs, and deer, but people only rarely. It makes animals very sick; they eventually recover from the symptoms—fever and blistered mouths and hooves—but never catch up in growth, weight, or vitality. Animals infected with this disease become useless as meat. The United States takes precautions against foot-and-mouth disease and has not experienced an outbreak since 1929. The last previous British epidemic occurred in the late 1960s. Since early 2000, however, the disease has been reported in Russia, five countries in Asia, seven in Africa, and five in South America. Once started, it is not easy to contain.[19] Thus, countries go to a great deal of trouble to eradicate foot-and-mouth disease and prevent its entry, and this disease is one of the main reasons why U.S. customs officials ask travelers whether they have recently visited farms.

A vaccine exists but poses its own international problems of trade and politics. Vaccinated animals could be carrying the virus but display no symptoms, and no country wants to import an infected animal or its products. Most countries refuse entry to meat or milk from vaccinated animals, and the rules of the European Union (EU) do not allow vaccination. Six weeks into the outbreak, however, the EU granted a waiver and allowed Britain to vaccinate animals against the disease. The British government chose not to do so, however. The Nestlé corporation, which controls much of the milk processing in the affected region, strongly opposed vaccination because it might have "potential massive negative impact on export of products to other countries."[20] Under pressure from this company and a food trade association, the government instead decided to follow standard procedures for dealing with foot-and-mouth disease outbreaks.

These procedures require officials to take three prompt actions: (1) destroy sick animals, (2) destroy healthy animals that might have come in contact with sick animals, and (3) quarantine people living in the vicinity of affected animals. Some countries confine farm families with animals that have the disease—or might have it—to what is effectively a war zone. In Holland, for example, officials did not permit members of such families to leave their property even to go to school, church, or the doctor. They permitted the besieged families to pick up supplies only at checkpoint barriers.[21]

Given the extent of this virus's contagion and its ability to disrupt the food supply and the lives of citizens, it is not difficult to imagine foot-and-mouth disease as an instrument of terror. Scientists may argue about whether it is better to vaccinate animals or destroy them promptly, but this disease can destroy food supplies, communities, and international trade as well as the confidence of a population in its government. The foot-and-mouth epidemic also pointed out gaps in food safety oversight.

While it was in progress, the United States banned import of meat from the European Union. Nevertheless, at least 750,000 pounds of prohibited meat entered U.S. warehouses after the ban, in part because of the inadequate inspection capability of federal agencies.[22]

Anthrax: A Bacterial Instrument of Terror?

Before a possible bioterrorist mailed letters laced with anthrax spores, biologists knew this microbe best as a prototype for Koch's Postulates, the rules developed in 1884 by Robert Koch, a German scientist, to prove that bacteria cause disease.[23] Anthrax bacteria (*Bacillus anthracis*) are common in soil and are eaten by grazing animals. They exist in two stages: rod-shaped *bacteria* that reproduce into long chains and form *spores* when food sources are depleted. The spores are exceptionally hardy; when eaten, they reconstitute into bacteria, invade the bloodstream, reproduce rapidly, and produce deadly toxins. When an infected animal dies, the bacteria turn into spores that eventually drop into the soil and continue the cycle.[24]

Anthrax is normally a veterinary problem. Infected animals are so visibly sick that farmers cull them before they get into the meat supply. Infected cows are too sick to produce milk, or they produce milk of unusable quality, which is why milk and cheese are not known sources of anthrax. Digestive acids and enzymes—and cooking—ordinarily kill the bacteria, and people seem to have some natural immunity. Because heavy bacterial infestations overcome these defenses and spores resist them, people occasionally acquire anthrax from eating undercooked meat from sick or downer water buffalo, goats, sheep, and cattle. Even so, foodborne anthrax is so rare that medical journals like to report the occasional cases. In August 2000, for example, Minnesota health officials described an outbreak of anthrax in a farm family whose members ate meat from a downer steer. When family members became ill, investigators discovered that the carcass was heavily infested with anthrax bacteria.[25]

Anthrax would be almost nonexistent in people if eating it were the only route of infection, but it also causes disease through the skin and lungs. The skin disease comes from handling infected carcasses. The lung disease comes from breathing in spores from infected animal skins or soil. These forms also are relatively rare. In the United States, health officials reported about 225 cases of the skin disease over the 50-year period from 1944 to 1994. In 2001, they added to this total a man in North Dakota who had disposed of five cows dead of anthrax. Officials logged only 18 cases of inhalation anthrax from 1900 to 1978, and just two from 1992 to 2000.[26]

Nevertheless, the hardiness and lethality of anthrax spores has long suggested their potential as agents of germ warfare, and numerous countries worked on secret anthrax bioweapons projects during the Cold War. Much of what is known about weapons-grade anthrax comes from studies of a single epidemic in the former Soviet Union in 1979. When the Soviet state collapsed, scientists were able to trace the epidemic to an accidental release of an aerosol of anthrax spores from a nearby germ weapons factory. Nearly all of the unlucky people and animals who developed the disease were downwind of the factory when the plume of invisible spores blew over.[27] Even before the U.S. anthrax mailings in 2001, experts on bioterrorism understood that anthrax is simple to grow, is durable, and is suitable for many forms of delivery, and that many countries had stockpiled spores: "The long-dreaded concern that chemical and biological weapons might reach terrorist hands is now a reality."[28] The United States worked on inhalation anthrax during the Cold War, and although it and numerous other countries signed a treaty in 1993 against this use, at least 10 countries are thought to be working on such projects. Ironically, because the spores mailed in 2001 were weapons-grade, some experts suspected they must have come from a U.S. military insider eager to demonstrate the need for more research on biological weapons. They were proven correct after a long, poorly handled investigation.[29]

The effects were devastating. During the following year, health officials logged 22 cases of anthrax caused by the mailings, among them five deaths. They investigated hundreds of reports of possible exposure and closed several government buildings to clear them of spores. As political commentator Daniel Greenberg explained, it had taken a "malevolently brilliant [attack] ideal to reach the ears and fears of the public." The attack focused attention on anthrax and induced political leaders to take action against bioterrorism. In 2002, President George W. Bush authorized $1.1 billion for bioterrorism control, much of it for strengthening the capacity of the public health system.[30]

Dealing with anthrax attacks, however, is no simple matter. As a preventive measure, officials treated 32,000 people who *might* have been exposed to anthrax with the protective antibiotic ciprofloxacin (cipro). Cipro is the most effective antibiotic against anthrax, largely because weapons programs deliberately created strains of the bacteria resistant to more common antibiotics such as penicillin. The drug produces unpleasant side effects—itching, swelling, and breathing problems—in nearly 20% of its takers. For this reason, and because of carelessness or inconvenience, many people stop taking the drug before completing the full course of treatment, thereby establishing conditions that favor the emergence of cipro-resistant anthrax—an utterly alarming scenario.[31]

Cipro has additional connections to food safety issues. It is a fluoroquinolone antibiotic closely related to another antibiotic, enrofloxacin, that is widely used to treat chickens and turkeys for respiratory ailments. The antibiotics are essentially the same; chickens metabolize enrofloxacin to cipro. Doctors have treated human infections with fluoroquinolone antibiotics since 1986, but resistance did not become a problem until 1996, when the FDA authorized use of these drugs to treat bacterial infections in poultry. As is customary, farmers fed the drug to entire flocks of chickens even if just a few were sick. Baytril, the enrofloxacin drug produced by Bayer, for example, is used on 128 million chickens worldwide and generates about $150 million in annual sales. By 1999, 18% of *Campylobacter* in chickens resisted enrofloxacin, and people exposed to such chicken bacteria could no longer be treated with cipro; 9,000 such cases were recorded that year. In 2000, the FDA proposed to ban the use of fluoroquinolone antibiotics in poultry feed. The other company making the poultry drug, Abbott Laboratories, agreed to discontinue using it in chickens, but Bayer contested the ban and keeps Baytril on the market. Bayer argues that the problem is overestimated and that withdrawing the drug would have little effect on the extent of antibiotic resistance. The company explains that using antibiotics in chickens is good for people as well as poultry: "If we are what we eat, we're healthier if they're healthier."[32] Drug companies may have little choice about giving up such drugs, however. Early in 2002, the three largest U.S. chicken producers, Tyson Foods among them, said they would reduce use of enrofloxacin, and McDonald's said it had decided a year earlier not to use meat from animals treated with fluoroquinolone antibiotics.[33]

Anthrax is not yet resistant to cipro, but it is likely to become so if the drug is given indiscriminately to large numbers of people who do not need it and do not complete the full course of treatment. The continued use of the analogous drug in chickens will almost certainly increase the numbers and kinds of resistant bacteria. In Taiwan, 60% of pathogenic *Salmonella* isolated from hospital patients have been shown to resist cipro; genetic techniques indicated that the resistant bacteria originated in herds of pigs treated with the drug. Scientists have now shown that giving cipro to chickens rapidly selects for resistant *Campylobacter*.[34]

These antibiotics connect to the issues discussed in this book in one other way. In yet another ironic twist, Bayer, the maker of enrofloxacin, acquired Aventis CropScience in December 2001 for €6 billion (euros), thereby becoming the owner of StarLink corn and other transgenic varieties. The merger unites the crop protection activities of Bayer and Aventis into a new company, Bayer CropScience, expected to generate more than €8 billion in annual sales by 2005.[35]

THE NEW POLITICS OF FOOD SAFETY: BIOTERRORISM

In revealing the vulnerability of the United States to harm from terrorists, the September 2001 attacks affected food safety issues in at least four ways. They (1) shifted the common use of the term *food security* to mean protection of the food supply against bioterrorism, (2) raised alarms about the ways food and biotechnology could be used as biological weapons, (3) encouraged more forceful calls for a single food agency to ensure food security, and (4) focused attention on the need for a stronger public health system to address food safety crises. Despite the apparent unity of purpose in dealing with the aftermath of the attacks, each of these effects displays the usual politics, to which we now turn.

A New Emphasis for Food Security: Safety from Bioterrorism

Prior to the terrorist attacks, food security in the United States had a relatively narrow meaning that derived from the need to establish criteria for deciding whether people were eligible to receive welfare and food assistance. In the 1980s, the U.S. government expanded its definition of "hunger" to include involuntary lack of access to food—the *risk* of hunger as well as the physical experience. By this definition, food security came to mean *reliable access to adequate food.*[36]

The international definition is broader, however. In 1948, the United Nations adopted the Universal Declaration on Human Rights, which said, "Everyone has the right to a standard of living adequate for the health and well-being of himself and of his family, including food, clothing, housing and medical care and the necessary social services, and the right to security in the event of unemployment, sickness, disability, widowhood, old age or other lack of livelihood in circumstances beyond his control."[37] Many interpret this provision to mean that people have a *right* to food security, in this case encompassing five elements: (1) reliable access to food that is not only (2) adequate in quantity and quality, but also (3) readily available, (4) culturally acceptable, and (5) safe. With respect to safety, the Geneva Convention of August 1949, an international agreement on the protection of civilians during armed conflict, expressly prohibited deliberate destruction or pollution of agriculture or of supplies of food and water. These broader meanings derived from work in international development, where it was necessary to distinguish the physical sensation of hunger (which can be temporary or voluntary), from the chronic, involuntary lack of food that results from economic inequities, resource constraints, or political disruption.[38]

The significance of the lack-of-access meaning of food security is evident from a health survey conducted in a remote region of Afghanistan just a few months prior to the September 2001 attacks. Not least because of decades of civil strife, Afghanistan is one of the poorest countries in the world, and its health indices are dismal: a life expectancy of 46 years (as compared to 77 years in the United States) and an infant mortality rate of 165 per 1,000 live births (as compared to 7).[39] At the time of the survey, the United Nations World Food Programme estimated that 3.8 million people in Afghanistan lacked food security and therefore required food aid. Investigators examined the health consequences of this lack and found poor nutritional status to be rampant in the population and a contributing factor in nearly all of the deaths that occurred during the survey period. Half of the children showed signs of stunted growth as a result of chronic malnutrition. Scurvy (the disease resulting from severe vitamin C deficiency) alone accounted for 7% of deaths among children and adults. Because visible nutrient deficiency diseases like scurvy are *late* indicators of malnutrition, the investigators viewed the level of food insecurity as a humanitarian crisis—less serious than in parts of Africa, but worse than in Kosovo during its 1999 upheavals.[40] After October 2001, when bombing raids led to further displacement of the population, the United Nations increased its estimate of the size of the food insecure population to 6 million and predicted that the number would grow even larger as humanitarian aid became more difficult to deliver.

In part to alleviate shortages caused by the bombings, resulting dislocations, and the collapse of civic order, the United States began a program of food relief through airdrops. The packages, labeled "Food gifts from the people of the United States of America," contained freeze-dried lentil soup, beef stew, peanut butter, jelly, crackers, some spices, and a set of plastic utensils, and provided one day's food ration for an adult—about 2,200 calories. Beginning in October 2001, airplanes dropped about

35,000 food packages a day. The quantities alone suggested that their purpose had more to do with politics than food security.[41] A British commentator did the calorie counts:

> If you believe, as some commentators do, that this is an impressive or even meaningful operation, I urge you to conduct a simple calculation. The United Nations estimates that there are 7.5 [million] hungry people in Afghanistan. If every ration pack reached a starving person, then one two hundredth of the vulnerable were fed by the humanitarian effort on Sunday. . . . But the purpose of the food drops is not to feed the starving but to tell them they are being fed. President Bush explained on Sunday that by means of these packages, "the oppressed people of Afghanistan will know the generosity of America and our allies.[42]

Even with a possible exaggeration of the extent of food insecurity, this comment suggests that food aid is a complicated business, and at best a temporary expedient. One problem is getting dropped food to the people who need it most. Figure 29 illustrates the fate of some of the food aid packages. As often happens, enterprising people collect the packages and sell them on the open market; this gets the food into public circulation, but at a price. In this instance, the packages also encountered unexpected safety hazards. The Pentagon warned that the Taliban might try to poison the packages or spread rumors of poisoning as a means of propaganda against the United States, but Taliban leaders denied this accusation: "No one can be that brutal and ignorant as to poison his own people."[43] The packages themselves presented hazards. They were packed in specially designed plywood containers that could be dropped from 30,000 feet without breaking, but several landed in the wrong place and destroyed people's homes. Children sent to collect the food packages died or lost limbs when they ran across fields planted with land mines. While the food drop was in progress, the political situation made it impossible for food aid to get into the country through conventional routes. Later, warlords stole shipments, and riots broke out when supplies ran out.[44] Political stability depends on food security, and food security is inextricably linked to political stability. Without such stability, food aid alleviates a small part of the humanitarian crisis—better than nothing, but never a long-term solution.[45]

Would increasing the amount of food aid alleviate the crisis? Former Senator George McGovern, U.S. ambassador to the World Food Programme said, "If these people have nourishment for healthy lives, this is less fertile territory for cultivation by terrorist leaders." Bringing in another issue germane to this book, he said that the war on hunger in

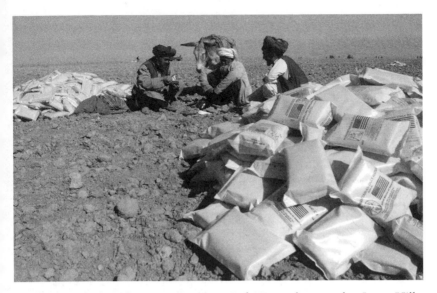

FIGURE 29. On October 13, 2001, *New York Times* photographer James Hill took this photograph of U.S. "Humanitarian Daily Rations" dropped over Afghanistan. The photograph appeared in the Week in Review section on October 21. Mr. Hill said the food packets were available in local markets for the equivalent of 60 cents each. (*Photographer's Journal: War Is a Way of Life*, November 19, 2001. Online: www.nytimes.com/photojournal. © 2001 New York Times Photo Archive. Used with permission.)

Afghanistan and elsewhere cannot be waged without *biotechnology*: "It is probably true that affluent countries can afford to reject scientific agriculture and pay more for food produced by so-called natural methods. But the 800 million poor, chronically hungry people of Asia, Africa and Latin America cannot afford such foods."[46] As we have seen, biotechnology is still a remote solution to food security problems, and it is difficult to imagine how it might have alleviated immediate food shortages in Afghanistan.

While aid agencies were attempting to deal with that situation, food security in the United States shifted to another aspect of its broader meaning: protecting the food supply against terrorists. Officials soon identified safe food and water as key components of "homeland security," as indicated by the rather frightening chart that appeared soon after the attacks (see figure 30). The chart demonstrates that security in this sense is no simple matter, as it requires the cooperation of nearly four-dozen federal bureaucracies to protect the nation's borders, nuclear power

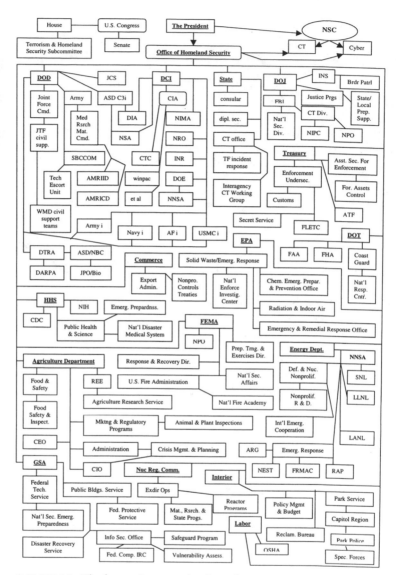

FIGURE 30. The byzantine organization of government units participating in the Office of Homeland Security. Agencies of the Department of Health and Human Services (shown here as HHS) appear
immediately above those of the Agriculture Department (USDA) on
the left side of the diagram. The Food and Drug Administration (of
DHHS) is conspicuously absent as a separate entity on this chart,
despite its responsibility for the safety of three-fourths of the food
supply, domestic and imported. (© 2001 Dr. Jay Jakub & The
Monterey Institute of International Studies. Used with permission.)

plants, and public facilities; fight bioterrorism; obtain intelligence; and protect food and water supplies. Whether this chart demonstrates the need for coordination—or its impossibility—is a matter of interpretation, but one aspect is striking: the minimal role allotted to the Department of Health and Human Services (DHHS). Although the DHHS secretary announced that his agency "was more fearful about the safety of the American food supply than anything else," one critical piece of his domain is noticeably missing: the FDA—the agency responsible for the safety of 75% of foods, domestic and imported. In contrast, the USDA receives detailed attention, perhaps indicating the relative degree to which the two agencies command the respect of Congress.[47]

Food as a Biological Weapon

A second result of the events of fall 2001 is heightened awareness of the possibility that terrorists might deliberately poison food and water supplies. Protection against food bioterrorism is difficult because of the long list of agents that can be used as bioweapons and the vast number of possibilities for delivering them. Experts point to the increasing centralization of the food supply as a factor increasing its vulnerability to sabotage. If, as mentioned in chapter 1, an accidental contamination of ice cream with *Salmonella* can make hundreds of thousands of people ill, it is easy to imagine the damage that could be caused by deliberate tampering.[48] The low rate of inspection of imported foods is an especially weak link in the chain of protection. Well before he was appointed director of the Office of Public Health Preparedness, Dr. Donald Henderson, an expert on infectious diseases, smallpox eradication, and now bioterrorism, wrote: "Of the weapons of mass destruction (nuclear, chemical, and biological), the biological ones are the most greatly feared, but the country is least well prepared to deal with them."[49]

Of particular concern is the role of biotechnology in developing weapons of bioterrorism. The research methods used to transmit desired genes into plants could easily be adapted for nefarious purposes: creating pathogenic bacteria resistant to multiple antibiotics or able to synthesize lethal toxins, or superweeds resistant to herbicides. As half the nation's soybeans resist Roundup, genetic mischief could do a great deal of damage. On this point, Dr. Henderson commented, "At least 10 countries are now engaged in developing and producing biological weapons. What with the growing power of biotechnology, one has to anticipate that this technology, like all others before it, will eventually be misused."[50]

Public health experts concerned about such possibilities cite prece-
dents, ancient and modern, for the use of poisoned food and drink to
achieve political ends. The Athenians forced Socrates to drink hemlock;
Shakespeare's Queen Gertrude succumbed to poisoned wine intended for
Hamlet; the Borgias were notorious for their deft poisoning of political
opponents. Medieval leaders of church and state employed tasters to protect against precisely such activities. As such examples demonstrate, foodborne biological weapons do not need to be confined to wartime but can
be used to achieve more personal political objectives.[51] Modern instances
also abound. In 1997, an evidently disgruntled U.S. laboratory employee
sent electronic mail messages inviting coworkers to partake of dough-
nuts; his message failed to mention that he had laced his treats with a
particularly virulent type of *Shigella,* and 45 people became ill. Also in
the U.S., during the 2001 December holidays, nearly 300,000 pounds of
ham products had to be recalled because an angry employee spiked them
with nails, screws, and other nonfood materials.[52] A review of such
episodes, published early in 2001, describes poisonings of water at German prisoner-of-war camps with arsenic, Israeli citrus fruit with mercury, and Chilean grapes with cyanide, suggesting that no food or drink
is invulnerable to such contamination.[53]

Far-fetched as it may seem, the single known case of food terrorism
designed to achieve political goals in the United States involved the deliberate poisoning of salad bars with *Salmonella.* This widely cited incident occurred in 1984 soon after followers of the Indian guru Bhagwan
Shree Rajneesh established communal headquarters in a small rural town
in Oregon. Followers were easily identifiable by their red clothing, red
beads, and aggressive interactions with neighbors, and they soon came
into conflict over issues related to land use and building permits. To keep
local residents from voting in an election for county commissioners who
might enforce zoning laws, members of the commune sprinkled *Salmonella* over salad bars and into cream pitchers at 10 restaurants, thereby
making at least 750 people sick.

This incident taught many lessons, not least that biological agents are
easy to use and to obtain: the commune clinic merely ordered them from
a biological supply house. Investigators had serious problems tracing the
source of contamination, however. For one thing, they could not imagine that the poisonings were deliberate; nobody claimed responsibility,
no motive was evident, and no such incident had been reported previously. They only were able to identify the perpetrators when one con-
fessed. Officials also decided that publicity about the outbreak might in-

cite copycat behavior and did not publish their findings until 1997. The incident became a classic example of how bioterrorism—even when causing no loss of life—can induce havoc. Although none of the victims died, 45 were hospitalized, and all but one of the affected restaurants soon went out of business.[54]

Beyond this example, the threat of food bioterrorism for political purposes remains theoretical. Nevertheless, fears of that possibility induce a wide range of responses, among them exploitation—the promotion and sale of unproved remedies. One practitioner, for example, suggests vitamin C as an alternative to vaccinations and antibiotics for bioterrorist-induced smallpox or anthrax: "Vitamin C . . . should prove highly effective against both of these conditions. I say 'should' only because their rareness has prevented any single vitamin C researcher from encountering enough cases to conduct a meaningful study and publish it. However, the likelihood that both of these conditions could be completely cured, even in their advanced stages, is compelling."[55] Largely as a result of such misleading suggestions, the National Center for Complementary and Alternative Medicine informs visitors to its Web site that no herbal or vitamin products can protect against bioterrorism, and the Federal Trade Commission sends warning letters to Web sites that make unsupportable claims that products such as oregano oil, coconut oil, or zinc mineral water protect against bioweapons.[56]

Although experts agree that such products are ineffective, they profoundly disagree about the degree of danger posed by food bioterrorism and the extent to which the country should devote resources to guard against it. Some believe that the food supply remains too diffuse to permit terrorists to harm very many people at one time, and that the water supply is even less vulnerable—for reasons of dilution, chlorination, sunlight, and filtration. They prefer to approach the problem from a public health standpoint and to determine the most important food safety risks and the ways those can best be addressed. They emphasize the vastly greater harm caused by foodborne microbes, tobacco, and inappropriate use of antibiotics in animal agriculture, and suggest that applying scarce resources to these problems—rather than to the frightening but much smaller risk of bioterrorism—will ultimately save more lives. As one group puts the matter, "Our security will be better enhanced by primary prevention of war and terrorism than by military counterattacks and reactive preparedness efforts. Instead of engendering fear of bioterrorism, let's build a health care system that can handle the real health crises that we face."[57] In this view, national preparedness against food bioterrorism inappropriately diverts resources from seeking solutions to more compelling food safety problems. Such perspectives are grounded in studies of risk communication. In their 1982 analysis of risk and culture referred to in the introductory chapter, Mary Douglas and Aaron Wildavsky said: "Risk aversion is a preoccupation with anticipating danger that leads to large-scale organization and centralization of power in order to mobilize massive resources against possible evils. The probability that any known danger will occur declines because of anticipatory measures. But the probability that if the unexpected happens it will prove catastrophic increases, because resources required for response have been used up in anticipation."[58]

Ensuring Food Security: A Single Food Agency

One repeated suggestion for a better method to address food safety problems is to centralize their oversight in a single administrative unit. Soon after the September 2001 events, officials throughout government agencies called on Congress to fund improvements in food safety and public health systems, especially those involving disease surveillance, food production quality control, food security (in the antibioterrorism sense), and inspection of imported foods.[59] The GAO pointed out that the threat of bioterrorism provided further evidence for the need to create a single food agency, and the Senate held hearings to debate that suggestion. While mulling over (or dismissing) the merits of this idea, Congress increased funding to allow the FDA to hire inspectors so the agency could double its capacity to oversee the safety of imported foods—from 1% to 2% of the total entering the country. The FDA asked for additional authority: to issue recalls, and to require food companies to increase preparedness against sabotage and demonstrate the traceability of ingredients and products. The consumer advocacy organization Center for Science in the Public Interest (CSPI) supported these requests, saying, "The success of such efforts would benefit from measures that CSPI has advocated for years—measures thwarted by the lobbying power of the food industry. If there has ever been a time to put safety before profits, it is now."[60]

At the Senate hearings, however, food industry officials flatly opposed such measures on the grounds that they would be expensive to implement and would force companies to open their books to federal regulators. One official of the Grocery Manufacturers of America said, "Before we scrap a system that is regarded as the best in the world, we should fully explore strategies to enhance the current system, through adequate funding, better coordination, and continued innovation"; another said, "I think we've already got the system in place to deal with terrorism. . . . We just need more information from the government to make sure we can address any potential threat."[61] Officials of the National Food Processors Association (NFPA) insisted that mandatory recall authority was not needed because its members were already recalling products. Instead, the only action needed is to

> heighten awareness of food security issues on the part of the food industry, across the board, while at the same time not increasing anxiety on the part of consumers. . . . Our current food safety system not only works, but works well. . . . We strongly believe that the best way to improve our nation's already admirable record on food safety is to continue progress towards a unified science- and risk-based food safety policy, including increased communications and improved coordination, rather than focusing on the creation of a new bureaucracy in the form of a single food agency.[62]

Instead, the NFPA preferred another strategy. It called on food industry trade groups to help create an Alliance for Food Security, a coalition of 80 food companies, government agencies, and public health groups united in encouraging federal agencies to cooperate and provide information about measures to enhance food safety. The alliance would develop guidance materials to help members "prevent—to the extent we can—threats from occurring to the safety of our nation's food supply . . . [and provide] a vital comprehensive, and cooperative forum for industry and government at all levels to effectively enhance and augment—where necessary—our food security systems."[62] At least 18 trade associations representing every conceivable facet of food processing and marketing used such arguments and alliances to try to persuade legislators to drop provisions in bioterrorism bills that might give the FDA further authority over domestic and imported foods.[63] While the bills were under consideration, both the FDA and USDA issued nonbinding guidelines for importers and domestic food producers, processors, transporters, and retailers. Table 14 summarizes just a few of the FDA's suggestions. Many of these measures seem more appropriate to penal institutions and are especially disturbing for what they conspicuously fail to mention—Pathogen Reduction: HACCP. Perhaps because following the advice is voluntary, the NFPA praised the FDA guidelines for "not identifying weaknesses in the system that could help terrorists and for giving companies flexibility in adopting security measures."[64]

In the early months of 2002, Congress worked on antibioterrorism legislation to increase the FDA's capacity to inspect imported food and

TABLE 14. FDA advice to food importers, producers, processors, transporters, and retailers about how to prevent problems with food security, 2002

Screen employees and check immigration status.

Establish an employee identification system.

Watch for unusual behavior (staying late, arriving early, removing documents, asking inappropriate questions).

Restrict personal items allowed (purses, lunches).

Inspect personal items.

Change locks when employees leave.

Inspect products for authenticity and package integrity.

Ensure that suppliers are known to practice appropriate food security measures.

Inspect incoming vehicles.

Secure and supervise mailrooms.

Restrict access by visitors.

Restrict access to computer systems.

Protect the perimeter; secure doors.

Notify authorities of evidence of unusual behavior, tampering, or sabotage.

SOURCE: FDA. *Food Security Preventive Measures Guidance,* January 9, 2002. Online: www.fda.gov.

allow the agency to detain suspect foods without a court order, and to require food companies to register and open their records to government inspectors. Industry groups such as the NFPA, the Grocery Manufacturers of America, and the Food Marketing Institute lobbied against these provisions and requested exemptions for their members, arguing that any new legislation would be "a vehicle for a huge expanse in federal power."[65] When the final bill sailed through the House and Senate, industry groups called it "much improved," no doubt because the bill required the FDA to put the new regulations through a standard rulemaking process and delay their implementation for another 18 months.[66]

Food Security as a Public Health Issue

Soon after the September 2001 terrorist attacks, commentators identified at least one cause of the nation's inability to respond adequately to such crises: years of neglecting the public health "infrastructure"—the oversight systems and personnel needed to track and prevent disease. The focus on "homeland security," they said, although perhaps politically necessary to allay public anxiety, diverted attention and resources away from basic public health needs. International actions also focused on matters other than public health, even when providing food aid. No responses to the crisis—domestic or international—were addressing "root causes"— the underlying social, cultural, economic, or environmental factors that might encourage terrorist activities. From the perspective of public health, bioterrorism may never entirely disappear, but it seems less likely to be used as a political weapon by people who have access to education, health care, and food, and who trust their governments to help improve their lot in life. If, as many believe, terrorism reflects frustration resulting from political and social inequities, it is most likely to thrive in countries that fail to provide access to basic needs, or that give lesser rights to ethnic, religious, or other minority groups. In such situations, public health can be a useful means to strengthen society as well as to avert terrorism.

The recent history of Afghanistan illustrates these points. Its health care system is poor by any standard, and its high infant mortality rate is approached by only one other country (Pakistan) outside of sub-Saharan Africa. As noted earlier, malnutrition is widespread, in part because only slightly more than one-tenth of the population has access to clean water supplies (contaminated water induces diarrheal and other infectious diseases that, in turn, contribute to malnutrition). In this situation, advised Richard Horton, editor of the *Lancet*, "Attacking hunger, disease, poverty, and social exclusion might do more good than air marshals, asylum restrictions, and identity cards. Global security will be achieved only by building stable and strong societies."[67]

Because a healthy population is an essential factor in economic development, the health effects of globalization—positive and negative— become important concerns. Globalization has improved the social, dietary, and material resources of many populations, but it has also heightened economic and health inequities. Globalization brings safe drinking water and antibiotics, but it also brings pressures to reduce food safety standards, protect intellectual property rights, and accept the marketing of high-profit "junk" foods. Food shortages are of particular concern for at least three reasons: their harm to health, their destabilizing effects on civil order and economic development, and, not least, their breach of the social contract in which food security—in every sense of the term— is a basic human right.[68]

With these ideas in mind, the American Public Health Association suggests short- and long-term strategies to prevent terrorism and its adverse health consequences: address poverty, social injustice, and disparities; provide humanitarian assistance; strengthen the ability of the public health system to respond to terrorism; protect the environment and food and water supplies; and advocate for control and eventual elimination of biological, chemical, and nuclear weapons.[69] Writer Laurie Garrett explains, "Public health is a bond—a trust—between a government and its people. . . . In return, individuals agree to cooperate by providing tax monies, accepting vaccines, and abiding by the rules and guidelines laid out by government public health leaders. If either side betrays that trust the system collapses like a house of cards." The value of public health approaches, in her view, is to bridge the inequities and help bring a sense of community in which the health of each individual depends on the health of others.[70] This idea makes sense, but it makes even more sense for societies to ensure safe and secure food for all citizens simply because it is the right thing to do.

ENSURING SAFE FOOD

I argue in this book that food safety is a political problem inextricably linked to matters of commerce, trade, and international relations. Ensuring food safety requires much more than following safe handling practices: it requires political action. We have seen how food companies often place commercial interests above those of consumer protection, and how government agencies often support business interests over those of public health. Today, the threat of food bioterrorism—the ultimate dread factor—reveals the importance of closing the long-standing gaps in oversight of food safety.

As consumers, we want to know that our government cares that the food we eat and the water we drink are safe (or safe enough). Given the topics discussed in this book, the FDA is less than reassuring when it tells us, "Consumers are final judges of the safety of the food they buy. . . . If there is any doubt about its safety, don't eat it."[60] Surely, we would feel better if we knew that food companies were doing everything possible to minimize food hazards, and that the government was looking out for our interests and making sure food companies were doing what they were supposed to. In the absence of such reassurance, we lose trust. In the absence of trust, we are most frightened by food hazards that we cannot control: genetically modified foods, mad cow disease, and food bioterrorism, for example.

If food safety is a matter of politics, what kinds of political actions are necessary to ensure safe food and restore trust in our food supply? Table 15 summarizes a few actions that we might demand of the food

TABLE 15. Suggestions for political actions to ensure safe food and improve trust in the food supply

The Food Industry

Accept responsibility for producing safe food.

Develop and follow Pathogen Reduction: HACCP plans at all stages of production, distribution, and service.

Disclose production processes on food labels.

Protect the environment at all stages of production and use.

Adhere to federal regulations for food production, distribution, and service.

Eliminate indiscriminate use of antibiotics in animal agriculture.

Promote high standards for food safety and environmental protection in international trade.

The Federal Government

Create a single food agency.

Institute mechanisms to include the views of consumers when making regulatory decisions.

Provide greater resources for food safety functions of regulatory agencies.

Move congressional funding authority for the FDA from agriculture to health committees.

Authorize regulatory agencies to recall unsafe foods

Require food companies to document the traceability of foods and ingredients.

Require labeling of genetically modified foods.

Support international treaties that protect the environment, public health, and food security (including the right to food as well as food safety).

Strengthen international treaties to prevent development of biological weapons; prohibit the use of genetic engineering for that purpose.

Actively develop and support international policies to promote public health, human rights, and food security in all countries.

The Public

Join consumer groups that promote food safety, environmental protection, and broader aspects of food security.

Advocate for domestic and international programs and policies to ensure safe food, protect the environment, support public health, and guarantee rights to food and food security.

Encourage others to join in such actions.

Elect officials committed to such actions.

industry, our government, and ourselves. We can begin with the food industry: What is reasonable for us to expect from companies that produce, prepare, and distribute our food? Like any other industry, the goals of the food industry are to maximize income by reducing costs and eliminating inconvenient regulatory intervention. It is unrealistic to trust food companies to keep the interests of consumers paramount, and we have seen that they are unlikely to pay much attention to consumer concerns unless forced to by government, public protest, or fear of poor public relations. If food companies want consumers to trust them, they must earn that trust by following the rules, disclosing production practices as well as nutrient contents, taking responsibility for lapses in safety, and telling the truth about matters of public interest. We would be more likely to trust the motives of food companies if they embraced Pathogen Reduction: HACCP, incorporated environmental protection into every stage of production and distribution, argued in international forums for stronger food safety and environmental standards, and worked with— not against—domestic and international regulatory policies.

The government also could do better to ensure safe food and restore trust in the food supply. Congress could help by putting consumer protection first and creating a single food agency with genuine authority over safety in the production and distribution of foods as well as over their effects on environmental and public health. Such an agency could be empowered to promote food security in all of its humanitarian aspects: reliable access, adequate quantity and quality, appropriate cultural relevance, and safety. While thinking about how to develop this agency, Congress could provide greater resources for food inspection, and give existing agencies the authority to enforce regulations, issue recalls, ensure traceability, and protect public health. One measure to reduce political influences on the FDA, for example, would be to transfer its funding decisions from agriculture committees to those devoted to health. Congress also could require genetically modified foods to be labeled— the issue that most inflames public distrust of the food biotechnology industry—and demand that the foods undergo examination of their safety and environmental effects before they are marketed.

On the international level, the government could sign and actively support treaties that promote food safety, environmental protection, and the right to food, as well as agreements to stop producing biological weapons, genetically modified or otherwise. If we are going to protect our country against bioterrorism, our government must become more actively involved in international policies to promote health and food security as human rights for everyone, everywhere.

What can we, as individuals, do to promote such actions? We can join consumer organizations that work for environmental protection, food assistance, public health, and human rights—all of which support food safety as a necessary component of food security. We can advocate for domestic and international programs and policies directed toward those goals, and we can elect officials committed to such purposes. We can explain to our friends and colleagues that the meaning of food safety extends well beyond "cook, chill, clean, separate." Food safety—and food security—are indicators of the integrity of our democratic institutions. They are worth our political commitment.

EPILOGUE

SINCE 2003, WHEN *SAFE FOOD* FIRST APPEARED, FOOD SAFETY ISSUES have evolved against a background of ongoing wars in Iraq and Afghanistan, the rise of China as an economic powerhouse, and deepening international concerns about climate change. Americans experienced revelations of abuses of corporate power, the deflation of the housing bubble, job losses, economic depression, and deep divisions in public opinion about abortion, immigration, and health care. If people now agree about anything, it is that they, as individuals, have little power to affect such events and divisions. In contrast, everyone can do something about food. The food revolution has arrived.

Signs of the food revolution are everywhere, fueled in large part by the writings of Eric Schlosser, Michael Pollan, Alice Waters, and Slow Food's Carlo Petrini. By the end of 2009, Pollan's *Omnivore's Dilemma* had been on the *New York Times* best-seller list for nearly one hundred twenty weeks. Food is now a respectable topic for academic study and much on the public agenda.[1] Food safety ought to be part of this movement. The 2008 election of President Barack Obama inspired hope that improvements in the nation's food system would at last be possible.

THE POLITICS OF FOOD BIOTECHNOLOGY: UPDATE

This book explores the disconnect between science- and value-based views of microbial contaminants and food biotechnology. With respect to genetically modified (GM) foods, what is most remarkable is how little has happened to resolve the disconnect. My shelf of books about GM foods gets longer each year, yet none of them has anything new to say. Agricultural biotechnology companies such as Monsanto and other proponents of GM foods continue to insist that use of this technology is essential for meeting the food needs of the world's expanding population, particularly in developing countries. Opponents continue to ask when the promises of food biotechnology will be fulfilled and to question its purported benefits and safety.[2] Although these conflicting views seem immovable, a few changes have occurred. Let's take a look.

Use of GM Crops

The FDA has been approving GM commodity crops since 1994, yet few are in production today. These few, however, are so widely adopted that virtually all of the corn (85 percent), cotton (88 percent), soybeans (91 percent), and sugar beets (95 percent) planted in the United States are varieties engineered to resist herbicides or insects.[3] Farmers prefer to plant GM varieties because such crops do not need to be treated with pesticides and herbicides as frequently as conventional crops. Farmers also believe that the yields of GM varieties are better. Whether such benefits are real and will last over time remains in dispute.

Despite continued international opposition, GM crops were grown in fifteen developing countries and ten industrial countries in 2008. In 2009, the European Union permitted farmers to plant only one GM crop: corn. Even so, Germany, France, Austria, Greece, Hungary, and Luxembourg banned GM corn, and Monsanto's production of GM wheat also was expected to elicit opposition in foreign markets.[4]

Since 1994, the FDA has approved several GM fruits and vegetables for production and marketing. But were these foods actually for sale in the produce sections of American supermarkets? When researching *What to Eat,* I found no regulator or advocate who knew. Most thought that production failures or consumer opposition kept GM produce off the market. The one GM food that seemed most likely to be available was Hawaiian papaya engineered to resist ringspot virus. In 2005, as I explained in *What to Eat,* I paid a biotechnology testing company, Genetic ID, to check several different kinds of supermarket papayas for modified genes. Indeed, the conventionally grown Hawaiian papayas tested positive. A certified organic Hawaiian papaya did not, and neither did a papaya grown in Jamaica. But because GM foods remain unlabeled, the public has no way to know.

Genetic "Pollution"

In chapter 8, I discuss the travails of the Berkeley plant biology professor Ignacio Chapela, whose article in *Nature* came under attack for demonstrating that genes from GM corn had drifted into native Mexican varieties and that these genes were more unstable than others. *Nature* wished it had never accepted the article and said so publicly. Berkeley denied tenure to Professor Chapela, but later granted it after extensive protest. That the criticism of his work was the result of politics—not science—became evident when *Nature* reported that other researchers had confirmed some of his findings. Eventually, *Nature* suggested, he would probably be proved right on all counts. Nevertheless, researchers who published more recent studies critical of agricultural biotechnology have also experienced unusually forceful attacks on the quality of their work by company and other pro-GM scientists.[5]

Roundup-Resistant "Superweeds"

Late in 2004, weeds resistant to Monsanto's herbicide Roundup began appearing in GM plantings in Georgia and soon spread to other Southern states. By 2009, more than one hundred thousand acres in Georgia were infested with Roundup-resistant pigweed. Planters were advised to apply multiple herbicides, thereby defeating the point of Roundup: to reduce chemical applications. In 2009, a supposedly inert surfactant in Roundup was found to kill human embryonic tissue cells. More than 250 environmental, health, and labor groups petitioned the EPA to take a closer look at the safety of solvents, preservatives, and surfactants in agricultural chemicals. "Inert" ingredients could no longer be considered benign.[6]

Golden Rice

Golden Rice (discussed in chapter 5) is the most prominent example of the public benefits of agricultural biotechnology, but ten years after its initial construction it remains a promise unfulfilled. Field trials began in 2008 and its developers hope they can produce the rice by 2011. In the interim, researchers reengineered the rice to contain higher levels of beta-carotene and demonstrated that people who ate it could, as expected, convert beta-carotene to vitamin A. Supporters of Golden Rice continue to complain about the impossible demands of regulators and antibiotechnology advocates. Advocates continue to argue that GM crops are unnecessary and threaten indigenous food security. The Gates Foundation is now the major funder of GM projects involving nutrient-enriched indigenous crops. Such technological approaches, advocates maintain, are doomed to fail unless they also address the underlying social causes of food insecurity and malnutrition.[7]

rBGH (Recombinant Bovine Growth Hormone)

Milk from cows treated with rBGH has become the flashpoint for concerns about GM foods and a major public incentive to choose organic dairy foods; the USDA's organic rules expressly forbid use of hormones and GM technology. Late in 2009, many countries continued to ban rBGH. In the United States, several states introduced legislation to allow GM-free labels, particularly on organic and other untreated dairy foods. In response, Monsanto organized a pro-rBGH public relations campaign that included its own "grassroots" organization. A spokesman for that group complained that critics of rBGH were backed by Consumers Union and PETA (People for the Ethical Treatment of Animals), "who make a profit, living and business by striking fear in citizens." Perhaps, but widespread public opposition to rBGH induced mainstream food processors and retailers such as Dannon, General Mills, and Walmart to stop buying rBGH-milk and to require suppliers to guarantee milk as GM-free: "We've done focus groups, and people don't want it."[8] Without a mass market for rBGH milk, use of this hormone seems unlikely to continue.

GM Labeling

As predicted, the failure to label GM foods continues to pose problems for the public and for industry. Because the vast majority of processed foods contain unlabeled GM oil, protein, or sweetener ingredients, organic foods are viewed as an increasingly attractive option. Organic suppliers such as Whole Foods, concerned that GM pollution might destroy consumer trust in organics, created the Non-GMO Project: "Our shared belief is that everyone deserves an informed choice about whether or not to consume genetically modified products." The Non-GMO Project seal guarantees a GM level of no more than 0.9 percent, the standard used in Europe, where higher percentages require labeling.[9]

In Europe, McDonald's has gone GM-free. In 2009, I collected McDonald's brochures in England and Italy that read, "We'd like to reassure you that we don't use any GM products or ingredients containing GM material in our food." In contrast, Hershey's British products use GM ingredients and say so. The company labels Reese's Nutrageous candy bars: "Contains: Peanuts, Genetically Modified Sugar, Soya and Corn."

Labeling may be a problem easily solved, but positions on GM foods are unlikely to budge until the benefits of food biotechnology are seen to accrue to the public as well as to the food biotechnology industry.

THE POLITICS OF MICROBIAL FOOD SAFETY: UPDATE

In contrast, since this book first appeared, value-based views of microbial contamination have shifted somewhat toward science-based views as a result of a seemingly unending series of outbreaks and recalls. Microbes continue to account for massive illness in the United States. Although noroviruses remain the leading cause, toxic forms of *Salmonella* and *E. coli* get far more attention, perhaps because they cause more serious harm to health and show up in the riskiest foods: meat, poultry, and produce.[10]

The Politics of Raw

The most prominent examples of recent clashes between science and values are those involving raw foods, particularly milk and oysters.

The Raw Milk Debates. Although dairy foods account for only 3 percent of reported cases of foodborne illness, a whopping 71 percent of those cases are caused by pathogens in raw milk.[11] Raw milk creates little dread or outrage in the public, but it enormously distresses health officials. Because pathogens are easily killed by pasteurization, deaths caused by pathogens in raw milk are easily prevented.

Safety scientists are baffled by the raw food movement, whose constituents believe—against all evidence—that raw milk is healthier and safer than pasteurized milk. To read the statements of raw milk advocates is to enter a parallel universe in which the usual standards of scientific judgment are thoroughly discounted. Such views are most prominently expressed by the Weston Price Foundation, named after the author of *Nutrition and Physical Degeneration* (1939). With considerable justification, Price argued that many of today's chronic diseases could be prevented by avoiding highly processed and refined foods.

The foundation, however, interprets this advice as "avoid pasteurization." It recommends "raw whole milk from grass-fed cows ... produced under clean conditions and promptly refrigerated." One would hope that by "clean conditions" the foundation means a HACCP plan (discussed in chapters 2 and 3), but it does not say so. Instead it says that "natural protective systems can be overwhelmed, and the milk contaminated, in situations conducive to filth and disease. Know your farmer!" Raw milk, it says, contains many antimicrobial and immune-supporting components (but, I would add, so does pasteurized milk). The foundation argues that grass feeding is healthier for cows, as well it may be. But researchers find grass-fed cattle capable of shedding almost as much *E. coli* O157:H7 as those in feedlots. To the question "Is it safe to consume raw milk?" the FDA's answer is blunt: "No. Raw milk is inherently dangerous and it should not be consumed by anyone at any time for any purpose."[12]

For proponents of raw milk, the issue is not safety; it is values and personal choice. Demand for raw milk is increasing and mail-order sales thrive. Although more than half the states allow raw milk to be sold within their territory, federal rules prohibit shipping of raw milk between states. Mail-order companies can get around this restriction by marketing raw milk as pet food. Raw milk is sold through pet food outlets and also through use of clandestine codes, cash transactions, secret drop-off points, buyers clubs, and cow-sharing programs. Are such programs safe? Although most raw milk does not cause illness, the CDC regularly reports outbreaks caused by pathogens in raw milk. Other values come into play when such pathogens are responsible for the death of a child fed raw milk from a cow share.[13] When belief systems are at stake, science-based arguments rarely work. A better strategy might be to legalize raw milk production but regulate its safety. Some raw milk producers voluntarily use HACCP plans. The FDA could require such plans and also require testing for pathogens. But doing so would undoubtedly elicit a level of opposition similar to that confronted by the FDA when it attempted to regulate the safety of raw oysters.

The Raw Oyster Debates. For more than a decade, the FDA has been trying to prevent deaths caused by *Vibrio vulnificus* bacteria that contaminate raw oysters grown in the Gulf of Mexico. These "flesh-eating" bacteria proliferate in warm months and are especially deadly; they kill half of the thirty or so people who develop infections from them each year. Such people tend to have weakened immune systems or chronic diseases, but often do not realize they are at risk.

In 2001, the oyster industry trade association, the Interstate Shellfish Sanitation Conference (ISSC), promised the FDA that the industry would substantially reduce *Vibrio* infections in oysters within seven years through a program of voluntary self-regulation and education aimed at high-risk groups. If this program failed to reduce the infection rate, the ISSC agreed that the FDA could require oysters to be treated after harvesting to kill pathogenic *Vibrio*.[14]

Treatment, in this case, means postharvest processing through techniques such as quick freezing, frozen storage, high hydrostatic pressure, mild heat, or low-dose gamma irradiation, any of which reduces *Vibrio vulnificus* to undetectable levels. By most reports, the effect of treatment on the taste and texture of oysters is slight, although raw oyster aficionados argue otherwise. In 2003, California refused to allow Gulf Coast oysters to enter the state unless they had undergone postharvest processing. The result? Sales of oysters remained the same but oyster-related deaths dropped to zero.

In contrast, states that did not require postharvest processing experienced no change in the number of deaths, meaning that the ISSC program had failed. Late in 2009, Michael Taylor, whom we met in chapters 2 and 7, reappeared in his newly appointed position as senior advisor to the FDA. In an almost exact reprise of his 1994 speech to the cattle industry about the need to regulate *E. coli* in ground beef, he informed participants at an ISSC meeting that the FDA intended to issue rules requiring postharvest processing of Gulf Coast oysters in summer months.[15]

But less than one month later, the FDA backed off. It said it would postpone the oyster-processing rules indefinitely:

> Since making its initial announcement, the FDA has heard from Gulf Coast oyster harvesters, state officials, and elected representatives from across the region about the feasibility of implementing post-harvest processing or other equivalent controls by the summer of 2011. These are legitimate concerns. It is clear to the FDA from our discussions to date that there is a need to further examine both the process and timing for large and small oyster harvesters to gain access to processing facilities or equivalent controls in order to address this important public health goal. Therefore, before proceeding, we will conduct an independent study to assess how post-harvest processing or other equivalent controls can be feasibly implemented in the Gulf Coast in the fastest, safest and most economical way.[16]

Apparently, fifteen or more *preventable* deaths every year are not enough to elicit preventive action by industry or the FDA. Despite years of warning and unmet promises, this industry was able to induce Congress to force the FDA to back down, thereby raising uncomfortable questions about the new administration's ability to improve the safety of the nation's food supply.

Outbreaks and Major Recalls

During the mid-2000s, the United States experienced an astonishing sequence of foodborne outbreaks, each with unique revelations of safety failures followed by calls for regulation, largely unheeded. Despite lack of recall authority, the FDA and the USDA frequently announced "voluntary" recalls. In July 2009, for example, the FDA announced fifty-six voluntary food recalls or market withdrawals because of health risk or mislabeling. The USDA announced four: pork skins (no inspection) and ground beef and dry milk contaminated with *Salmonella* or *E. coli* O157:H7. Some outbreaks involved hundreds of cases of illness dispersed among many states. These required the CDC to conduct intense investigations, not always successfully.[17]

Table 16 summarizes some of the most prominent incidents from 2006 to 2009. Each of these incidents reveals key flaws in the present food safety system and the need for legislative measures to address these flaws.

2006: Spinach (E. coli O157:H7). This outbreak was notable for the trouble it caused and its source. Of the 205 people who became ill, about 30 developed hemolytic uremia syndrome, and three died. The source was a widely distributed Dole brand of bagged baby spinach packed by Natural Selection Foods, a company run by Earthbound Farms, a leading supplier of organic vegetables. Because the packing plant washed the spinach thoroughly, the company and growers were shocked to learn that washing was insufficient to remove the pathogen. Growers also were shocked by the subsequent losses of sales, estimated at $100 million. By 2009, spinach sales had not yet returned to pre-outbreak levels.[18]

Investigators traced the spinach to a particular field in the middle of a cattle ranch one mile away from a stream used by the free-range cattle as a crossing. They isolated the outbreak *E. coli* strain from stream water, cattle feces, and the feces of wild boar at the crossing, but found none in the spinach field. Contaminated water from the cattle crossing seemed a likely source, as did wild boar. Investigators sampled wild animals in the area and found the outbreak strain in cattle (34 percent of samples), wild boar (15 percent), water, and soil, but in no other animals. Later, the California Department of Fish and Game found the strain in only one of 184 wild boar. Investigators concluded that "no definitive determination could be made regarding how *E. coli* O157:H7 pathogens contaminated spinach in this outbreak."[19]

But how had the bacteria survived washing? The packing plant used state-of-the-art washing procedures under a HACCP plan. Investigations revealed only minor procedural flaws. Although this was the twentieth *E. coli* O157:H7 outbreak from leafy greens in recent years, nobody seemed to have come to grips with how firmly these bacteria adhere to leaf surfaces. They can be incorporated into lettuce or spinach leaves just under the surface and form tightly adhering biofilms.[20]

Although the spinach was marketed as conventional, industrial growers immediately blamed the outbreak on manure-based fertilizers used in organic production. In October 2006, I wrote an opinion piece for the *San Jose Mercury News* listing the obvious lessons taught by the outbreak—prevention is essential, voluntary never works, industrial agriculture has its down side—among them, "don't blame organics this time."[21] A vegetable grower in California soon set me straight. He knew that the spinach was in the second year of the three-year transition required for organic certification. Even so, manure was probably not the source, as no trace of the outbreak strain appeared on the spinach field.

Early in 2007, I visited Earthbound Farms and its packing plant and met with its microbiological consultant. The company had instituted test-and-hold procedures to prevent contaminated produce from coming into or leaving the plant. Such practices should be standard for this industry. California now requires the leafy greens industry to use good manufacturing practices (GMPs), but these are voluntary. The FDA, which had been advising lettuce growers to use GMPs for years, extended its voluntary guidance to spinach.[22]

In spring 2007, I attended a meeting of California vegetable producers at which Bill Marler, an attorney who represents victims of foodborne illness, challenged growers to "put me out of business." He warned that voluntary actions would not succeed and nothing short of mandatory federal regulations would be effective, not least because of the high human costs of foodborne illness. One of his spinach clients spent 51 days in the hospital and 18 days on dialysis, with medical bills of $500,000.[23]

Regulations are politically unpopular. They are difficult to implement, generate costs, and are not always applied fairly or consistently. But without accountability and enforcement, nothing stops outbreaks from occurring. Without a congressional mandate to take stronger action, the FDA again in July 2009 issued guidance to the producers of lettuce and spinach, necessarily voluntary and nonbinding.[24]

TABLE 16. Selected examples of food recalls and outbreaks of foodborne illness in the United States, 2006–2009

Year	Product (Manufacturer)	Contaminant	Health Consequences	Scope
2006	Spinach, fresh (Dole, packed by Natural Selection Foods, San Juan Bautista, CA)	*E. coli* O157:H7	205 illnesses: 103 hospitalizations, 3 deaths	26 states
	Iceberg lettuce, Taco Bell restaurants	*E. coli* O157:H7	71 illnesses: 53 hospitalizations	5 states
2007	Pet food (Menu Foods, Canada)	Melamine	Illnesses and deaths of undetermined numbers of cats and dogs	60 million cans and pouches
	Ground beef (Cargill)	*E. coli* O157:H7	At least 13 illnesses	4 states 845,000 lbs (first recall); 1,084,000 lbs (second recall)
2008	Beef, raw and frozen (Hallmark/Westland)	Mad cow disease (nonambulatory cattle)	None recorded	143 million lbs
	Jalapeño peppers (maybe tomatoes)	*Salmonella* Saintpaul	1,442 illnesses	43 states, DC, Canada
2009	Peanut butter (Peanut Corporation of America, Blakely, GA)	*Salmonella* Typhimurium	714 illnesses: 171 hospitalizations, ~9 deaths	~4,000 products 46 states, Canada
	Pistachio nuts (Setton Pistachio, Terra Bella, CA)	*Salmonella* (multiple strains)	None recorded	~2 million pounds, 664 products
	Raw cookie dough (Nestlé Toll House)	*E. coli* O157:H7	80 illnesses: 35 hospitalizations	31 states
	Ground beef (Beef Packers, Inc, Fresno, CA, owned by Cargill)	*Salmonella* Newport (antibiotic-resistant)	28 illnesses	3 states 826,000 lbs

2006: Iceberg Lettuce, Taco Bell (E. coli O157:H7). This incident exposed the challenges faced by investigators looking for the source of outbreaks caused by restaurant meals. Late in 2006, nine of eleven people in New Jersey who became ill from foodborne *E. coli* said they had eaten at a Taco Bell restaurant. Because meat is cooked—a kill step—investigators focused on foods eaten raw: cilantro, cheese, green onions, yellow onions, tomatoes, and shredded lettuce. These came from a central distributor and were difficult to trace, but Taco Bell reported finding *E. coli* O157:H7 in green onions from a California supplier. It removed the onions from its restaurants and stopped the supply chain.[25]

The company also launched a public relations offensive. It bought full-page advertisements, sent out news releases, and conducted nearly a thousand interviews with the media. Its president explained, "Neither the health department nor we know what caused [the outbreak]. Not everybody that got sick ate at Taco Bell." A manager said, "We're losing money for no reason. . . . Nobody found anything and nobody proved anything."[26]

What food was the source? Federal investigators did their own testing, cleared green onions, and identified the outbreak strain in one sample of yellow onions. The CDC identified foods eaten more frequently by people who had become ill—lettuce, cheddar cheese, and ground beef—and guessed that lettuce was the most likely source. Because multiple Taco Bell outlets were involved, the lettuce must have been contaminated early in the distribution chain. With that uncertain speculation, the CDC investigations concluded.[27]

Calls for regulation followed. Eric Schlosser wrote, "Aside from industry lobbyists and their Congressional allies, there is little public support for the right to sell contaminated food. Whether you're a Republican or a Democrat, you still have to eat." A *New York Times* editorial said, "Surely it is time to give government regulators the power and resources they need to ensure the safety of fresh fruits and vegetables."[28] Representatives introduced food safety bills in Congress. None passed.

2007: Pet Foods (Melamine). In March 2007, Menu Foods, a Canadian pet food manufacturer, recalled a record-breaking sixty million cans and pouches sold under ninety-five brand names.[29] Although this incident involved pet, not human, food, it was such a stunning example of safety systems gone awry that I thought it deserved book-length analysis: *Pet Food Politics: The Chihuahua in the Coal Mine* (University of California Press, 2008).

To summarize: Menu Foods obtained two ingredients commonly used to increase the protein content of pet foods, wheat gluten and rice protein concentrate, through a supply chain that began in China. There, manufacturers fraudulently added an industrial chemical, melamine, to wheat flour and sold it as wheat and rice proteins. Melamine is 67 percent nitrogen. Because tests for protein in food actually measure nitrogen, not protein itself, melamine fooled the test and boosted the apparent protein content.

Melamine, a constituent of plastic dinnerware, is toxic only when consumed in large amounts. But when mixed with one of its by-products, cyanuric acid, even small amounts spontaneously form crystals in the urinary tracts of dogs and cats. More than six thousand pet owners participated in class-action lawsuits and were awarded $30 million in judgments. The FDA, which regulates pet food as animal feed, was overwhelmed by calls from distraught pet owners, but its main concern was whether melamine had entered the human food supply, and for good reason. Some of the melamine-tainted pet food had been fed to pigs and chickens, and the false rice protein went into fish feed.

My conclusion: we have only one food supply for pets, people, and farm animals, and it is global. In researching the book, I uncovered a long history of fraudulent use of melamine in fish and animal feed, as well as in pet food in modern China. In *Pet Food Politics,* I argued that safety problems with pet food must be addressed immediately. Otherwise, we must expect similar problems with human food. Hence the book's subtitle, *The Chihuahua in the Coal Mine.*

Nonetheless, even I was taken aback when melamine turned up in Chinese infant formula and caused at least 300,000 illnesses, 50,000 hospitalizations, and six deaths. Chinese manufacturers so commonly used melamine as an adulterant that investigators discovered the chemical in a vast array of milk drinks, coffee drinks, crackers, cookies, and chocolates distributed throughout Asia and elsewhere.[30]

The pet food and infant formula scandals induced the Chinese government to punish perpetrators, sometimes with death sentences, and to enact new food safety laws. Pet food companies initiated routine testing for melamine. The usual calls for regulation followed. Yet two years later, a government review of the FDA's handling of the pet food recalls merely suggested that the agency consider seeking legislative action to give it more effective methods for dealing with recalls.[31]

2007: Ground Beef Products (E. coli O157:H7). This particular recall focused attention on the devastation to affected individuals. It resulted in a $100 million lawsuit filed against Cargill on behalf of an affected young dancer, Stephanie Smith, whose travails were covered extensively by the *New York Times* and other media. But it also focused attention on the meat industry's resistance to pathogen testing as well as to its cozy relationships with USDA inspectors.

As explained in chapter 1, hamburger is typically made from trimmings from multiple animals (sometime hundreds) slaughtered in any number of states. To ensure safety, companies ought to test for pathogens but have little incentive to do so. If they test and find pathogens, they land in "a regulatory situation." As a company official explained to the *New York Times:* "One, I have to tell the government, and two, the government will trace it back to them [the slaughterhouse]. So we don't do that." The USDA, in turn, uses a "restrained approach" to regulation. A USDA official said his agency has the power to require pathogen testing but does not use it. Why not? Because the USDA also takes the companies' needs into consideration: "I have to look at the entire industry, not just what is best for public health."[32]

2008: Ground Beef (Mad Cow Disease). Sometimes, ground beef induces revulsion as well as illness. The "largest to date" recall record set by pet foods did not last long. In February 2008, the Hallmark/Westland Beef Packing Company recalled more than 143 million pounds of raw and frozen beef products produced over a two-year period. An employee of the Humane Society infiltrated the plant and secretly filmed a video ("WARNING: Contains graphic footage") displaying the slaughter of "downer" cows for food as well as other violations of USDA rules.[33]

Older, nonambulatory cattle are at risk for mad cow disease, or BSE (discussed in chapter 8). The USDA secretary said, "It is extremely unlikely that these animals were at risk for BSE because of the multiple safeguards; however, this action is necessary because plant procedures violated USDA regulations." A particular source of concern was that Hallmark/Westland produced ground meat for federal school meals. Although BSE had never been found in U.S. cows, the incident demonstrated links between inhumane treatment of animals and public health.[34]

It also highlighted inadequacies in the USDA's meat inspection system. Insiders complained that inspectors who cite slaughterhouse violations get in trouble with the USDA and are told not to record violations. Representative George Miller (Dem-CA) said the recall "raises alarming questions about the U.S. Department of Agriculture's ability to monitor the safety of meat that is being shipped to our nation's schools. It is outrageous that it took a non-governmental organization to shed light on the egregious abuses that were happening right under the USDA's nose. . . . [The USDA] still can't tell us exactly which schools may have received this tainted meat, or how much of it has already been consumed or re-processed into other foods."[35] Lawsuits followed. Legislation did not.

2008: Peppers, not Tomatoes (Salmonella). This outbreak demonstrated how entire industries can be damaged in the search for a source of foodborne illness. On May 22, 2008, the New Mexico Health Department notified the CDC that several people had been infected with *Salmonella* Saintpaul. Some cases clustered in the Navajo Nation and investigations by the Indian Health Service suggested tomatoes as the likely source. The FDA warned residents of New Mexico and Texas not to eat local raw tomatoes and soon expanded the warning nationally. Restaurant chains stopped serving tomatoes, consumers stopped buying them, and tomato growers lost $200 million in sales.[36]

To verify the source, the CDC conducted seven epidemiologic and environmental investigations, none easy to interpret. Salsa and guacamole were mentioned frequently by people who became ill; these foods contained tomatoes and either raw jalapeño or Serrano peppers. CDC investigators found the outbreak strain in peppers from Mexico. But they continued to consider tomatoes as a possible source until the end of June and did not lift the tomato warning until July 17. By that time, the domestic tomato industry had been virtually destroyed. Also destroyed was a good deal of public confidence in the safety of fresh produce and in government oversight.[37]

Federal officials explained their error: "Local, state, tribal, and federal response capacity often is strained during large and complex outbreaks. . . . This can cause delays."[38] Perhaps, but an analysis of the events by the Pew Charitable Trusts came to tougher conclusions. It questioned why safety officials from two federal and three state agencies insisted that tomatoes were the vector and spoke publicly "with significant variations in facts and messages." It said officials should have learned from previous recalls and charged that despite repeated calls for action, "the establishment of mandatory, enforceable safety standards for the growing, harvesting, processing, and distribution of fresh fruits and vegetables has not happened."[39]

2009: Peanut Butter (Salmonella). Late in 2008, the CDC became aware of clusters of illness caused by *Salmonella* Typhimurium in young and old people in schools or long-term care facilities. In interviews, 86 percent said they had eaten chicken and 77 percent said they had eaten peanut butter. Because frequencies in the general population are 85 percent for eating chicken and 59 percent for eating peanut butter, peanut butter seemed the more likely source. In January 2009, King Nut Companies, a distributor of peanut butter manufactured by the Peanut Corporation of America (PCA), recalled five-pound tubs of the PCA product.[40]

Because peanuts destined for peanut butter are roasted, the contamination must have occurred *after* processing. The plant shipped two kinds of peanut butter: bulk intended for institutions, and ingredients intended for food processors. Samples of both were found to contain the outbreak strain. Eventually, companies recalled nearly four thousand food products containing peanut butter, among them crackers, frozen chicken, emergency disaster rations, and pet foods—so many that the FDA produced an online "widget" to keep track of them.

The politics of this particular incident were especially telling. Investigations revealed that the PCA plant knowingly shipped peanut butter contaminated with *Salmonella*. When tests came back positive, PCA retested the samples. The company operated under GMPs, not HACCP. It had been inspected recently, evidently rather casually.[41]

PCA was involved with regulatory agencies in one other way: the company produced peanuts for export. For reasons of history (see chapter 1), the USDA is responsible for the safety of exported peanuts that might contain aflatoxin. Under pressure from peanut producers, the 2002 Farm Bill specifically exempted the USDA's Peanut Standards Board from conflict-of-interest rules. This exemption permitted the head of PCA to be appointed to that board in 2008 for a term ending in 2011 (he resigned in the wake of the recall). PCA soon filed for bankruptcy, thereby avoiding claims and lawsuits.

Oddly, PCA's plants in Texas and Georgia had organic certification; the organic inspector had issued violation notices but had no authority to close the plants. The FDA asked one recipient of PCA peanuts, WestCo Fruit and Nut Co., to voluntarily recall its products; WestCo refused. The FDA had to serve the company with a warrant and eventually seize the products. This took weeks. In March, the FDA issued after-the-fact advice to the peanut industry—voluntary and nonbinding, of course— about how to produce peanuts safely.[42] Given the casual safety practices of food industries and the overall regulatory vacuum, the satirical newspaper *The Onion* proposed a creative solution to the *Salmonella* problem. It is shown in figure 31.

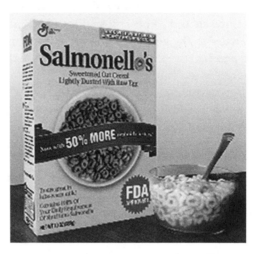

FIGURE 31. "FDA Approves Salmonello's."
Reprinted with permission of *The Onion*.
Copyright © 2009 by Onion, Inc., www
.theonion.com.

This particular recall induced President Obama to signal that his administration intended to take food safety more seriously. In reference to his then seven-year-old daughter, he said: "At bare minimum, we should be able to count on our government keeping our kids safe when they eat peanut butter. That's what Sasha eats for lunch, probably three times a week, and you know I don't want to have to worry about whether she is going to get sick as a consequence of having her lunch."[43]

The new leadership of the FDA also commented on the implications of the peanut butter recalls: "From our vantage point, the recent salmonella outbreak linked to contaminated peanut butter represented far more than a sanitation problem at one troubled facility. It reflected a failure of the FDA and its regulatory partners to identify risk and to establish and enforce basic preventive controls. And it exposed the failure of scores of food manufacturers to adequately monitor the safety of ingredients purchased from this facility."[44]

2009: Pistachios (Salmonella). Late in March 2009, the FDA announced that Setton Pistachios was voluntarily recalling about a million pounds of nuts. The FDA learned about the *Salmonella* problem from Kraft Foods, which sells a pistachio trail mix. Kraft obtained the mix from a small nut company in Illinois, Georgia's Nut, which evidently uses a HACCP plan; the company routinely tests for *Salmonella* and found it in Setton pistachios. Georgia Nut recalled its products and notified Kraft. Kraft informed the FDA and issued its own recall—just the way the food safety system is supposed to work.[45]

Other aspects worked less well. Although its packing plant had passed recent inspections with relatively minor violations, Setton knew it had *Salmonella* problems. When tests came back positive, Setton reheated the nuts but shipped them out without testing to confirm that the bacteria had been killed. The reheated pistachios often were processed on lines used for raw, potentially contaminated nuts. Setton also had a surprising method for handling the recalled nuts: it repackaged them and shipped them out. Other pistachio companies reacted to these revelations by establishing a Web site listing products that had not been recalled.[46]

In this instance, the FDA asked for voluntary recalls before anyone became ill, suggesting that the new management team was serious about prevention. The FDA warned food companies that it expected them to follow voluntary GMPs, explained how to do recalls, and issued guidance to pistachio growers about avoiding contaminants. But without congressional authority to force recalls and stop shipments of potentially contaminated products, the FDA could do little more.[47]

2009: Nestlé's Toll House Cookie Dough (E. coli *O157:H7).* This outbreak demonstrated the inadequacy of warning labels and the compelling need for preventive controls. Cookie dough is not supposed to be eaten raw; it is intended to be baked. Packages are labeled with warnings, usually along the lines of "Bake before enjoying" or, as Nestlé's post-recall packages now say, "Do not consume raw cookie dough." But let's be honest: raw cookie dough is irresistibly delicious. A *Consumer Reports* survey found that 39 percent of respondents admitted to eating dough when they make cookies; surely this underestimates the true percentage.[48]

Companies know that customers eat raw dough. Nestlé said it took special precautions as a result, and investigators were able to identify only minor violations at the plant. Although they found *E. coli* O157:H7 in one dough sample, it was not the outbreak strain. Investigations linked cases of illness to eating the Nestlé dough, but "conclusions could not be made with regard to the root cause of the contamination." The recall cost Nestlé more than $30 million.[49]

To people who became ill after eating raw cookie dough, unsolved mysteries and corporate costs hardly matter. Bill Marler, the lawyer mentioned earlier, describes another client: "I spent most of last week being supportive, but feeling helpless, as a client who ate *E. coli* O157:H7–tainted Nestlé Toll House Cookie Dough, may well be slowly dying after spending over 100 days in the hospital (still there), losing her large intestine and gall bladder, and spending weeks on dialysis. It is crazy that people think a foodborne illness is a 'tummy ache.' "[50]

2009: Ground Beef (Antibiotic-Resistant Salmonella). Throughout the summer of 2009, Colorado health officials were dealing with cases of *Salmonella* infections caused by eating ground beef. The most serious were caused by a strain of *Salmonella* Newport highly resistant to a wide range of common antibiotics. Investigators traced the illnesses to ground beef produced by Beef Packers, Inc., a subsidiary of Cargill. The nearly 826,000-pound recall was especially complicated because the company repackaged the meat into small retail-size units. The USDA's list of receiving retailers fills twenty-four pages.[51]

Beyond generic food safety, this incident raised concerns about additional public health issues: humane treatment of animals, the safety of school meals, and antibiotic resistance in food pathogens. A year earlier, USDA investigators had observed workers at this plant using cattle prods to render animals unconscious so they could be dragged into the slaughterhouse. Use of cattle prods is legal; dragging unconscious and potentially contaminated animals is not. Cargill said "the animals balked because there were too many auditors present that day."[52] Even if true, a statement like this is unlikely to reassure anyone that the meat is safe.

Beef Packers is a major supplier of meat to the USDA's school lunch program. The recall covered meat sent to retailers, not schools. Investigative reporters for *USA Today* discovered that while the recall was in progress, the USDA bought 450,000 pounds of ground beef produced by Beef Packers during the dates covered by the recall and sent several lots to schools. The USDA knew that Beef Packers had a history of positive *Salmonella* tests, but did not disclose that information. An official told *USA Today* that if it did, it "would discourage companies from contracting to supply product for the National School Lunch Program and hamper our ability to provide safe and nutritious foods to American school children.[53]

As for antibiotic resistance: in this instance, the USDA was faced with a new possibility. Could the agency consider antibiotic-resistant *Salmonella* to be an adulterant, thereby making the meat subject to immediate recall? In August, an official announced to a meat industry conference that the USDA still considered *E. coli* O157:H7 to be an adulterant and was considering other such controls, some of them involving *Salmonella*. This was a warning that the new administration at the USDA—if not its inspectors—also intended to take foodborne illness more seriously.[54]

The multiple antibiotic resistance of this *Salmonella* strain raised particular alarms. As discussed in chapters 1 and 6, most antibiotics in the United States are fed to farm animals for nontherapeutic purposes, a practice that selects for antibiotic-resistant bacteria. This problem was the focus of a Pew Commission investigation (in which I participated), which recommended immediate reduction in the use of nontherapeutic antibiotics in animal agriculture.[55]

Congress considered legislation, but the meat industry opposed it. The American Meat Institute said restrictions on antibiotic use "will jeopardize the industry's ability to protect animal health, animal welfare and the food supply." A coalition of twenty meat producer organizations wrote the White House that antibiotics were vital to livestock and poultry production, and restrictions "are not supported by any conclusive scientific evidence." The American Veterinary Medical Association also opposed restrictions. The Pew report, it said, "contains significant flaws and major deviations from both science and reality. These missteps lead to dangerous and under-informed recommendations about the nature of our food system—and shocking recommendations for interventions that are scarcely commensurate with risk."[56] Despite the evident importance of antibiotics to human health, self-interest politics makes this issue—as well as the others discussed here—difficult to resolve.

Taken together, these incidents ought to have provided all the evidence Congress might need to enact food safety legislation. Collectively, they demonstrate that without such legislation, food companies are likely to continue to cut safety corners, lobby against having to produce food safely, and collude with federal agencies to overlook safety hazards—regardless of threats to public health. And because animal wastes (USDA-regulated) are the ultimate source of pathogens on leafy greens and raw cookie dough (FDA-regulated), these incidents also argue for regulation by one agency, not two.

TOWARD A MORE EFFECTIVE FOOD SAFETY SYSTEM

In 2004, Tommy Thompson announced his resignation as secretary of health and human services with these now famous words: "I, for the life of me, cannot understand why terrorists have not attacked our food supply because it is so easy to do." Fears of bioterrorism induced Congress to require the FDA to implement rules about registration and import shipments, but that was all.[57]

You might think, as I do, that the surest way to prevent food bioterrorism would be to enact a comprehensive food safety system. Such a system would not only protect against microbial biohazards, but also those that might be posed by old and new technologies such as mercury in fish from coal-burning power plants, the cloning of food animals, genetic modification of animals and fish, chemicals leaching from plastics, and nanotechnology.

You also might think that the recent spate of outbreaks and recalls would have induced Congress to take action. In 2007, Michael Taylor told Congress, "The sad truth is that we have no system for managing multi-state foodborne illness outbreaks. . . . Congress must act to solve this problem." How? By enacting what food safety advocates in and out of government had been recommending for years: a single food agency responsible for overseeing mandatory HACCP (or its euphemistic equivalent, "preventive controls") for all foods, from farm to table.[58]

With Congress unwilling to take on this challenge, the alternative is to try a stepwise approach, beginning with fixing the FDA. In the wake of the 2007 pet food recalls, the FDA's Science Board released a scathing report on the agency's lack of scientific and financial resources. It pointed out that from 1988 to 2007, Congress had enacted 123 statutes that increased the FDA's regulatory responsibilities but granted few additional resources. The FDA issued a Food Protection Plan attempting to set forth priorities but almost everything it suggested would require new legislation. Even so, critics of the plan such as Michael Taylor pointed out that it failed to treat food safety as a farm-to-table problem or to hold the food industry responsible and accountable.[59]

At the time he made these statements, Taylor was a professor at George Washington University. Because of his previous connection to Monsanto, antibiotechnology advocates considered him the prime example of how the revolving door favors corporate over public interests. In 2009, despite such concerns, he was reappointed to the FDA with responsibility for implementing whatever food safety legislation Congress chose to enact. Congress was considering bills aimed at fixing the FDA. Because of Taylor's work in the mid-1990s, the USDA's rules did not need much fixing; they mostly needed to be enforced.

In the interim, the FDA did what it could to unblock regulations put on hold by the previous administration. In 2009, it implemented rules for shell eggs first proposed in 2004, issued guidance (still voluntary) for melons, tomatoes, and leafy greens, and speeded up its warning systems. It also showed hopeful signs of collaborating with the USDA on common food safety problems. The USDA does not usually deal with the safety of leafy greens, for example, but large growers asked the USDA to establish a marketing agreement to "facilitate the practical application" of the FDA voluntary guidance. Producers who signed on to the agreement would be obliged to follow GMPs. This might appear to be real progress, but never underestimate politics. Small growers strongly opposed the marketing agreement on the grounds that adhering to GMPs puts them at a competitive disadvantage.[60]

Overall, safety practices remain voluntary as of early 2010. For mandatory food safety, Congress would have to act. As this book goes to press, creating a food safety system that unites the functions of the FDA and the USDA seems politically unfeasible. Instead, Congress seems likely to pass legislation designed to strengthen the FDA. The bills authorize the FDA to require science-based (HACCP-like) safety standards for all foods from farm to table, and to demand recalls, retain contaminated products, and conduct other long-awaited enforcement measures. As might be expected, these bills were vigorously opposed by industrial food producers. But they also were opposed by producers of local, organic, and sustainable foods who, understandably, wanted regulations more appropriate to their smaller scale of operations.[61]

No matter how these issues resolve, the proposed legislation falls far short of what is needed. The many industry critics of a unified food safety system argue that a single agency and mandatory requirements will not end foodborne illness; as long as humans prepare food, accidents will happen. Yes, but the single agency idea is worth pursuing because neither the separate agencies nor voluntary actions by food companies have been able to prevent more frequent and deadly outbreaks. We only have one food system, and it makes sense to put one agency in charge of it. At issue is how to achieve an effective food safety system. For this, we need a much higher level of public dread and outrage. It is time for food safety to join the food revolution.

THE SCIENCE OF PLANT BIOTECHNOLOGY

IN WRITING THIS BOOK, I TRIED TO MAKE THE SCIENTIFIC ISSUES accessible to general readers, omitting technical details but retaining accuracy. The purpose of this appendix is to provide a bit more information about the underlying science of food biotechnology. Although it is not necessary to know very much about this science in order to understand its political implications, a grasp of fundamental concepts, approaches, and interpretations can help bridge the gap between science-based and value-based approaches to evaluating risk. At the very least, this information helps to explain why some scientists have difficulty understanding public distrust of genetically engineered foods.

Science has much to teach us about the biological and physical worlds we inhabit, and its methods and approaches are useful tools for investigating such matters. The basic concepts are not difficult to understand, but the methods—and especially the vocabulary—can be intimidating. Here, I extend the discussion of plant biotechnology given in chapter 5 and offer further details, still nontechnical, about the methods used to introduce new genes into plants, particularly those for synthesis of beta-carotene in Golden Rice. Let's begin with a brief overview of basic biological principles having to do with DNA and its functions in bacteria and plants.

A (VERY) QUICK REMINDER ABOUT DNA, GENES, AND PROTEINS

DNA (deoxyribonucleic acid) is the principal determinant of the genetic characteristics of most living organisms: humans, animals, plants, bacteria, and many viruses. One of its functions is to specify the structure of proteins. The details of the processes through which DNA reproduces itself and carries out its functions appear immensely complicated—always a good sign that they are incompletely understood. They are also abstract. DNA and proteins are submicroscopic; their actions must be inferred. Furthermore, scientists (like specialists in any field) typically describe molecular actions in a vocabulary impenetrable to the uninitiated.[1]

Fortunately, we need to use only a few of the most familiar terms: DNA and its subunits (DNA bases, of which there are 4), and protein and its subunits (amino acids, of which there are 20).[2]

No matter what organism it comes from, DNA is composed of just four subunits—the DNA bases. These differ in size and shape and are arranged on the DNA molecule like beads on a string. The *sequence* of stringing constitutes a four-letter code that contains the genetic information of the cells that make up body organs and tissues. To summarize the basic details:

- Sequences of DNA bases (DNA segments) arranged in a specified order constitute genes.
- Some gene DNA sequences specify the structure of proteins.
- Other DNA sequences specify the structure of molecules that signal where genes begin and end.
- Gene DNA sequences specify the order in which amino acids link to make specific proteins; a sequence of three DNA bases specifies 1 of the 20 amino acids (this is the *genetic code*).
- Proteins are composed of various combinations of the 20 different amino acids linked in a specific order defined by the gene DNA sequence.
- Proteins do the work of cells, muscles, and other organs as structural components, signals, or enzymes.
- Enzymes catalyze biochemical reactions in the body.
- The structure of DNA is helical; its two strands are twisted around each other in a double helix.
- Proteins differ from one another in structure; they fold into specific three-dimensional shapes that depend on the sequence of their amino acids (and other components that may be introduced during or after protein synthesis).
- The structure of a protein determines its function.

These biological features operate in the same way in most organisms. Differences among species depend on the specific order of base sequences in their DNA and, therefore, in the sequence of amino acids in their proteins. When scientists extract genes from bacteria, they are taking segments of DNA that contain the same DNA bases that are already in plants—just arranged in a different sequence. The commonality of DNA bases among organisms is the main reason why many scientists are perplexed by public anxieties about genetic engineering; DNA is DNA—its base subunits are the same—no matter where it comes from or where it goes.

MORE ABOUT MAKING RICE GOLDEN: PLASMIDS

As noted in chapter 5, the genetic engineering of beta-carotene into rice represents an extraordinary technical achievement. The "foreign" genes must be identified and reproduced, inserted into the plant's DNA, and made to function in the plant and reproduce in its seeds. How all of this is accomplished is quite remarkable, as the methods take advantage of the unique and rather bizarre properties of a species of common soil bacteria, *Agrobacterium tumifaciens*. Table 17 outlines the use of this system to put genes for beta-carotene into rice; it describes the *less* complicated of the two approaches used for this purpose.[3,4]

Agrobacteria can infect a variety of plants that have been scratched, torn, or "wounded" in some way. At the wound site, the bacteria induce the plant to form swellings—crown galls—a form of plant cancer. The bacteria do not actually penetrate into the plant's tissues. Instead, they attach to the wound site and transfer a special piece of their DNA into the plant. This piece, called transfer-DNA (T-DNA), contains genes and DNA base sequences that enable it to enter the plant cells, find the plant's DNA, integrate into it, and specify the production of proteins that cause plant cells to make crown galls. Why might *Agrobacterium* do this? The most likely explanation is that the T-DNA also contains genes that cause crown galls to produce unusual amino acid derivatives called opines. Opines are not normally made by plants and do nothing for them. Instead, they serve as a preferential food for *Agrobacteria*, giving them a competitive edge in the ecological world of soil bacteria.

What makes *Agrobacterium tumifaciens* uniquely qualified to transfer genes from other organisms to plants is that the T-DNA is not really part of its own DNA. Instead, the T-DNA is carried on a small, entirely separate, circular piece of DNA called a *plasmid*. Most bacteria contain plasmids (but without T-DNA) Plasmids are self-replicating, which means that they contain genes that specify their own reproductive functions; they multiply independently of the bacterial chromosome—the structure that contains the bacteria's DNA.

Typically, plasmids carry genes for traits that are useful—but not essential—for bacterial growth or reproduction. *Agrobacterium tumifaciens* plasmids, for example, carry T-DNA and its genes for crown gall. Other bacteria contain plasmids with genes for a variety of functions highly germane to issues discussed in this book: the ability to fix atmospheric nitrogen, synthesize the *Bacillus thuringiensis* (*Bt*) toxin, produce pathogenic toxins (*E. coli* O157:H7 and *Bacillus anthracis*), resist certain antibiotics, and—most important—infect other bacteria. Plasmid genes for these last two characteristics, for example, are often responsible for the widespread dissemination of resistance to antibiotics within a bacterial species, and from one kind of bacteria to another.

Agrobacterium plasmids are unique in containing T-DNA. On these plasmids, the T-DNA is flanked by DNA base sequences that mark its borders. As the T-DNA enters the plant, any DNA that lies between its border regions will be transferred into the plant's cells, regardless of where that DNA came from. *Agrobacterium* plasmids, therefore, solve a major technical problem: how to get desirable genes from bacteria or other foreign sources inserted into the cells of food plants.

Plant biotechnologists select the genes they want from any organism, get rid of unwanted T-DNA genes responsible for crown gall and opines, insert desired genes and regulatory DNA sequences between the T-DNA border regions, and use the *Agrobacterium* system to inject the newly constructed T-DNA into plant

TABLE 17. Highlights of one of the methods used to genetically engineer beta-carotene into Golden Rice*

Obtain the starting vector

Obtain a previously constructed *Agrobacterium* plasmid vector containing a transfer-DNA (T-DNA) from which the gene segments for crown gall and opines have been removed.

Construct the transfer-DNA

Using enzymes that split and reattach DNA at specific points, introduce into the T-DNA, one step at a time (not necessarily in this order):

- The daffodil gene for one enzyme in the pathway for making beta-carotene
- The gene from bacteria that specifies the other missing enzymes in the beta-carotene pathway
- Genes from peas and bacteria for proteins that will transport the new enzymes to the rice endosperm
- A marker gene for resistance to the antibiotic hygromycin (which blocks protein synthesis in rice and other plants)
- Regulatory DNA segments from cauliflower mosaic virus
- DNA segments that mark places where genes are to be inserted and removed
- Marker genes for resistance to other antibiotics
- DNA regulatory segments that enable the new genes to function in rice endosperm

Construct the new plasmid vector

Insert the plasmid with its new T-DNA "construct" into *Agrobacterium* by mixing them together in the presence of an electric current (electroporation), a process that makes the bacteria more permeable.

---

cells. This system does not work efficiently, and only a rare plant accepts the T-DNA. To identify the successful transfers, scientists add marker genes to the T-DNA, usually for resistance to antibiotics. The constructed plasmid—with the original genes for infectivity (but with crown gall functions removed), and the desired genes, regulatory elements, and markers inserted into the T-DNA— is called a *transmission vector*. When the system works, the bacteria containing the vector attach to the plant and actively transfer the T-DNA to the plant's cells. Once in the plant, the T-DNA genes and sequences integrate into the plant's DNA; the integrated genes specify the production of the desired proteins; the proteins move to the appropriate places in the plant's cells; and the plant displays the new characteristic.[5]

But that is not all. Constructing T-DNA sequences with foreign genes that actually function in plants requires the action of numerous enzymes that break DNA molecules at specific sites ("restriction" enzymes), enzymes that reattach split pieces (ligases), and a great many steps carried out in a specific order. For the

TABLE 17. (*continued*)

Prepare rice embryos for growth in tissue culture

Grow rice plants until they just set seeds; collect the immature seeds.

Remove the embryos from the seeds, and grow them in tissue culture (a medium containing nutrients and plant hormones).

Remove the sheath (plant material) that surrounds the embryos to make them more permeable; continue growing them in tissue culture.

Transfer plasmid T-DNA into rice embryos

Collect the unsheathed rice embryos growing in tissue culture and immerse them in a suspension of *Agrobacterium* containing the beta-carotene T-DNA plasmid vector.

Grow the vector-treated embryos in tissue culture.

Select the rare rice embryos able to accept the plasmid T-DNA

Add the antibiotic hygromycin to the growth medium, and continue growing the rice embryos; only those with the T-DNA containing the gene for resistance to hygromycin survive.

Test the surviving rice embryos to make sure they contain the genes for beta-carotene.

Grow the successfully transformed embryos in a rooting medium; grow the plants to maturity in a greenhouse; allow the plants to set seeds to maturity.

Harvest the rice seeds, and test them for beta-carotene. The rice grains that contain beta-carotene are yellow (hence: Golden Rice).

SOURCE: Ye X, et al. *Science* 2000;287:303–305.
*Refer to figure 13, page 156.

system to work in rice, for example, the scientists also must successfully grow rice cells in tissue culture (an artificial medium containing nutrients and growth factors), infect the rice cells, grow them back into rice plants, and have the rice breed true under greenhouse conditions. Each one of these steps presents its own set of technical difficulties. Thus, genetic engineering requires a "feel" for how to make all of the steps work, which transforms the technology into an art as well as a science. The artistic aspects add to the difficulty of explaining the science to nonspecialists.

BRIDGING THE GAP

At issue is what is to be done to bridge the gap in knowledge and outlook between scientists and nonscientists. In a preliminary draft of this appendix (now much revised), I argued that scientists must work harder to explain their methods, approaches, and findings to the public, and that the public must take responsibility for demanding such explanations. One of the scientists who commented on that draft said that if I am asking people to demand explanations, I must also insist that they *listen* to the explanations, and with an open mind. He also mentioned that people like me who attempt to provide understandable explanations of science have a responsibility to ensure that the explanations are reasonably complete. I have tried to do this but have also tried to explain the ways in which science is political and inextricably linked to its social context and consequences.

NOTES

This section contains reference citations along with occasional notes. Citations follow the spare, unpunctuated "Vancouver" style used by most biological science journals, as described in *JAMA* 1993;269:2282–2286 (translation: *Journal of the American Medical Association,* 1993, volume 269, pages 2282 to 2286). Sometimes, issue numbers follow the volume in parentheses. Thus, *Food Technology* 1991;45(5):248–253 refers to an article published in the fifth (in this case, May) issue. As is customary in this style, text citations sometimes appear out of numerical order; these are space-saving cross-references to material cited earlier in the *same* chapter. Also to save space, references to multiple quotations or facts in a paragraph are listed in order under one note at its end; references to U.S. government reports omit their place and publisher (Washington, DC: U.S. Government Printing Office); and citations to articles in professional journals signed by multiple authors list only the first three followed by et al. Except as otherwise noted, documents obtained from Internet sources were available at the cited addresses in February 2010.

For clarity, most references give the full name of organizations, government agencies, and the titles of journals and publications, but certain frequently used terms are abbreviated as follows:

Am	American
APHIS	Animal and Plant Health Inspection Service (of USDA)
CDC	Centers for Disease Control and Prevention (of DHHS)
CFSAN	Center for Food Safety and Applied Nutrition (of FDA)
CNI	Community Nutrition Institute
CSPI	Center for Science in the Public Interest
DHHS	U.S. Department of Health and Human Services
EPA	Environmental Protection Agency

ERS   Economic Research Service (of USDA)

FCN   *Food Chemical News*

FDA   Food and Drug Administration (of DHHS)

FIFRA   Federal Insecticide, Fungicide and Rodenticide Act

FR   *Federal Register*

FSIS   Food Safety and Inspection Service (of USDA)

GAO   General Accounting Office (of Congress) (since 2004, the Government Accountability Office)

J   *Journal, Journal of, Journal of the*

JAMA   *Journal of the American Medical Association*

MMWR   *Morbidity and Mortality Weekly Report* (of CDC)

NEJM   *New England Journal of Medicine*

NYT   *New York Times*

OTA   Office of Technology Assessment (formerly of Congress, now defunct)

Suppl   Supplement

USDA   U.S. Department of Agriculture

WSJ   *Wall Street Journal*

INTRODUCTION: FOOD SAFETY IS POLITICAL

1. Kaufman M. Biotech critics cite unapproved corn in taco shells. *Washington Post*, September 18, 2000:A2. Freese B. *The StarLink Affair.* Washington, DC: Friends of the Earth, July 2001, at www.foodallergyangel.com/documents/GMO/StarlinkReport.pdf. *Food Traceability Report. StarLink: Lessons Learned.* Washington, DC: FCN Publishing, 2001. Taylor MR, Tick JS. *The StarLink Case: Issues for the Future.* Washington, DC: Pew Initiative on Food and Biotechnology, October 2001, at www.pewtrusts.org/our_work_report_detail.aspx?id=33384. Goldberg RA. *Aventis CropScience and StarLink Corn.* Boston: Harvard Business School (Case N9-902-411), November 5, 2001.

2. Lambert B, Buysse L, Decock C, et al. A *Bacillus thuringiensis* insecticidal crystal protein with a high activity against members of the family Noctuidae. *Applied and Environmental Microbiology* 1996;62:80–86.

3. O'Reilly B. Reaping a biotech blunder. *Fortune*, February 19, 2001:156–164.

4. EPA. Assessment of scientific information concerning StarLink corn Cry9C *Bt* corn plant-pesticide; notice. *FR* 65:65246–65251, October 31, 2000. This notice gives a particularly clear account of how corn gets commingled in grain elevators and dry mills (corn meal and flour) and wet mills (corn starch, sweeteners, protein, fiber, and alcohol).

5. EPA. Allergenicity assessment of Cry9C *Bt* corn plant pesticide. *FR* 64:71452–71453, December 21, 1999. EPA. *FIFRA Scientific Advisory Panel Meeting, November 28, 2000* (SAP Report No. 2000-06), at www.epa.gov/scipoly/SAP/meetings/2000/112800_mtg.htm.

6. FDA. *FDA Evaluation of Consumer Complaints Linked to Foods Allegedly*

Containing StarLink™ Corn, June 13, 2001, at www.epa.gov/scipoly/SAP/meet ings/2001/july/fda.pdf. CDC. *Investigation of Human Health Effects Associated with Potential Exposure to Genetically Modified Corn,* June 11, 2001, at www .cdc.gov/nceh/ehhe/cry9creport/pdfs/cry9creport.pdf.

7. EPA. *FIFRA Scientific Advisory Panel Meeting, July 17–18, 2001* (SAP Report No. 2001-09), at www.epa.gov/scipoly/sap/meetings/2001/071701_mtg.htm.

8. Kaufman M. Biotech corn fuels a recall. *Washington Post,* September 23, 2000:A1,A6. Pollack A. Aventis gives up license to sell bioengineered corn. *NYT,* October 13, 2000:C5.

9. Kaufman M. Biotech grain is in 430 million bushels of corn, firm says. *Washington Post,* March 18, 2001:A8. Lin W, Price GK, Allen E. StarLink: impacts on the U.S. corn market and world trade. In *Feed Situation and Outlook Yearbook* (USDA/ERS, FDS-2001), April 2001:40–48. Kilman S. Regulators are urged to permit bioengineered corn to be in food. *WSJ,* October 26, 2000:B23.

10. Pollack A. Aventis tries a new tack on StarLink corn. *NYT,* April 24, 2001:C4. Durbin D. Review of EPA Documents Shows Agency Had Knowledge in 1998 of Possible Biotech Contamination (press release). Washington, DC: U.S. Senate, December 1, 2000.

11. Barboza D. Gene-altered corn changes dynamics of grain industry. *NYT,* December 11, 2000:A1,A24.

12. Winter G. Taco Bell's core customers seem undaunted by shell scare. *NYT,* October 3, 2000:C6. Kaufman M. Biotech corn may be in various foods. *Washington Post,* October 19, 2000:A1. Barboza D. Negligence suit is filed over altered corn. *NYT,* December 4, 2000:C2.

13. Pollack A. Kraft recalls taco shells with bioengineered corn. *NYT,* September 23, 2000:C1,C15.

14. Mendelson J, Blackwelder B, Ritchie M, et al. Letter to the Honorable William Jefferson Clinton re: Kraft recall of taco shells and genetically engineered food, September 27, 2000, at http://pirg.org/ge/GE.asp?id2=4785&id3=ge&.

15. Aventis battles consumer groups at EPA hearing to decide GE corn's safety. *Nutrition Week,* December 1, 2000:1–2.

16. Kaufman M. U.S. will buy back corn seed: firms to be compensated for batches mixed with biotech variety. *Washington Post,* March 8, 2001:A3. Hansen M. Starlink-Cry9C Protein (Consumers Union comments, EPA Docket number OPP-00688), November 28, 2000, at www.consumersunion.org/pub/core_food _safety/002294.html. Lueck S. Aventis is criticized over biotech corn. *WSJ,* October 27, 2000:B2.

17. Carroll J. Judge will approve settlement on use of StarLink corn. *WSJ,* March 7, 2002:A4.

18. Institute of Medicine. *Ensuring Safe Food: From Production to Consumption.* Washington, DC: National Academy Press, 1998.

19. Snow CP. *Two Cultures and the Scientific Revolution: The Rede Lecture.* London: Cambridge University Press, 1959.

20. Geertz C. Empowering Aristotle (book review). *Science* 2001;293:53.

21. Handler P. Some comments on risk assessment. In: *National Research Council Current Issues and Studies* (annual report). Washington, DC: National Academy of Sciences, 1979. Cited in Douglas and Wildavsky (note 26):32.

22. Groth E. Communicating with consumers about food safety and risk issues. *Food Technology* 1991;45(5):248–253.

23. Massey A. Crops, genes, and evolution. *Gastronomica* 2001;1(3):21–29.

24. DHHS. *Determining Risks to Health: Federal Policy and Practice*. Dover, MA: Auburn House, 1986.

25. DHHS. *Healthy People 2010*, Vol 1, January 2000. Online: www.health.gov/healthypeople/.

26. Douglas M, Wildavsky A. *Risk and Culture: An Essay on the Selection of Technical and Environmental Dangers*. Berkeley: University of California Press, 1982. Quotation: 73,80–81.

27. Fischler C. Raison et déraison dans la perception des risques alimentaires. *Cahiers de Nutrition et de Diététique* 1998;33:297–300. Fischler writes: "Si l'on est ce que l'on mange et que l'on ne sait plus ce que l'on mange, sait-on encore ce que l'on est?" Also see, of course: Lévi-Strauss C. *The Raw and the Cooked*, Vols. 1–3. Chicago: University of Chicago Press, 1968–1969.

28. Slovic P. *The Perception of Risk*. London: Earthscan, 2000. Lowrance WW. *Of Acceptable Risk: Science and the Determination of Safety*. Los Altos, CA: William Kaufmann, 1976. Scherer CW. Strategies for communicating risks to the public. *Food Technology* 1991;45(10):110–116. Bennett P, Calman K, eds. *Risk Communication and Public Health*. New York: Oxford University Press, 1999:3–19.

29. Burros M. Congress moving to revamp rules on food safety: reducing federal role. *NYT*, July 3, 1995:1,28. Thonney PF, Bisogni CA. Government regulation of food safety: interaction of scientific and societal forces: a scientific status summary. *Food Technology* 1992:46 (1):73–80.

30. Sandman PM. Risk communication: facing public outrage. *EPA J* 1987;13(9):21–22. Frewer L. Risk perception, social trust, and public participation in strategic decision making: implications for emerging technologies. *Ambio* (Sweden) 1999;28:569–574.

31. Commission of the European Communities. *Communication from the Commission on the Precautionary Principle*. Brussels, February 2, 2000, at http://portal.unesco.org/shs/en/ev.php-URL_ID=6615&URL_DO=DO_PRINT PAGE&URL_SECTION=201.html.

32. Foster KR, Vecchia P, Repacholi MH. Science and the precautionary principle. *Science* 2000;288:979–981. Groth E. *Science, Precaution and Food Safety: How Can We Do Better?* (discussion paper for the US Codex Delegation), February 2000, at www.consumersunion.org/food/codexcpi200.htm.

33. Montague P. The precautionary principle. *Rachel's Environment & Health Weekly*, 586, February 19, 1998, at www.seismo.unr.edu/htdocs/academic/ANDERSON/Papers/Precaution/Montague_PrecautionaryPrinciple.pdf.

34. *The EU-U.S. Biotechnology Consultative Forum: Final Report*. Brussels, December 2000, at http://europa.eu/rapid/pressReleasesAction.do?reference=IP/00/1484&format=HTML&aged=0&language=EN&guiLanguage=en.

35. Whelan EM. Our "stolen future" and the precautionary principle. *Priorities for Health* 1996;8(3), at www.acsh.org/healthissues/newsID.712/health issue_detail.asp. Also see: Paarlberg RL. *The Politics of Precaution: Genetically Modified Foods in Developing Countries*. Baltimore: Johns Hopkins University Press, 2001.

PART 1. RESISTING FOOD SAFETY

1. Mead PS, Slutsker L, Dietz V, et al. Food-related illness and death in the United States. *Emerging Infectious Diseases* 1999;5:607–625. CDC. Preliminary FoodNet data on the incidence of foodborne illnesses—selected sites, United States, 2000. *MMWR* 2001;50 (April 6):241–246.

2. Fox N. *Spoiled: the Dangerous Truth About a Food Chain Gone Haywire.* New York: Basic Books, 1997:66–67.

3. Brown J, Byers T, Thompson K, et al. Nutrition during and after cancer treatment: a guide for informed choices by cancer survivors. *CA: Cancer J for Clinicians* 2001;51(3):153–187.

CHAPTER 1. THE POLITICS OF FOODBORNE ILLNESS: ISSUES AND ORIGINS

1. Smith RJ. Institute of Medicine report recommends complete overhaul of food safety laws. *Science* 1979;203:1221–1224. Although warning labels are no longer required, the role of saccharin in human cancer is still under debate. A 1998 review by the World Cancer Research Fund (*Food, Nutrition, and the Prevention of Cancer: A Global Perspective.* Washington, DC: American Institute for Cancer Research, 1998:356–358) concluded that saccharin "probably has no relationship with the risk of bladder cancer in the amounts obtainable from normal diets." For a more cautious view, see: Corcoran L, Jacobson M. Saccharin: bittersweet. *Nutrition Action Healthletter* 1998;25(3):11–13. My assessment: if saccharin does affect cancer risk, it does so weakly.

2. Kessler DA. Food safety: revising the statute. *Science* 1984;223:1034–1040. Kramer CS, Penner KP. Food safety: consumers report their concerns. *National Food Review* 1986;9(spring):21–24. Stevens WK. Officials call microbes most urgent food threat. *NYT*, March 28, 1989:C1,C11.

3. U.S. food safety defense weakening; needs bolster. *CNI Weekly Report*, May 31, 1984:4–5. Carlson M. Do you dare to eat a peach? *Time*, March 27, 1989:24–38. Warning! Your food, nutritious and delicious, may be hazardous to your health. *Newsweek*, March 27, 1989:16–25. Jacobson MF, Lefferts LY, Garland AW. *Safe Food: Eating Wisely in a Risky World.* Los Angeles: Living Planet Press, 1991.

4. Burros M. New urgency fuels effort to improve safety of food. *NYT*, May 7, 1990:A1,D11.

5. Wolf ID. Critical issues in food safety, 1991–2000. *Food Technology* 1992;46(1):64–70. Lynch S, Lin C-TJ. Food safety: meal planners express their concerns. *FoodReview* 1994;17(2):14–18. Food safety concerns addressed by editors, members of public. *Illinois Agrinews*, October 3, 1997:A14.

6. Mead PS, Slutsker L, Dietz V, et al. Food-related illness and death in the United States. *Emerging Infectious Diseases* 1999;5:607–625.

7. Chicken: what you don't know can hurt you. *Consumer Reports*, March 1998:12–18. Dahl E, DeWaal CS. *Scrambled Eggs: How a Broken Food Safety System Let Contaminated Eggs Become a National Food Poisoning Epidemic.* May 1997. Online: www.cspinet.org/reports/eggs.html.

8. Archer DL, Kvenberg JE. Incidence and cost of foodborne diarrheal dis-

ease in the United States. *J Food Protection* 1985;48:887–894. Council for Agricultural Science and Technology. *Foodborne Pathogens: Risks and Consequences*. Ames, IA, September 1994.

9. CDC. Incidence of foodborne illnesses—FoodNet, 1997. *JAMA* 1998;280: 1651–1652. GAO. *Food Safety: Information on Foodborne Illnesses* (GAO/RCED-96-96), May 8, 1996.

10. Institute of Medicine. *Ensuring Safe Food: From Production to Consumption*. Washington, DC: National Academy Press, 1998. Its appendix B reviews the history of changes in federal food safety responsibilities.

11. CDC. Preliminary FoodNet data on the incidence of foodborne illnesses—selected sites, United States, 2001. *MMWR* 2002;51 (April 19):325–329.

12. Roberts T, van Ravenswaay E. The economics of food safety. *National Food Review* 1989;12(3):1–8. Buzby JC, Roberts T. ERS estimates U.S. foodborne disease costs. *FoodReview* 1995;18(3):37–42. Buzby JC, Roberts T, Lin C-TJ, et al. *Bacterial Foodborne Disease: Medical Costs and Productivity Losses*. USDA/ERS, August 1996. Buzby JC, Roberts T. ERS updates U.S. foodborne disease costs for seven pathogens. *FoodReview* 1996;19(3):20–25. GAO. *Food Safety: Federal Efforts to Ensure the Safety of Imported Foods Are Inconsistent and Unreliable* (GAO/RCED-98-103), April 1998. Buzby JC. Children and microbial foodborne illness. *FoodReview* 2001;24(2):32–37.

13. Gilchrist A. *Foodborne Disease & Food Safety*. Chicago: American Medical Association, 1981.

14. DeWaal CS, Barlow K, Alderton L, et al. *Outbreak Alert! Closing the Gaps in Our Federal Food Safety Net*. Washington, DC: CSPI, October 2001. DeWaal CS, Dahl E. *Dine at Your Own Risk*. CSPI, November 1996.

15. Linnan MJ, Mascola L, Lou XD, et al. Epidemic listeriosis associated with Mexican-style cheese. *NEJM* 1988;319:823–828.

16. Buchanan RL, Doyle MP. Foodborne disease significance of *Escherichia coli* O157:H7 and other enterohemorrhagic *E. coli*. *Food Technology* 1997;51(10): 69–76. The numbers and letters distinguish the strain of *E. coli*. The letter O refers to a somatic antigen (protein on the bacterial body that elicits an immune response), and *H* refers to an antigen on the bacterial flagella. (The variant is pronounced as it is spelled: E co-lie O one five seven H seven.) Grabowski EF. The hemolytic-uremic syndrome—toxin, thrombin, and thrombosis. *NEJM* 2002;346:58–61.

17. Gansheroff LJ, O'Brien AD. *Escherichia coli* O157:H7 in beef cattle presented for slaughter in the U.S.: higher prevalence rates than previously estimated. *Proceedings of the National Academy of Sciences* 2000;97:2959–2961. Mead PS, Griffin PM. *Escherichia coli* O157:H7. *Lancet* 1998;352:1207–1212.

18. CDC reports *E. coli* cases exceed previous estimates. *Nutrition Week*, December 11, 1998:3,6. Marks S, Roberts T. *E. coli* O157:H7 ranks as the fourth most costly foodborne disease. *FoodReview* 1993;16(3):51–59.

19. MacDonald JM, Ollinger ME, Nelson KE, et al. *Consolidation in U.S. Meatpacking* (Agricultural Economic Report No. 785). USDA/ERS, February 2000. Heffernan W. *Consolidation in the Food and Agriculture System: Report to the National Farmers Union*. Columbia : University of Missouri, February 5, 1999. GAO. *Dairy Industry: Information on Milk Prices and Changing Market Structure* (GAO-01-561), June 2001.

20. Tyson Foods. Tyson and IBP Agree on Merger Terms (press release), June 27, 2001, at www.accessmylibrary.com/coms2/summary_0286–26709621_ITM.

21. Sierra Club. *The Rap Sheet on Animal Factories,* August 2002. Online: www.sierraclub.org.

22. Goodman PS. An unsavory byproduct: runoff and nutrient pollution. *Washington Post,* August 1, 1999:A1. Five additional articles in this series followed on August 2 and 3.

23. Armstrong GL, Hollingsworth J, Morris JG. Emerging foodborne pathogens: *Escherichia coli* O157:H7 as a model of entry of a new pathogen into the food supply of the developed world. *Epidemiologic Reviews* 1996;18:29–51.

24. Hennessy TW, Hedberg CW, Slutsker L, et al. A national outbreak of *Salmonella enteritidis* infections from ice cream. *NEJM* 1996;334:1281–1286.

25. Levy SB, FitzGerald GB, Macone AB. Changes in intestinal flora of farm personnel after introduction of a tetracycline-supplemented feed on a farm. *NEJM* 1976;295:583–588. An entertaining (and accurate) source, far ahead of its time, is Schell O. *Modern Meat: Antibiotics, Hormones, and the Pharmaceutical Farm.* New York: Random House, 1984.

26. Burros M. F.D.A. proposal on meat safety draws criticism. *NYT,* June 8, 1983:C1. Wright K. The policy response: in limbo. *Science* 1990;249:24.

27. National Research Council. *The Use of Drugs in Food Animals: Benefits and Risks.* Washington, DC: National Academy Press, 1999:9.

28. Leonard R. Drugs as feed additives increase risk to health. *Nutrition Week,* August 7, 1998:4–5. For the science behind these arguments, see: Smith KE, Besser JM, Hedberg CW, et al. Quinolone-resistant *Campylobacter jejuni* infections in Minnesota, 1992–1998. *NEJM* 1999;340:1525–1532. Witte W. Medical consequences of antibiotic use in agriculture. *Science* 1998;279:996–997. Levy SB. Private arsenals and public peril. *NEJM* 1998;338:1375–1378.

29. Federal policy statements: FDA. *Guidance for Industry. Consideration of the Human Health Impact of the Microbial Effects of Antimicrobial New Animal Drugs Intended for Use in Food-Producing Animals,* December 13, 1999, at www.fda.gov/OHRMS/DOCKETS/98fr/122399d.txt. GAO. *Food Safety: The Agricultural Use of Antibiotics and Its Implications for Human Health* (GAO/RCED-99-74), April 1999. CDC. *Draft—A Public Health Action Plan to Combat Antimicrobial Resistance,* June 2000, at www.cdc.gov/drugresistance/actionplan/aractionplan.pdf. Three papers in the October 18, 2001, *NEJM* describe the supermarket findings (2001;345:1147–1166), as does an accompanying editorial: Gorbach S. Antimicrobial use in animal feed—time to stop. *NEJM* 2001;345:1202–1203.

30. Mellon M, Benbrook C, Benbrook KL. *Hogging It! Estimates of Antimicrobial Abuse in Livestock.* Washington, DC: Union of Concerned Scientists, 2001. Barza M, Gorbach S, DeVincent SJ, eds. The need to improve antimicrobial use in agriculture: ecological and human health consequences. *Clinical Infectious Diseases* 2002;34 Suppl 3:71–143. Osvath R. Bill would phase out fluoroquinolones, other antibiotics. *FCN,* March 4, 2002:6–7.

31. Brody JE. Studies find resistant bacteria in meats. *NYT,* October 18, 2001:A12.

32. Ferber D. Livestock feed ban preserves drugs' power. *Science* 2002;295:27.

Burros M. Poultry industry quietly cuts back on antibiotic use. *NYT,* February 10, 2002:A1,A26.

33. Couzin J. Cattle diet linked to bacterial growth. *Science* 1998;281:1578–1579. Diez-Gonzalez F, Callaway TR, Kizoulis MG, et al. Grain feeding and the dissemination of acid-resistant *Escherichia coli* from cattle. *Science* 1998;281:1666–1668. Beers A. Feed supplement can reduce *E. coli* shedding, study shows. *FCN,* April 29, 2002:15. Crump JA, Sulka AC, Langer AJ, et al. An outbreak of *Escherichia coli* O157:H7 infections among visitors to a dairy farm. *NEJM* 2002;347:555–560.

34. Friedland WH. The new globalization: the case of fresh produce. In: Bonnano A, Busch L, Friedland WH, et al., eds. *From Columbus to ConAgra: The Globalization of Agriculture and Food.* Lawrence: University Press of Kansas, 1994:210–231. For statistics on food imports, see: USDA/ERS. *Vegetables and Specialties Yearbook,* at http://usda.mannlib.cornell.edu/MannUsda/viewTaxon omy.do?taxonomyID=6.

35. Burros M. Salad bars: how clean are they? *NYT,* August 25, 1999:F1,F9.

36. Holler T. The iron rule in Omaha's jungle. *Social Policy* 2002;32(4):21–27. Schlosser E. *Fast Food Nation.* New York: Houghton Mifflin, 2001.

37. Morris JG, Potter M. Emergence of new pathogens as a function of changes in host susceptibility. *Emerging Infectious Diseases* 1997;3:335–344.

38. Hearn L. Haceldama. *Cincinnati Commercial,* September 5, 1875. Reprinted in: Cott J. *Wandering Ghost: The Odyssey of Lafcadio Hearn.* New York: Alfred A. Knopf, 1991:61–69. Cott defines *haceldama* as a New Testament word meaning "field of blood."

39. Smith MS, Roth DM. *Chronological Landmarks in American Agriculture* (Agricultural Information Bulletin No. 425). USDA/ERS, November 1990. Brady RP, Cooper RM, Silverman RS, eds. *Fundamentals of Law and Regulation: An In-Depth Look at Foods, Veterinary Medicines, and Cosmetics.* Washington, DC: Food and Drug Law Institute, 1997.

40. Goodwin LS. *The Pure Food, Drink, and Drug Crusaders, 1879–1914.* Jefferson, NC: McFarland, 1999. Coppin CA, High J. *The Politics of Purity: Harvey Washington Wiley and the Origins of Federal Food Policy.* Ann Arbor: University of Michigan Press, 1999. The authors argue that Wiley's interests in promoting pure food legislation had more to do with self-interest in expanding his bureau than with public health.

41. Sinclair U. *The Jungle,* 1906 (Bantam Classic edition, 1981). The introduction by Morris Dickstein explains the genesis of the book. The five quotations are from pages 135, 275, 135, 99, and 36, respectively.

42. Congress immediately amended the 1906 Meat Inspection Act (the Beveridge Amendment) and reenacted it as the Meat Inspection Act of 1907. This book uses 1906 as the relevant date.

43. National Research Council. *Meat and Poultry Inspection: The Scientific Basis of the Nation's Program.* Washington, DC: National Academy Press, 1985.

44. *Congressional Record—Senate,* June 30, 1906:9791–9792 (Vol. 40, Part 10, 59th Congress, 1st Session). CDC. Achievements in public health, 1900–1999: safer and healthier foods. *MMWR* 1999;48(40):905–913.

45. *Congressional Record—House*, June 29, 1906:9735–9740 (Vol. 40, Part 10, 59th Congress, 1st Session).

46. Wiley HW. *1001 Tests of Foods, Beverages and Toilet Accessories Good and Otherwise: Why They Are So*. New York: Hearst's International Library, 1914:ix–xix.

47. Robinson RA. *Food Safety and Security: Fundamental Changes Needed to Ensure Safe Food* (GAO-02-47T), October 10, 2001.

48. GAO. *Food Safety and Quality: Who Does What in the Federal Government* (GAO/RCED-91-19A and GAO/RCED-91-19B), December 1990.

49. GAO. *Food Safety and Quality: Uniform, Risk-based Inspection System Needed to Ensure Safe Food Supply* (GAO/RCED-92-152), June 1992.

50. GAO. *Food Safety: U.S. Lacks a Consistent Farm-to-Table Approach to Egg Safety* (GAO/RCED-99-184), July 1999. Bäumler AJ, Hargis BM, Tsolis RM. Tracing the origins of *Salmonella* outbreaks. *Science* 2000;287:50–52.

51. National Research Council. *Poultry Inspection: The Basis for a Risk-Assessment Approach*. Washington, DC: National Academy Press, 1987. USDA/FSIS. Enhanced poultry inspection: proposed rule. *FR* 59:35639–35657, July 13, 1994. GAO. *Food Safety: Weaknesses in Meat and Poultry Inspection Pilot Should Be Addressed before Implementation* (GAO-02-59), December 2001.

52. Putnam J, Allshouse J. Imports' share of U.S. diet rises in late 1990s. *FoodReview* 2001;24(3):15–22. FDA, USDA, EPA, CDC. *Food Safety from Farm to Table: A National Food Safety Initiative: Report to the President*, May 1997. Online: vm.cfsan.fda.gov/-dms/fsreport.html.

CHAPTER 2. RESISTING MEAT AND POULTRY REGULATION, 1974–1994

1. Morgan D. Trying to lead the USDA through a thicket of politics. *Washington Post*, July 5, 1978:A8.

2. Foreman CT. Unequal protection, unfair competition: the cause and effect of different standards for food safety and nutrition (speech). Washington, DC: Consumer Federation of America's Consumer Assembly, March 1991 (revised June 10, 1991).

3. Jacobson M. *Nutrition Scoreboard*. New York: Avon Books, 1974. Sarasohn J. Ex-USDA chief Glickman joins Akins group. *Washington Post*, February 8, 2001:A21.

4. Center for Public Integrity. *Safety Last: The Politics of E. coli and Other Food-Borne Killers*. Washington, DC, 1998. Quotation: 52. Also see: *Food Safety and Government Regulation of Coliform Bacteria*. Hearing before the Subcommittee on Agricultural Research, Conservation, Forestry, and General Legislation. 103rd Congress, 1st Session, February 5, 1993:69–70. Mulkern AC. Is USDA too close to meat industry? *Denver Post*, August 11, 2002:A1.

5. *American Public Health Association et al. v. Earl Butz, Secretary of Department of Agriculture et al.* 511 F. 2d 331 (DC Circuit Court of Appeals), December 19, 1974.

6. Gilchrist A. *Foodborne Disease & Food Safety*. Chicago: American Medical Association, 1981:95–98.

7. Sugarman C. The road to food safety? How the government's new rules

will (and won't) protect your dinner. *Washington Post,* October 29, 1997:E1,E11. Lachance PA. Development of stored food and water systems. *Environmental Biology and Medicine* 1971;1:205–228. I am indebted to George Pillsbury and James Behnke for explaining this history.

8. USDA/FSIS. Pathogen reduction: Hazard Analysis Critical Control Point (HACCP) systems: final rule with request for comments. *FR* 61:38806–38989, July 25, 1996.

9. USDA/FSIS. Generic HACCP models and guidance materials available for review and comment. *FR* 61:32053–32054, June 12, 1997.

10. National Research Council. *Meat and Poultry Inspection: The Scientific Basis of the Nation's Program.* Washington, DC: National Academy Press, 1985:159.

11. National Research Council. *An Evaluation of the Role of Microbiological Criteria for Food and Food Ingredients.* Washington, DC: National Academy Press, 1985.

12. *USDA's "Discretionary Inspection" Plan for Meat and Poultry Processing Plants.* House of Representative Committee on Government Operations. Hearing before the Human Resources and Intergovernmental Relations Subcommittee. 101st Congress, 1st Session, April 11, 1989. Quotations: Carol Tucker Foreman, 59–60; Delmer Jones, 4; Thomas Devine, 66.

13. National Advisory Committee on Microbiological Criteria for Foods. *Hazard Analysis and Critical Control Point System.* Washington, DC: USDA and FDA, March 20, 1992. Waites WM, Arbuthnott JP. Foodborne illness: an overview. *Lancet* 1990;336:722–725.

14. GAO. *Food Safety and Quality: Uniform, Risk-Based Inspection System Needed to Ensure Safe Food Supply* (GAO/RCED-92-152), June 1992. USDA/FSIS. Streamlined inspection system: cattle and staffing standards. *FR* 53:48262–48275, November 30, 1988.

15. Crutchfield S. Food safety at a glance. *FoodReview* 1998;21(3):34–35.

16. Committee on Evaluation of USDA Streamlined Inspection System for Cattle (SIS-C). *Cattle Inspection.* Washington, DC: National Academy Press, 1990:4.

17. CDC. Update: Multistate outbreak of *Escherichia coli* O157:H7 infections from hamburgers—Western United States, 1992–93. *JAMA* 1993;269:2194–2196. Bell BP, Goldoft M, Griffin PM, et al. A multistate outbreak of *Escherichia coli* O157:H7–associated bloody diarrhea and hemolytic uremic syndrome from hamburgers: the Washington experience. *JAMA* 1994;272:1349–1353.

18. Egan T. Tainted hamburger raises doubts on meat safety. *NYT,* January 27, 1993:A10.

19. Tolchin M. Clinton orders hiring of 160 meat inspectors. *NYT,* February 12, 1993:A23.

20. Nugent RJ. *Statement on Food Safety and Government Regulation of Coliform Bacteria.* Hearing before the Subcommittee on Agricultural Research, Conservation, Forestry, and General Legislation of the Committee on Agriculture, Nutrition, and Forestry. 103rd Congress, 1st Session :34, February 5, 1993. Mr. Nugent was president of Jack in the Box (headquarters: San Diego, CA).

21. Pollack A. A battle-scarred burger warrior. *NYT,* October 3, 1999:A2.

Schneider K. Clinton proposes to change the way meat is inspected. *NYT*, March 17, 1993:A1,A18.

22. Modernizing meat inspections (editorial). *NYT*, April 2, 1993:A32.

23. Altman LK. Lessons are sought in outbreak of illness from tainted meat. *NYT*, February 9, 1993:C3. Sullivan A. Machines speed testing of food for bacteria. *WSJ*, July 15, 1996:B1.

24. Wachsmuth IK. *Escherichia coli* O157:H7—harbinger of change in food safety and tradition in the industrialized world. *Food Technology* 1997;51(10):26.

25. Burros M. Agriculture dept. policy blamed for tainted food. *NYT*, March 3, 1993:C1,C4.

26. Quoted in Fox N. *Spoiled: The Dangerous Truth About a Food Chain Gone Haywire*. New York: Basic Books, 1997:256–57. Later quotation: 245.

27. Beyond Beef, USDA agree on meat handling labels. *Nutrition Week*, May 7, 1993:3.

28. Burros M. U.S. intends to require label on meat's cooking. *NYT*, May 6, 1993:A18.

29. Burros M. Agriculture dept. unveils cooking labels for meat. *NYT*, August 12, 1993:A18. Most safety labeling on meat is postponed. *NYT*, October 10, 1993:25. DeWaal C. Remarks to the Association of Food Journalists, Washington, DC, September 7, 1997.

30. Sugarman C. Court blocks safety labels on meat products. *Washington Post*, October 15, 1993:A11.

31. Egan T. A year later, raw meat still lacks labels. *NYT*, December 20, 1993:A1,D10.

32. Baquet D, Johnston D. U.S. expanding scope in review of gifts to Agriculture secretary. *NYT*, August 7, 1994:A1,A24. Johnston D. Agriculture chief quits as scrutiny of conduct grows. *NYT*, October 4, 1994:A1,A16.

33. Greenhouse L. High court voids theory used to press independent counsel's cases over gifts to Espy. *NYT*, April 28, 1999:A26.

34. Burros M. Agriculture dept. scraps poultry bacteria plan. *NYT*, October 27, 1994:A20.

35. Van Natta D, Lacey M. Access proved vital in last-minute race for Clinton pardons. *NYT*, February 25, 2001:A1,A14.

36. Cross HR. Testimony before Senate Agriculture Committee, February 5, 1993. Quoted in: Foreman CT. *Hearing statement before the House Committee on Science, Space and Technology, Subcommittee on Technology, Environment and Aviation*, 103rd Congress, 2nd Session, May 5, 1994:5.

37. Taylor MR. Change and opportunity: harnessing innovation to improve the safety of the food supply (speech). American Meat Institute annual convention, San Francisco, CA, September 29, 1994.

38. Beers A. FSIS expands *E. coli* O157:H7 adulteration policy. *FCN*, January 18, 1999:3,17,18.

39. American Meat Institute. Meat and supermarket industries say USDA "misleading consumers" (press release). Washington, DC, November 1, 1994.

40. Donnelly J. As *E. coli* sampling commences, lobbyists throw down gauntlet. *Food & Drink Daily*, October 25, 1994.

41. Food industry opposes food safety initiative. *Nutrition Week*, November 4, 1994:7.

42. The meat industry's bad beef (editorial). *NYT*, November 20, 1994:A14.

43. Judge upholds USDA program to test meat. Archived: *The Victoria Advocate*, December 14, 1994 at http://news.google.com/newspapers?nid=861&dat=19941214&id=sTMKAAAAIBAJ&sjid=MUsDAAAAIBAJ&pg=4778,2876108. *Texas Food Industry Association, et al. v. Mike Espy, et al.*, 870 F. Supp. 143 (W.D. Tex. 1994).

44. Pratt, S. Some unsavory questions for meat industry group. *Chicago Tribune*, November 3, 1994:1,10.

45. Heersink M. Memo to Safe Food Coalition (leaflet). November 2, 1994. Mary Heersink was a founder of Safe Tables Our Priority (STOP). Her son survived infection with *E. coli* O157:H7.

46. USDA/FSIS. HACCP-based meat and poultry inspection concepts. *FR* 62:31553–31562, June 10, 1997. Ingersoll B. Meat industry spurred to revise policies. *WSJ*, August 27, 1997:A3.

CHAPTER 3. ATTEMPTING CONTROL OF FOOD PATHOGENS, 1994–2002

1. DeWaal CS, Barlow K, Alderton L, et al. *Outbreak Alert! Closing the Gaps in Our Federal Food Safety Net*. Washington, DC: CSPI, October 2001. FDA. Development of Hazard Analysis Critical Control Points for the food industry: request for comments. *FR* 59:39888–39896, August 4, 1994. Quote: 39889–39890. See: www.fda.gov/Food/FoodSafety/HazardAnalysisCriticalControlPoints HACCP/default.htm.

2. FDA/CFSAN. *Second Interim Report of Observations and Comments: Hazard Analysis and Critical Control Point (HACCP) Pilot Program for Selected Food Manufacturers. HACCP: A State-of-the-Art Approach to Food Safety* (FDA Backgrounder). FDA/CFSAN, August 1999, at http://vm.cfsan.fda.gov/~comm/haccpoth.html.

3. FDA. New egg safety steps announced, safe-handling labels and refrigeration will be required. *HHS News*, July 1, 1999. Also see: FDA. Procedures for the safe and sanitary processing and importing of fish and fishery products; final rule. *FR* 60:65095–65202, December 18, 1995. FDA. Consumers advised of risks associated with raw sprouts. *HHS News*, July 9, 1999.

4. GAO. *Food Safety: Federal Oversight of Seafood Does Not Sufficiently Protect Consumers* (GAO-01-204), January 2001. GAO. *Food Safety: Federal Oversight of Shellfish Safety Needs Improvement* (GA)-0-702), July 2001. Abboud L. Bad fish slips through FDA's safety net. *WSJ*, October 9, 2002: D1,D2.

5. USDA/FSIS. Pathogen Reduction: Hazard Analysis Critical Control Point (HACCP) systems: proposed rule. *FR* 60:6774–6889, February 3, 1995. USDA/FSIS. Final rule with request for comments. *FR* 61:38806–38989, July 25, 1996. USDA documents on food safety are online at: www.fsis.usda.gov.

6. *U.S. Meat and Poultry Inspection Issues*. Joint hearings before the Subcommittee on Department Operations and Nutrition and the Subcommittee on Livestock. 103rd Congress, 2nd Session, April 19, 1994. Statement of Bruce Tompkin, vice president, Product Safety, Armour Swift-Eckrich: 114.

7. American Meat Institute. Meat and Supermarket Industries Say USDA "Misleading Consumers" (press release). Washington, DC, November 1, 1994. Foreman CT. Statement (press conference), National Press Club, Washington DC, May 30, 1995.

8. Schulte B. Inspection changes for meat assailed. *Philadelphia Inquirer*, June 16, 1995:A3. Meat and Poultry Processors Use "Bare-Knuckled Tactics" to Delay Food Safety Reforms (press release). CSPI, June 22, 1995.

9. Morgan D. Industry finds a way around budget cutters: House Appropriations Panel proves friendlier to corporate subsidies. *Washington Post*, June 26, 1995:A1.

10. Jouzaitis C. Food safety regulations face challenge. *Chicago Tribune*, July 10, 1995:A1. Cushman JH. Narrow defeat for a measure on bad meat. *NYT*, July 13, 1995:B9. Burros M. Congress moving to revamp rules on food safety: reducing federal role. *NYT*, July 3, 1995:1,28. The Dole bill was S. 343, 104th Congress.

11. The Republican assault on meat safety (editorial). *NYT*, June 22, 1995:A26. Jacobson MJ, DeWaal CS. GOP rhetoric masks an attack on overdue clean-meat rules. *San Francisco Examiner*, June 27, 1995:A15.

12. Rogers D. House panel slows food-safety rules, maintains ban on offshore oil drilling. *WSJ*, June 28, 1995:A4.

13. Herbert B. Let them eat poison. *NYT*, July 3, 1995:21.

14. Meat safety rules back on track—USDA's Glickman (news release). *Reuters News Service*, July 19, 1995.

15. Meat Industry Agenda Fails Again (press release). Washington, DC: S.T.O.P. (Safe Tables Our Priority), July 20, 1995.

16. Jouzaitis C. Rollback of meat testing stalls in House. *Chicago Tribune*, July 20, 1995:3. DeWaal C. Remarks before the Association of Food Journalists Convention (speech). Washington, DC, September 7, 1997.

17. USDA/FSIS. Generic HACCP models and guidance materials available for review and comment. *FR* 61:32053–32054, June 12, 1997.

18. Burros M. Plan for food safety panel is criticized. *NYT*, April 1, 1996:A14.

19. Ingersoll B. Meat inspectors omit duties as work grows. *WSJ*, May 23, 1996:B1,B6. Center for Public Integrity. *Safety Last: The Politics of* E. coli *and Other Food-Borne Killers*. Washington, DC, 1998.

20. GAO. *Food Safety: New Initiatives Would Fundamentally Alter the Existing System* (GAO-RCED-96-81), March 1996.

21. Purdum TS. Meat inspections facing overhaul, first in 90 years. *NYT*, July 7, 1996:A1,A11.

22. Buzby JC, Crutchfield SR. USDA modernizes meat and poultry inspection. *FoodReview* 1997;20(1):14–17. Crutchfield S, Buzby JC, Roberts T, et al. *An Economic Assessment of Food Safety Regulations: The New Approach to Meat and Poultry Inspection* (Agricultural Economic Report No. 755), USDA/ERS, July 1997.

23. Belluck P. Juice-poisoning case brings guilty plea and a huge fine. *NYT*, July 24, 1998:A12.

24. Questions of pasteurization raised after E. coli is traced to juice. *NYT*, November 4, 1996:A17.

25. Drew C, Belluck P. Deadly bacteria a new threat to fruit and produce in the U.S. *NYT*, January 4, 1998:1,14. Clay T, Goldberg R. *Odwalla, Inc* (case study). Boston: Harvard Business School, November 5, 1997:30.

26. Belluck P. Accord is reached in food-poisoning case: juice maker's multi-million-dollar settlement may be a landmark. *NYT*, May 27, 1998:A16.

27. Coca-Cola will buy Odwalla, maker of fruit drinks. *NYT*, October 31, 2001:C4. Odwalla provides ongoing financial reports on its Web site: www .odwalla.com.

28. Food labeling: warning and notice statement; labeling of juice products: final rule. *FR* 63:37030–37056, July 8, 1998. The term "5-logs" means 5 logarithmic units, indicating a 100,000-fold reduction. FDA deemed a reduction of this size to indicate that there would be no significant microbiological hazard during the shelf life of the product.

29. Richards B. Odwalla's woes are a lesson for natural-food industry: FDA seeks tighter quality controls as *E. coli* outbreak raises concerns. *WSJ*, November 4, 1996:B4.

30. FDA. Hazard Analysis and Critical Control Point (HACCP); procedures for the safe and sanitary processing and importing of juice: final rule. *FR* 66:6137–6202, January 19, 2001.

31. USDA/FSIS. Generic *E. coli* testing for sheep, goats, equine, ducks, geese, and guineas: proposed rule. *FR* 62:59305–59310, November 3, 1997.

32. Morganthau T. *E. coli* alert. *Newsweek*, September 1, 1997:26–32.

33. Stout D. 5 million hamburger patties may be tainted, US warns. *NYT*, August 16, 1997:1,7. Janofsky M. 25 million pounds of beef is recalled. *NYT*, August 22, 1997:A1,A18.

34. Belluck P. The tangled trail that led to a beef recall. *NYT*, August 24, 1997:1,24.

35. Burger King. A letter to our customers about hamburgers, food safety and flame broiling. *NYT*, August 25, 1997:A11. Whelan EM. Safe meat: there is a better way (editorial). *WSJ*, August 26, 1997:16.

36. Ingersoll B. Meat industry spurred to revise policies. *WSJ*, August 27, 1997:A3.

37. Drew C. Search widens to find source of tainted beef. *NYT*, September 11, 1997. Belluck P. U.S. indicts producer of contaminated beef. *NYT*, December 17, 1998:A24. FSIS to review food recalls. *Nutrition Week*, April 8, 2002:1. USDA/FSIS. Recall Information at www.fsis.usda.gov/FSIS_Recalls/index.asp.

38. Becker E. 19 million pounds of meat recalled after 19 fall ill. *NYT*, July 20, 2002:A1,A9. Winter G. Democrats say slow meat recall threatened consumers. *NYT*, July 27, 2002:A9. Burros M. Federal audit faults department's meat and poultry inspection system. *NYT*, July 10, 2002:A15. GAO. *Meat and Poultry: Better USDA Oversight and Enforcement of Safety Rules Needed to Reduce Risk of Foodborne Illnesses* (GAO-02-292), August 2002.

39. Leonard RE. Hudson Foods, Inc: a risk management disaster. *Nutrition Week*, August 29, 1997:4–5.

40. Grey J. U.S. seeks new power to regulate meat safety. *NYT*, October 9, 1997:A28.

41. Sugarman C. Building a safer burger. *Washington Post*, September 3, 1997:E1,E10.

42. Armstrong GL, Hollingsworth J, Morris JG. Emerging foodborne pathogens: *Escherichia coli* O157:H7 as a model of entry of a new pathogen into the

food supply of the developed world. *Epidemiologic Reviews* 1996;18(1):29–51. Gansheroff LJ, O'Brien AD. *Escherichia coli* O157:H7 in beef cattle presented for slaughter in the U.S.: higher prevalence rates than previously estimated. *Proceedings of the National Academy of Sciences* 2000;97:2959–2961.

43. USDA/FSIS. Beef products contaminated with *Escherichia coli* O157:H7. *FR* 64:2803–2805, January 19, 1999.

44. Beers A. FSIS expands *E. coli* O157:H7 adulteration policy. *FCN*, January 18, 1999:3,17,18.

45. Glickman D. Letter to Rosemary Mucklow, executive director, National Meat Association, USDA, January 28, 1999. Copies of this letter circulated widely through electronic mail. See: Meat Industry Internet Newsservice. Glickman cancels speech after meat group's comment, January 29, 1999. Online: www.spcnetwork.com/mii/1999/990176.htm.

46. USDA/FSIS. *E. coli* O157:H7 contamination of beef products. *FR* 67:62325–62334, October 7, 2002.

47. Burros M. New U.S. standards for meat are snared in a court fight. *NYT*, December 4, 1999:A11. Ingersoll B. USDA is set to present new evidence Supreme Beef failed to meet standards. *WSJ*, December 10, 1999:A6.

48. Meat trade groups support Supreme Beef in lawsuit. *Food Regulation Weekly*, January 10, 2000:8–9. Burros M. Judge gives meat plant a reprieve from closing. *NYT*, December 11, 1999:A12.

49. Burros M. Ground beef is recalled for *E. coli*. *NYT*, December 26, 1999:A14.

50. A threat to meat inspection (editorial). *NYT*, May 26, 2000:A18.

51. Supreme Beef refuses USDA request to halt production. *Food Regulation Weekly*, June 19, 2000:12–13.

52. Beers A. Supreme Beef prepares to battle USDA in court over performance standards. *FCN*, November 27, 2000:3–4. USDA takes aim at Supreme Beef in latest round. *FCN*, March 19, 2001:18–19.

53. *Supreme Beef Processors, Inc. v. USDA*, 275 F. 3d432 (5th Cir. 2001).

54. Murphy D. Commentary: Salmonella Ruling—Can USDA's Loss Be Turned into Industry's Gain? *Meat Marketing & Technology*, December 14, 2001. Online: www.meatingplace.com (but no longer available).

55. A threat to meat inspection (editorial). *NYT*, December 26, 2001: A28.

56. Murano E. Ensuring meat safety (letter). *NYT*, January 2, 2002:A14. Ms. Murano was USDA undersecretary for food safety.

57. Movement on meat safety (editorial). *NYT*, February 9, 2002:A18.

58. Beers A. USDA won't appeal Supreme ruling, may seek regulatory changes. *FCN*, February 18, 2002:1,24. More legal challenges to *Salmonella* standard? *FCN*, June 17, 2002:1,13.

59. Bills seek to restore power for federal *Salmonella* tests. *NYT*, March 15, 2002:A12. Beers A. Harkin bill gets tougher on pathogen contamination. *FCN*, March 18, 2002:1,17,18.

60. USDA/FSIS. HACCP-based meat and poultry inspection concepts. *FR* 62:31553–31562, June 10, 1997. USDA/FSIS. *Backgrounder: HACCP-Based Inspection Models*, July 1998.

61. *American Federation of Government Employees v. Glickman*, 215 F.3d 7 (D.C. Cir. 2000).

62. HACCP appears to be in jeopardy as court rules against inspection system. *Nutrition Week*, July 7, 2000:1–2.

63. *American Federation of Government Employees v. Glickman*, 127 F.Supp. 2d 243 (D.D.C. 2001). Beers A. Union once again appeals HIMP ruling. *FCN*, February 19, 2001:4.

64. GAO. *Food Safety: Weaknesses in Meat and Poultry Inspection Pilot Should Be Addressed before Implementation* (GAO-02-59), December 2001. Quotations: 5,33–34.

65. USDA/FSIS. *An Overview of the HACCP-Based Inspection Models Project* (backgrounder), January 2002.

66. Beers A. Appeals court sides with USDA on HIMP—for now. *FCN*, April 8, 2002:1,13,14. Beers A. New HIMP data shows previously unrevealed problems. *FCN*, June 10, 2002:1,20,21.

67. Schlosser E. *Fast Food Nation*. New York: Houghton Mifflin, 2001.

68. The *West County Times* (Contra Costa, CA) tracked this story: Lyons C, Holbrook D. Three killed at sausage factory. (June 22, 2000:A1,A16). Marshall S, Jokelson A, Holbrook D, et al. State says plant is unlicensed. (June 23, 2000:A1,A16.) A grand jury indicted Mr. Alexander for murder in September 2000. He was tried, given a death sentence, but died in prison in 2005.

69. Anderson B. Beefed-up authority eyed for state inspectors. *West County Times*, June 30, 2000:A4. Association of Technical and Supervisory Professionals calls for Billy's resignation. *FCN*, July 31, 2000:4–5. USDA officials call for end to workplace violence. *The Food Safety Educator* (USDA/FSIS) 2000;5(3):2.

70. Hazelkorn B. Inspector abuse: how bad is it? MeatNews.com No. 381, July 19, 2000. Eye for an eye: abusive inspectors (No 477, October 11, 2000). Why we can't just get along (No. 510, November 8, 2000). It's all about communication (No. 740, January 30, 2001). Online: www.meatnews.com/index.cfm?fuseaction=Article&artNum=381 (477, 510, 740). No longer available.

71. Beers A. Number of reported workplace violence incidents increasing, USDA data shows. *FCN*, May 20, 2002:22–23. USDA expands scope of workplace violence directive. *FCN*, June 24, 2002:28–29.

72. Milbank Memorial Fund. *Conflict and Violence in the Food Safety Workplace: A Report on Meetings*, September 2000, at www.milbank.org/0107 foodsafety.html.

CHAPTER 4. ACHIEVING SAFE FOOD: ALTERNATIVES

1. USDA. *U.S. Imports of Agricultural, Fish, and Forestry Products, All Countries, 2000*, at www.fao.org/docrep/008/y7867e/y7867e00.htm. Friedland WH. The new globalization: the case of fresh produce. In: Bonnano A, Busch L, Friedland, WH, et al., eds. *From Columbus to ConAgra: The Globalization of Agriculture and Food*. Lawrence: University Press of Kansas, 1994:210–231.

2. GAO. *Food Safety: Federal Efforts to Ensure the Safety of Imported Foods Are Inconsistent and Unreliable* (GAO/RCED-98-103), April 1998. Wasik JF. How safe is your produce? *Consumers Digest*, September/October 1998:61–66.

3. Chazan G. Moscow lets U.S. poultry back in. *NYT*, April 15, 2002:A13.

4. GAO. *U.S. Agricultural Exports: Strong Growth Likely but U.S. Export Assistance Programs' Contribution Uncertain* (GAO/NSIAD-97-260), September 1997.

5. FAO and WHO. *Understanding the Codex Alimentarius.* Rome, 2006, at ftp://ftp.fao.org/codex/Publications/understanding/Understanding_EN.pdf.

6. Avery N, Drake M, Lang T. *Cracking the Codex: An Analysis of Who Sets World Food Standards.* London: National Food Alliance, 1993.

7. Gerth J, Weiner T. Imports swamp U.S. food-safety efforts. *NYT,* September 29, 1997:A1,A10.

8. Daniels RW. Home food safety. *Food Technology* 1998;52(2):54–56.

9. DHHS. *Healthy People 2000: National Health Promotion and Disease Prevention Objectives* (conference edition), 1990:339–341. DHHS. *Promoting Health, Preventing Disease: Objectives for the Nation,* 1980:58.

10. DHHS. *Healthy People 2010: Understanding and Improving Health* (conference edition, Vol. 1), 2000:10-1 to 10-17.

11. Glickman D (USDA Secretary), Shalala D (DHHS Secretary). "Dear Colleague" letter on Partnership for Food Safety Education letterhead, September 1997.

12. Mokhiber R, Weissman R. *Which way, CFA?* Focus on the Corporation, June 8, 2000, at www.mail-archive.com/ctrl@listserv.aol.com/msg44112.html.

13. Partnership for Food Safety Education. *Fight BAC! A National Public Education Campaign to Reduce the Risk of Foodborne Illness,* 1998. Online: www.fightbac.org.

14. USDA/FSIS. *Backgrounder: Food Safety Education: Making a Difference in Improving Public Health,* October 1998.

15. American Dietetic Association and ConAgra Foundation. *Home Food Safety . . . It's in Your Hands.* Chicago, IL, 2000.

16. Barboza D. Meatpackers' profits hinge on pool of immigrant labor. *NYT,* December 21, 2001:A26. Tyson Foods indicted in plan to smuggle illegal workers. *NYT,* December 20, 2001:A1,A32.

17. Osterholm MT. No magic bullet: more inspectors is fine and dandy. But don't kid yourself: government can't "solve" the problem of food safety. *Newsweek,* September 1, 1997:33. At the time, Mr. Osterholm was chief of epidemiology, Minnesota Department of Health.

18. Olson DG. Irradiation of food. *Food Technology* 1998;52(1):56–62. *Radiation Pasteurization of Food* (Issue paper No. 7). Ames, IA: Council for Agricultural Science and Technology, April 1996. GAO. *Food Irradiation: Available Research Indicates That Benefits Outweigh Risks* (GAO/RCED-00-217), August 2000.

19. Morrison RM. Food irradiation still faces hurdles. *FoodReview* 1992;15(2):11–15.

20. USDA. Fruits and vegetables from Hawaii: proposed rule. *FR* 67:35932–35936, May 22, 2002.

21. Meat industry pushes irradiation. *Illinois Agrinews,* November 21, 1997:C3. Grey J. U.S. seeks new power to regulate meat safety. *NYT,* October 9, 1997:A28.

22. Whelan EM. Safe meat: there is a better way (editorial). *WSJ,* August 26, 1997:16.

23. Produce Marketing Association. Fact Sheet: Irradiation. Newark, DE, No-

vember 1997. The association's mission is to "create a favorable, responsible environment that advances the marketing" of fresh fruits, vegetables, and flowers sold by its 2,500 members. O'Connor T. FDA approves irradiation for beef. *Illinois Agrinews*, December 12, 1997:C3. Mr. O'Connor was executive vice president of the Illinois Beef Forum, a trade association for the state beef industry.

24. Food and Drug Modernization Act of 1997, Public Law 105-115, 105th Congress, 1st Session, November 21, 1997, 111 Stat. 2296. Section 306: Disclosure of irradiation. Section 307: Irradiation petition.

25. FDA. Irradiation in the production, processing, and handling of food. *FR* 62:64107–64121, December 3, 1997. Kolata G. Irradiating red meat approved as a means to kill deadly germs. *NYT*, December 3, 1997:A1,A33.

26. Leonard RE. 1997: the year of living dangerously. *Nutrition Week*, February 6, 1998:4–5. Chicken: what you don't know can hurt you. *Consumer Reports*, March 1998:12–18.

27. Farm Security and Rural Investment Act of 2002. Public Law 107-171, 107th Congress, 2nd Session, May 13, 2002. 116 Stat. 134. Liddle AJ. DQ field tests irradiated burgers as farm bill relaxes labeling law. *Nation's Restaurant News*, May 20, 2002:3,234.

28. Kolata G, Drew C. Long quest for safer food revisits radiation method. *NYT*, December 4, 1997:A1,A24.

29. Frenzen PD, Majchrowicz A, Buzby JC, et al. Consumer acceptance of irradiated meat and poultry products. *Issues in Food Safety Economics* (Agriculture Information Bulletin No. 757), USDA/ERS, August 2000.

30. *Consumers' Views on Food Irradiation*. Washington, DC: Food Marketing Institute and Grocery Manufacturers of America, 1998. These are trade organizations for grocery retailers, wholesalers, and food and beverage product companies.

31. Expert Panel on Food Safety and Nutrition. Irradiation of food. *Food Technology* 1998;52:56–62. Morrison RM, Buzby JC, Lin C-TJ. Irradiating ground beef to enhance food safety. *FoodReview* 1997;20(1):33–37. Buzby JC, Morrison RM. Food irradiation—an update. *FoodReview* 1999;22(3):21–22.

32. Fulmer M. Hum of interest builds around irradiated food. *Los Angeles Times*, November 20, 2001:C1.

33. Leonard R. Food safety mismanagement puts consumer health at risk. *Nutrition Week*, April 16, 1999:4–5.

34. DeWaal CS, Barlow K, Alderton L, et al. *Outbreak Alert! Closing the Gaps in Our Federal Food-Safety Net*. Washington, DC: CSPI, October 2001.

35. Headrick ML, Korangy S, Bean NH, et al. The epidemiology of raw milk–associated foodborne disease outbreaks reported in the United States, 1973 through 1992. *Am J Public Health* 1998;88:1219–1221. CDC. Outbreak of *Listeriosis* associated with homemade Mexican-style cheese—North Carolina, October 2000–January 2001. *MMWR* 2001;50:560–562. Cody SH, Abbott SL, Marfin AA, et al. Two outbreaks of multidrug-resistant *Salmonella* serotype typhimurium DT104 infections linked to raw-milk cheese in Northern California. *JAMA* 1999;281:1805–1810. Villar RG, Macek MD, Simons S, et al. Investigation of multidrug-resistant *Salmonella* serotype typhimurium DT104 infections linked to raw-milk cheese in Washington State. *JAMA* 1999;281:1811–1816.

36. Keene WE. Lessons from investigations of foodborne disease outbreaks. *JAMA* 1999;281:1845–1847.

37. Wakin DJ. New scrutiny of cheese offends refined palates. *NYT*, July 14, 2000:B1,B9.

38. American Cheese Society. Platform of the American Cheese Society Regarding Mandatory Pasteurization (flyer). Distributed at the National Association for the Specialty Food Trade Fancy Food Show, New York, July 11–14, 1999. The society, which promotes American-made specialty cheeses, is headquartered in Louisville, Kentucky. Online: www.cheesesociety.org.

39. USDA/FSIS. Pathogen reduction: Hazard Analysis Critical Control Point (HACCP) systems: proposed rule. *FR* 60:6774–6889, February 3, 1995.

40. Sara Lee pleads guilty to selling adulterated meat from Michigan plant. *Detroit Free Press*, June 23, 2001, at www.accessmylibrary.com/coms2/summary _0286–8343460_ITM. USDA/FSIS. Owners of Texas Firm Sentenced for Selling Adulterated Meat Products (press release), January 2, 2002.

41. Steinhauer J. Number of victims of *E. coli* poisoning in upstate New York grows to nearly 300. *NYT*, September 9, 1999:B5. Barstow D. A wholesome tradition tainted: *E. coli* takes terrible toll on families and fair's future. *NYT*, September 20, 1999:B1,B6.

42. Institute of Medicine. *Ensuring Safe Food: From Production to Consumption.* Washington, DC: National Academy Press, 1998. Quotations: v–vi, 12–13.

43. Food Marketing Institute. *Long-Range Priorities for Food Safety* (adopted by the FMI Board of Directors). Washington, DC, October 28, 1988. Also see: *White House Conference on Food, Nutrition, and Health, Final Report,* 1970:129–141. Smith RJ. Institute of Medicine report recommends complete overhaul of food safety laws. *Science* 1979;203:1221–1224. Institute of Food Technologists. Guiding principles for optimum food safety oversight and regulation in the United States. *Food Technology* 1998;52(5):30,50,52.

44. GAO. *Food Safety and Quality: Uniform, Risk-Based Inspection System Needed to Ensure Safe Food Supply* (GAO/RCED-92-152), June 1992:6.

45. Harman JW. *Food Safety: A Unified, Risk-Based System Needed to Enhance Food Safety* (GAO/T-RCED-94-71), November 4, 1993.

46. Dyckman LJ. *Food Safety: U.S. Needs a Single Agency to Administer a Unified, Risk-Based Inspection System* (GAO/T-RCED-99-256), August 4, 1999.

47. Kessler DA (FDA Commissioner). Memorandum to the Secretary of DHHS. Washington, DC: DHHS, March 12, 1993.

48. Burros M. Clinton to battle foodborne illness. *NYT*, January 25, 1997:A1,A7. Marwick C. Putting money where the U.S. mouth is: initiative on food safety gets under way. *JAMA* 1997;277:1340–1342.

49. FDA, EPA, CDC. *Food Safety from Farm to Table: A National Food Safety Initiative: Report to the President.* FDA/EPA/CDC, May 1997, at www.foodsafety .gov/~dms/fsreport.html.

50. Broder JM. Clinton to seek additional money for food safety. *NYT*, December 28, 1997:A1,A17.

51. Burros M. President to push for food safety: seeks more money, and power to tighten import controls. *NYT*, July 4, 1998:A1,A9.

52. GAO. *Food Safety: Opportunities to Redirect Federal Resources and Funds Can Enhance Effectiveness* (GAO/RCED-98-224), August 1998.

53. Leonard R. Food safety proposals may be a health hazard. *Nutrition Week,* August 28, 1998:4–5.

54. Molotsky I. Clinton to appoint council to oversee safety of food. *NYT,* August 25, 1998:A15. In response to NAS report Clinton appoints a food safety council; no czar. *Nutrition Week,* August 28, 1998:1,6.

55. USDA, DHHS, EPA. President's national food safety initiative. *FR* 63:45922–45923, August 27, 1998.

56. DHHS, USDA. *Backgrounder: 2000 President's Food Safety Initiative.* DHHS/USDA, February 25, 1999. Federal food safety documents are available online: www.foodsafety.gov. Endicott RC. 46th annual report: 100 leading national advertisers. *Advertising Age,* September 24, 2001:s1–s26.

57. Draft food safety strategic plan offers no surprises. *Food Regulation Weekly,* January 17, 2000:6–7.

58. Food Safety Council strategic plan will get "real," Levitt promises. *Food Regulation Weekly,* February 14, 2000:11.

59. USDA/FSIS. Performance standards for the production of processed meat and poultry products; proposed rule. *FR* 66:12589–12636, February 27, 2001. Bush administration blocks proposed rule on *Listeria* testing. *Nutrition Week,* January 26, 2001:1–2. USDA released proposed *Listeria* rule from chokehold. *Nutrition Week,* February 23, 2001:6. Burros M. New meat-testing regulation wins backing of White House. *NYT,* February 27, 2001:A21.

60. Burros M. U.S. proposed end to testing for *Salmonella* in school beef. *NYT,* April 5, 2001:A1,A14. Becker E. Agriculture chief disavows plan to eliminate test on school beef. *NYT,* April 6, 2001:A1,A19. Beers A. USDA reinstates *Salmonella* testing of school-lunch beef. *FCN,* April 9, 2001:3–4.

61. Jackson D. School lunches: illness on menu, and Jackson D, Dougherty G. Meat from troubled plants sold to U.S. lunch program. *Chicago Tribune,* December 9, 2001:C1,C17.

62. GAO. *Food Safety: Continued Vigilance Needed to Ensure Safety of School Meals* (GAO-02-669T), April 30, 2002.

63. Taylor MR. Reforming food safety: a model for the future. *Food Technology* 2002;56(5):190–194.

64. Weber W. The road ahead for the European Food Authority. *Lancet* 2001;358:650.

65. GAO. *Food Safety: Experiences of Four Countries in Consolidating Their Food Safety Systems* (GAO/RCED-99-80), April 1999.

PART 2. SAFETY AS A SURROGATE:
THE IRONIC POLITICS OF FOOD BIOTECHNOLOGY

Some parts of these chapters are drawn from articles published previously and are used with their publishers' permission: Nestle, M. Allergies to transgenic foods—questions of policy, *NEJM* 1996;334:726–728 (Massachusetts Medical Society); Food biotechnology: labeling will benefit industry as well as consumers, *Nutrition Today* 1998;33(1):6–12 (Lippincott Williams & Wilkins);

Food biotechnology: politics and policy implications. In: Kiple KF, Ornelas-Kiple CK, eds. *The Cambridge World History of Food and Nutrition*, Vol. II. Cambridge: Cambridge University Press, 2000:1643–1662; Agricultural biotechnology, policy, nutrition. In: Murray TH, Mehlman MJ, eds. *Encyclopedia of Ethical, Legal, & Policy Issues in Biotechnology*. New York: John Wiley & Sons, 2000:66–76.

1. Agricultural Biotechnology: The Road to Improved Nutrition & Increased Production? (conference). Boston, MA: Tufts University School of Nutrition Science and Policy, November 1–2, 2001.

2. For the origin of *Frankenfoods*, see Safire W. On language. *NYT Magazine*, August 13, 2000:23. Mr. Safire notes that biotechnophobes needed a frightening metaphor, "and the Franken-prefix did the trick." He credits the term to this letter from Paul Lewis, an English professor at Boston University: "Ever since Mary Shelley's baron rolled his improved human out of the lab, scientists have been bringing just such good things [genetically modified tomatoes] to life. If they want to sell us Frankenfood, perhaps it's time to gather the villagers, light some torches, and head to the castle" (*NYT,* June 16, 1992:A24).

3. Gaull GE, Goldberg RA, eds. *New Technologies and the Future of Food and Nutrition.* New York: John Wiley & Sons, 1991.

4. Fraley R. Sustaining the food supply. *Bio/Technology* 1992;10:40–43.

5. I am indebted to my NYU colleague Dorothy Nelkin for her discussion of these ideas. See: Nelkin D. *Selling Science: How the Press Covers Science and Technology.* San Francisco: W.H. Freeman, 1995.

CHAPTER 5. PEDDLING DREAMS: PROMISES VERSUS REALITY

1. GAO. *Genetically Modified Foods: Experts View Regimen of Safety Tests as Adequate, but FDA's Evaluation Process Could Be Enhanced.* (GAO-02-566), May 2002. Greenpeace. *How to Avoid Genetically Engineered Food: True Food Shopping List.* Washington, DC, October 2000.

2. Mann CC. Crop scientists seek a new revolution. *Science* 1999;285:310–314.

3. Gaull GE, Goldberg RA, eds. *New Technologies and the Future of Food and Nutrition.* New York: John Wiley & Sons, 1990:97,150. Angell PS. Playing God in the garden (letter). *NYT Magazine*, November 15, 1998:26.

4. Feldbaum CB. *The Transfer of Agricultural Biotechnology to Developing Countries: A Series of Case Studies.* Washington, DC: Biotechnology Industry Organization, 1996.

5. Conversion of potatoes (cheap) into potato chips (more expensive, higher profit) is an example of adding value, as is the addition of vitamins to sugar-coated cereals.

6. Ollinger M, Pope L. *Plant Biotechnology: Out of the Laboratory and into the Field* (Agricultural Economic Report No. 697), USDA, 1995. Leary W. Cornucopia of new foods is seen as policy on engineering is eased. *NYT,* May 27, 1992:A1. Brownlee S. Dollars for DNA: biotech seems near to living up to its

hype. *US News & World Report*, May 25, 1998:48,50. Agricultural biotechnology. *Nature Biotechnology* 2000;18(suppl):IT59–IT61.

7. Vidal J. Special report: GM food debate. *Guardian* (London), August 28, 2001. The planting figures may be conservative; Monsanto alone claimed 103 million acres in 2000.

8. A group called Syracuse Cultural Workers produces a t-shirt satirizing the original Monsanto slogan as *Lies, Death, Profits*, at http://syracuseculturalworkers.com/aboutus.

9. Monsanto. *2000 Annual Report*. Online: www.monsanto.com. Pharmacia divested its 84% stake in Monsanto in 2002.

10. Enriquez J, Goldberg R. *Gene Research, the Mapping of Life, and the Global Economy* (case study). Boston: Harvard Business School, October 16, 1998.

11. Caswell MF, Fuglie KO, Klotz CA. *Agricultural Biotechnology: An Economic Perspective* (Agricultural Economic Report No. 687). USDA, 1994. Pennisi E. A bonanza for plant genomics. *Science* 1998;282:652–654.

12. Bokanga M. Biotechnology and cassava processing in Africa. *Food Technology* 1995;49:86–90. Knorr D. Improving food biotechnology resources and strategies in developing countries. *Food Technology* 1995;49:91–93. Messer E. Sources of institutional funding for agrobiotechnology for developing countries. *Advanced Technology Assessment Systems* 1992;9:371–378.

13. Beachy R. Transferring genes. In: Burke WS, ed. *Symbol, substance, science: the societal issues of food biotechnology* (proceedings of a conference, July 28–29, 1993). Research Triangle Park, NC: USDA Office of Agricultural Biotechnology and North Carolina Biotechnology Center, 1993:45–51,61. Beachy RN. Facing fear of biotechnology. *Science* 1999;285:335. Dr. Beachy is now president of the Donald Danforth Plant Science Center in St. Louis, MO. Although the center is listed on the Monsanto Web site as a partner, Dr. Beachy says he has not been funded by Monsanto since 1991 (see letters to the editor: *Science* 1999;285:1489).

14. Sommer A, West KP. *Vitamin A Deficiency: Health, Survival, and Vision*. New York: Oxford University Press, 1996. Sommer A. *Vitamin A Deficiency and Its Consequences: A Field Guide to Detection and Control*. 3rd ed. Geneva: World Health Organization, 1995.

15. Yoon CK. Stalked by deadly virus, papaya lives to breed again. *NYT*, July 20, 1999:F3.

16. Hamilton JO. Biotech: an industry crowded with players faces an ugly reckoning. *Business Week*, September 26, 1994:84–92.

17. Wambugu F. Biotechnology: protesters don't grasp Africa's need. *Los Angeles Times*, November 11, 2001:M1. Wambugu FM. *Modifying Africa: How Biotechnology Can Benefit the Poor and Hungry, A Case Study from Kenya*, Nairobi, 2001.

18. Monsanto. Meeting the World's Needs with Fewer Resources (press release). St. Louis, MO, 1996. Council for Biotechnology Information. Biotechnology and the Developing World (leaflet). The council's public relations materials appear online at www.whybiotech.com.

19. Ye X, Al-Babili S, Klöti A, et al. Engineering the provitamin A (β-carotene)

biosynthetic pathway into (carotenoid-free) rice endosperm. *Science* 2000;287: 303–305. Heldt H-W. *Plant Biochemistry and Molecular Biology.* Oxford: Oxford University Press, 1997.

20. Dary O, Mora JO. Food fortification to reduce vitamin A deficiency: International Vitamin A Consultative Group recommendations. *J Nutrition* 2002; 132:2927s–2933s.

21. Normile D. Rockefeller to end network after 15 years of success. *Science* 1999;286:1468–1469. Christensen J. Golden Rice in a grenade-proof greenhouse. *NYT,* November 21, 2000:F1,F5. Normile D. Monsanto donates its share of Golden Rice. *Science* 2000;289:843–845. The scientists describe the patent and legal issues in: Beyer P, Al-Babili S, Ye S, et al. Golden Rice: introducing the β-carotene biosynthesis pathway into rice endosperm by genetic engineering to defeat vitamin A deficiency. *J Nutrition* 2002;132:506s-510s.

22. Nash JM. Grains of hope. *Time,* July 31, 2000:39–46.

23. Potrykus I. Nutritionally enhanced rice to compete [*sic*] malnutrition disorders of the poor (handout). From Agricultural Biotechnology: The Road to Improved Nutrition and Increased Production? (conference), Boston, Tufts University School of Nutrition Science and Policy, November 2, 2001.

24. Potrykus I. Golden Rice and beyond. *Plant Physiology* 2001;125:1157–1161.

25. Greenpeace. Background information: the false promise of genetically engineered rice. February 2001. Haverlin B. GE rice is fool's gold, February 9, 2001. Khoo M. Greenpeace demands false biotech advertising be removed from TV, February 9, 2001, at www.greenpeace.org/usa.

26. The Potrykus group said the rice contained 1.6 micrograms (µg) beta-carotene per gram (g), but thought 2 µg/g realistic. The U.S. standard for vitamin A is 300 µg per day for children aged one to three years, 700 µg for adult women, and 900 µg for adult men. At a conversion rate of 12 µg beta-carotene to 1 µg vitamin A, the beta-carotene standard is 3,600 (12 × 300) µg for young children; 8,400 (12 × 700) µg for women; and 10,800 (12 × 900) µg for men. If Golden Rice contains 2 µg per g beta-carotene, the amounts are halved. Children would need to eat 1,800 g rice (4 lb); women 4,200 g (9 lb); and men 5,400 g (12 lb) a day to meet the U.S. standard for vitamin A. Rice is cooked in twice its volume of added water (example: 1 cup raw rice plus 2 cups water to yield 3 cups cooked rice). Therefore, the amounts of *cooked* rice are 12, 27, and 36 lb per day, respectively. Lower conversion ratios reduce these amounts.

27. Institute of Medicine. *Dietary Reference Intakes for Vitamin A, Vitamin K, Arsenic, Boron, Chromium, Copper, Iodine, Iron, Manganese, Molybdenum, Nickel, Silicon, Vanadium, and Zinc.* Washington, DC: National Academy Press, 2001:65–126.

28. Potrykus I. "Genetically engineered 'Golden Rice' is fool's gold": response from Prof. Ingo Potrykus. Ag BioTech InfoNet, February 10, 2001. Online: www.biotech-info.net/IP_response.html.

29. Conway G. Grain of hope. *Guardian* (London), March 21, 2001. Online: www.guardian.co.uk.

30. Olson JA. Carotenoids. In: Shils ME, Olson JA, Shike M, et al., eds. *Modern Nutrition in Health and Disease,* 9th ed. Philadelphia: Lippincott Williams

& Wilkins, 1998:525–541. Also: Torun B, Chew F. *Protein-Energy Malnutrition* (1998:963–988).

31. Nestle M. Genetically engineered "golden" rice unlikely to overcome vitamin A deficiency (letter). *J Am Dietetic Association* 2001;101:289–290. This letter points out that beta-carotene itself raises questions. Food sources of beta-carotene protect against cancer and heart disease, but supplements do not and may be harmful or beneficial depending on circumstances. The health effects of adding this single nutrient to rice endosperm are uncertain.

32. Filteau SM, Tomkins AM. Promoting vitamin A status in low-income countries. *Lancet* 1999;353;1458–1460. Summer A, Davidson FR, Ramakrishnan U, et al. Twenty-five years of progress in controlling vitamin A deficiency: looking to the future. Proceedings of the XX International Vitamin A Consultative Group Meeting, Hanoi, Vietnam, February 12–15, 2001. *J Nutrition* 2002;132(9 suppl):2843s–2990s.

33. Potrykus I. Golden Rice and the Greenpeace dilemma. Ag BioTech InfoNet, February 15, 2001. Online: www.biotech-info.net/2_IP_response.html.

CHAPTER 6. RISKS AND BENEFITS: WHO DECIDES?

1. Pew Initiative on Food and Biotechnology. *Public Sentiment about Genetically Modified Food*, June 21–23, 2001, at www.pewtrusts.org/news_room_detail.aspx?id=32822. The survey included 1,231 adults.

2. International Food Information Council. *U.S. Consumer Attitudes toward Food Biotechnology*, November 2001. Wirthlin Group Quorum conducted five surveys from 1997 to 2001; Cogent Research conducted the September 2001 telephone survey of about 1,000 adults.

3. OTA. *New Developments in Biotechnology: Public Perceptions of Biotechnology* (OTA-BP-BA-45), 1987. Also see: Zimmerman L, Kendall P, Stone M, et al. Consumer knowledge and concern about biotechnology and food safety. *Food Technology* 1994;48:71–77. Wie SH, Strohbehn CH, Hsu CHC. Iowa dietitians' attitudes toward and knowledge of genetically engineered and irradiated foods. *J Am Dietetic Association* 1998;98:1331–1333. *Genetically Modified Foods: Are You Afraid of Eating Them?* (Poll, December 1999).

4. Hoban TJ. Consumer acceptance of biotechnology: an international perspective. *Nature Biotechnology* 1997;15:232–234. Aerni P. Public attitudes towards agricultural biotechnology in developing countries: a comparison between Mexico and the Philippines. Cambridge, MA: Center for International Development, Harvard University, October 1, 2001, at www.inai.org.ar/ogm/Public%20Attitudes%20towards%20Agricultural%20Biotechnology%20in%20developing%20countires.pdf.

5. Barling D, de Vriend H, Cornelese JA, et al. The social aspects of food biotechnology: a European view. *Environmental Toxicology and Pharmacology* 1999;7:85–93. Frewer L. Public perceptions of genetically modified foods in Europe. *J Commercial Biotechnology* 1999;6:108–115. Thompson PB. *Food Biotechnology in Ethical Perspective*. London: Blackie Academic & Professional, 1997.

6. HRH, the Prince of Wales. Seeds of disaster. *Daily Telegraph* (London), June 8, 1998. Reprinted in *Ecologist* 1998;28(5):252–253.

7. Smith G, Gruner P. "Scaremonger" but Charles is right to call for debate. *Evening Standard* (London), June 8, 1998:4.

8. Thavis J. Vatican experts OK plant, animal genetic engineering. *St. Louis Review*, October 22, 1999:E1. Lyman E. Pope expresses opposition to GMOs: cites need for "the respect of nature." Bureau of National Affairs, No. 221, November 15, 2000, at http://online.sfsu.edu/~rone/GEessays/PopeGMO.htm.

9. Genetically modified food: food for thought. *Economist*, June 19, 1999: 19–21.

10. Frederickson DS. *The Recombinant DNA Controversy: A Memoir: Science, Politics, and the Public Interest 1974–1981*. Washington, DC: American Society for Microbiology, 2001. For another view, see: Krimsky S. *Genetic Alchemy: The Social History of the Recombinant DNA Controversy*. Cambridge, MA: MIT Press, 1994.

11. Commoner B. Unraveling the DNA myth: the spurious foundation of genetic engineering. *Harper's*, February 2002:39–47.

12. Fuchs RL, Astwood JD. Allergenicity assessment of foods derived from genetically modified plants. *Food Technology* 1996;50(2):83–88. Metcalfe DD, Fuchs RL, Townsend R, et al., eds. Allergenicity of foods produced by genetic modification. *Critical Reviews in Food Science and Nutrition* 1996;36(suppl): S1–S186.

13. Consumer & Biotechnology Foundation. *Genetically Modified Foods and Allergenicity: Safety Aspects and Consumer Information* (workshop proceedings), May 28–29, 1999. Den Haag. *The Netherlands: Stichting Consument en Biotechnologie*, 1999.

14. Buchanan BB. Genetic engineering and the allergy issue. *Plant Physiology* 2001;126:5–7.

15. Burks AW, Fuchs RL. Assessment of the endogenous allergens in glyphosate-tolerant and commercial soybean varieties. *J Allergy and Clinical Immunology* 1995;96:1008–1110.

16. Winslow R. Allergen is inadvertently transferred to soybean in bioengineering test. *WSJ*, March 14, 1996:B6.

17. Nordlee JA, Taylor SL, Townsend JA, et al. Identification of a Brazil-nut allergen in transgenic soybeans. *NEJM* 1996;334:688–692.

18. FDA. Statement of policy: foods derived from new plant varieties. *FR* 57:22984–22986, May 29, 1992.

19. FDA. Food labeling: food derived from new plant varieties. *FR* 58:25837–25841, April 28, 1993. BIO favors limited notification on biotech food 3-year sunset. *FCN*, May 16, 1994:7–8.

20. EPA. *FIFRA Scientific Advisory Panel Meeting, November 28, 2000* (SAP Report No. 2000-06), December 1, 2000. EPA Scientific Advisory Panel (SAP) reports are online at: www.epa.gov/scipoly/sap [Note: search by date].

21. Nestor EW, Roberts CE, Pearsall NN, et al. *Microbiology: A Human Perspective*. 2nd ed. Boston: WCB/McGraw-Hill, 1998.

22. Holmberg SD, Osterholm MT, Senger KA, et al. Drug-resistant *Salmonella* from animals fed antimicrobials. *NEJM* 1984;311:617–622. Tacket CO,

Dominguez LB, Fisher HJ, et al. An outbreak of multiple-drug-resistant *Salmonella* enteritis from raw milk. *JAMA* 1985;253:2058–2060. White DG, Zhao S, Sudler R, et al. The isolation of antibiotic-resistant *Salmonella* from retail ground meats. *NEJM* 2001;345:1147–1154.

23. FDA. Secondary direct food additives permitted in food for human consumption; food additives permitted in feed and drinking water of animals; aminoglycoside 3'-phosphotransferase II: final rule. *FR* 59:26700–26711, May 23, 1994. The kanamycin (neomycin) resistance gene specifies the enzyme, aminoglycoside 3'-phosphotransferase II.

24. FDA. Guidance for industry: use of antibiotic-resistance marker genes in transgenic plants: draft guidance. September 4, 1998. FDA documents on antibiotic resistance are available at http://vm.cfsan.fda.gov/~dms/opa-armg.html.

25. FDA Task Force on Antimicrobial Resistance. *Key Recommendations and Report.* FDA, December 2000. FDA. HHS releases action plan to combat antimicrobial resistance (press release). January 18, 2001.

26. Goldburg R, Rissler J, Shand H, et al. *Biotechnology's Bitter Harvest: Herbicide-Tolerant Crops and the Threat to Sustainable Agriculture.* Washington, DC: Biotechnology Working Group, 1990. Rissler J, Mellon M. *The Ecological Risks of Engineered Crops.* Cambridge, MA: MIT Press, 1996.

27. Kaiser J. Pests overwhelm *Bt* cotton crop. *Science* 1996;273:423.

28. Benson S, Arax M, Burstein R. A growing concern: as biotech crops come to market, neither scientists—who take industry money—nor federal regulators are adequately protecting consumers and farmers. *Mother Jones,* 1997; January/February:36–43,66,68,71.

29. Kling J. Could transgenic supercrops one day breed superweeds? *Science* 1996;274:180–181. Also see: Mikkelsen TR, Anderson B, Jorgensen RB. The risk of crop transgene spread. *Nature* 1996;380:31.

30. Scott SE, Wilkinson MJ. Low probability of chloroplast movement from oilseed rape (*Brassica napus*) into wild *Brassica rapa*. *Nature Biotechnology* 1999;17:390–393. Saxena D, Flores S, Stotzky G. Insecticidal toxin in root exudates from *Bt* corn. *Nature* 1999;402:480. Kuiper HA, Kleter GA, Noordam MY. Risks of the release of transgenic herbicide-resistant plants with respect to humans, animals, and the environment. *Crop Protection* 2000;19:773–778.

31. Benbrook C. Do GM crops mean less pesticide use? *Pesticide Outlook* 2001;October:204–207.

32. Reichhardt T. US sends mixed message in GM debate . . . as questions emerge over cost effectiveness. *Nature* 1999;400:298. Wolfenbarger LL, Phifer PR. The ecological risks and benefits of genetically engineered plants. *Science* 2000;290:2088–2093.

33. Carpenter JE. *Case Studies in Benefits and Risks of Agricultural Biotechnology: Roundup Ready Soybeans and Bt Field Corn.* Washington, DC: National Center for Food and Agriculture Policy, January 2001. Fernandez-Cornejo J, McBride WD. *Adoption of Bioengineered Crops* (Ag. Econ. Rep. No. AER810), USDA/ERS, May 2002. Benbrook CM. *The Bt Premium Price: What Does it Buy?* Minneapolis, MN: Institute for Agriculture and Trade Policy, February 2002, at www.gefoodalert.org/library/admin/uploadedfiles/Bt_Premium_Price_What_Does _It_Buy_The.pdf.

34. Simon S. Biotech soybeans plant seed of risky revolution. *Los Angeles Times,* July 1, 2001:A1.

35. Technical points: To construct soybeans resistant to Roundup, Monsanto scientists selected variants of *Agrobacterium* resistant to glyphosate, isolated the gene for the resistant enzyme, and introduced that *Agrobacterium* gene into soybeans (see appendix). Glyphosate is the common name for N-phosphonomethyl glycine, an amino acid analog that inhibits the enzyme 5-enolpyruvylshikimate-3-phosphate synthase (alternatively called 3-phoshoshikimate 1-carboxyvinyltransferase), which catalyzes synthesis of aromatic amino acids—tryptophan, phenylalanine, and tyrosine—in plant, bacterial, and fungal (but not animal) cells. See: Cobb A. *Herbicides and Plant Physiology.* London: Chapman & Hall, 1992:6.1–6.3. Rogers SG. Biotechnology and the soybean. *Am J Clinical Nutrition* 1998;68(suppl):1330s–1332s.

36. Monsanto. Responses to questions raised and statements made by environmental/consumer groups and other critics of biotechnology and Roundup Ready soybeans, April 21, 1997, at http://db.zs-intern.de/uploads/1190982382-mon santoGlyphosateResistantWeeds1997.pdf.

37. Paoletti MG, Pimentel D. Environmental risks of pesticides versus genetic engineering for agricultural pest control. *J Agricultural and Environmental Ethics* 2000;12:279–303.

38. Cox C. Glyphosate: Part 1: toxicology. Part 2: human exposure and ecological effects. *J Pesticide Reform* 1995;15(3):14–21 and 1995;15(4):14–20.

39. Coghlan A. Splitting headache: Monsanto's modified soya beans are cracking up in the heat. *New Scientist,* November 20, 1999:25.

40. CDC. Eosinophilia-myalgia syndrome—New Mexico. *JAMA* 1989; 262:3116. Mayeno AN, Gleich GJ. Eosinophilia-myalgia syndrome and tryptophan production: a cautionary tale. *Trends in Biotechnology* 1994;12:346–352. Philin RM, Hill RH, Flanders WD, et al. Tryptophan contaminants associated with eosinophilia-myalgia syndrome. *Am J Epidemiology* 1993;138:154–159.

41. Kilbourne EM, Philen RM, Kamb ML, et al. Tryptophan produced by Showa Denko and epidemic eosinophilia-myalgia syndrome. *J Rheumatology* 1996;23(suppl 46):81–88. Also see: Sternberg EM. Intimidation of researchers by special-interest groups (letter). *NEJM* 1997;337:1316. In response, the editor of *J Rheumatology,* D.A. Gordon, said that the Showa Denko–sponsored "reports and our editorial process qualify as unbiased peer review" (1316–1317).

42. Pusztai A. *Report of the Project Coordinator on Data Produced at the Rowett Research Institute,* SOAEFD (Scottish Office, Agriculture Environment & Fisheries Department) Flexible Fund Project RO 818, October 22, 1998, at www.rowett.ac.uk/gmo.

43. Enserink M. Institute copes with genetic hot potato. *Science* 1998;281: 1124–1125. Biotech: the pendulum swings back. *Rachel's Environment & Health Weekly,* May 16, 1999. Health risks of genetically modified foods (letters). *Lancet* 1999;353:1811.

44. Berger A. Hot potato. *British Medical J* 1999;318:611.

45. Bourne FJ, Chesson A, Davies H, et al. *Audit of Data Produced at the Rowett Research Institute,* SOAEFD (Scottish Office, Agriculture Environment & Fisheries Department) Flexible Fund Project RO 818, August 21, 1998, at www .rowett.ac.uk/gmoarchive/gmaudit.pdf. Enserink M. Preliminary data touch off

genetic food fight. *Science* 1999;283:1094–1095. Christie B. Scientists call for moratorium on genetically modified foods. *British Medical J* 1999;318:483.
    46. Coghlan A, Concar D, MacKenzie D. Frankenfears. *New Scientist*, February 20, 1999:4.
    47. Ewen WB, Pusztai A. Health risks of genetically modified foods (letter). *Lancet* 1999;354:684.
    48. The Royal Society. *Review of Data on Possible Toxicity of GM Potatoes*, May 18, 1999, at http://royalsociety.org/displaypagedoc.asp?id=6170. Hoge W. Britons skirmish over genetically modified crops. *NYT*, August 23, 1999:A3. Ellison S. U.K. study dismisses research faulting genetically altered food. *WSJ*, May 19, 1999:A19.
    49. Ewen SWB, Pusztai A. Effect of diets containing genetically modified potatoes expressing *Galanthus nivalis* lectin on rat small intestine. *Lancet* 1999;354:1353–1354. Fenton B, Stanley K, Fenton S, et al. Differential binding of the insecticidal lectin GNA to human blood cells. *Lancet* 1999;354:1354–1355. Kuiper HA, Noteborn HPJM, Peijnenburg AACM. Adequacy of methods for testing the safety of genetically modified foods. *Lancet* 1999;354:1315–1316.
    50. Horton R. Genetically modified foods: "absurd" concern or welcome dialogue? *Lancet* 1999;354:1314–1315.
    51. Flynn L, Gillard MS. Pro-GM food scientist "threatened editor." *Guardian* (London), November 1, 1999, at www.guardian.co.uk/science/1999/nov/01/gm .food. See: Correspondence: GM food debate. *Lancet* 1999;354:1725–1729. Enserink M. The *Lancet* scolded over Pusztai paper. *Science* 1999;286:656.
    52. Losey JE, Rayor LS, Carter ME. Transgenic pollen harms monarch larvae. *Nature* 1999;399:214.
    53. Stix G. The butterfly effect: new research findings and European jitters could cloud the future for genetically modified crops. *Scientific American,* August 1999:28–29. The finding inspired a book: Jack A. *Imagine a World without Monarch Butterflies: Awakening to the Hazards of Genetically Altered Foods.* Becket, MA: One Peaceful World Press, 1999. Kucinich DJ. *Statement before the Senate Committee on Agriculture, Nutrition, and Forestry.* 106th Congress, 1st Session, October 7, 1999, at http://agriculture.senate.gov/Hearings/Hearings _1999/kuc99107.htm.
    54. Steyer R. Scientists discount threat to butterfly from altered corn. *St. Louis Post-Dispatch*, November 2, 1999:A5.
    55. Biotechnology Industry Organization. Scientific symposium to show no harm to monarch butterfly (press release). Chicago, November 2, 1999.
    56. Yoon CK. No consensus on effect of genetically altered corn on butterflies. *NYT*, November 4, 1999:A20.
    57. Wraight CL, Zangerl AR, Carroll MJ, et al. Absence of toxicity of *Bacillus thuringiensis* pollen to black swallowtails under field conditions. *Proceedings of the National Academy of Sciences* 2000;97:7700–7703. Milius S. Bt corn variety OK for black swallowtails. *Science News* June 10, 2000:372.
    58. Yoon CK. New data in duel of biotech corn vs. butterflies. *NYT,* August 22, 2000:D2. Jesse LC, Obrycki JJ. Field deposition of *Bt* transgenic corn pollen: lethal effects on the monarch butterfly. *Oecologia* 2000;125:241–248.

59. Kaplan JK. *Bt* corn not a threat to monarchs. *Agricultural Research* 2002;50:16–18.

60. Sears MK, Hellmich RL, Stanley-Horn DE, et al. Impact of *Bt* corn pollen on monarch butterfly populations: a risk assessment. *Proceedings of the National Academy of Sciences* 2001;98:11937–11942 (other papers, 11908–11936). The journal posted the papers online prior to publication at www.pnas.org. Pollack A. Data on genetically modified corn: reports say threat to monarch butterflies is "negligible." *NYT,* September 8, 2001:C2.

61. EPA. Biotechnology corn approved for continued use (press release), October 16, 2001, at http://yosemite1.epa.gov/opa/admpress.nsf/b1ab9f485b09897 2852562e7004dc686/8db7a83e66e0f7d085256ae7005d6ec2.

62. GAO. *Genetically Modified Foods: Experts View Regimen of Safety Tests as Adequate, but FDA's Evaluation Process Could Be Enhanced* (GAO-02-566), May 2002. Office of Science and Technology Policy. Proposed federal actions to update field test requirements for biotechnology derived plants and to establish early food safety assessments for new proteins produced by such plants. *FR* 67:50577-50580, August 2, 2002. National Research Council. *Environmental Effects of Transgenic Plants: The Scope and Adequacy of Regulation.* Washington, DC: National Academy Press, 2002. National Research Council. *Animal Biotechnology: Science-Based Concerns,* August 20, 2002. Online: www.nap.edu/books/0309084393/html.

CHAPTER 7. THE POLITICS OF GOVERNMENT OVERSIGHT

1. OTA. *A New Technological Era for American Agriculture* (OTA-F-475), 1992. Office of Science and Technology Policy. Coordinated framework for regulation of biotechnology: announcement of policy and notice for public comment. *FR* 51:23302–23393, June 26, 1986.

2. USDA/APHIS *Questions and Answers on Biotechnology Permits for Genetically Engineered Plants and Microorganisms* (APHIS 21-35-001), April 1991. Also see: MacKenzie DR. Agricultural biotechnology, law, APHIS regulation. In: Murray TH, Mehlman MJ, eds. *Ethical, Legal, and Policy Issues in Biotechnology.* Vol. 1. New York: John Wiley & Sons, 2000:56–66.

3. Institute for Food Technology. IFT expert report on biotechnology and foods: introduction. *Food Technology* 2000;54(8):124–136. Also see: 54(9):53–61 (safety evaluation), 54(9):62–74 (labeling), and 54(10):61–79 (benefits and concerns).

4. Kilman S. Growing pains: genetic engineering's biggest impact may eventually be in agriculture. The key word: eventually. *WSJ,* May 30, 1994:R7. OTA. *Biotechnology in a Global Economy* (OTA-BA-494), 1991. Thomas JA. Biotechnology: therapeutic and nutritional products. In: Thomas JA, ed. *Biotechnology and Safety Assessment.* 2nd ed. Philadelphia: Taylor & Francis, 1998:283–300.

5. Bauman DE, DeGeeter MJ, Peel CJ, et al. Effect of recombinantly derived bovine growth hormone (BGH) on lactational performance of high yielding dairy cows (Abstract P 86). *J Dairy Science* 1982;65(suppl):121. Pell AN, Tsang DS, Howlett BA, et al. Effects of a prolonged-release formulation of Sometribove (n-methionyl bovine somatotropin) on Jersey cows. *J Dairy Science* 1992;75:3416–

3431. Liebhardt WC, ed. *The Dairy Debate: Consequences of Bovine Growth Hormone and Rotational Grazing Technologies*. Davis: University of California Sustainable Agriculture Research and Education Program, 1993.

6. Violand BN, Schlittler MR, Lawson CQ, et al. Isolation of *Escherichia coli* synthesized recombinant eukaryotic proteins that contain ε-N-acetyllysine. *Protein Science* 1994;3:1089–1097. This amino acid replaced lysine in a "significant portion" of rBGH proteins.

7. Brody JE. Of Luddites, cows, and biotechnology miracles. *NYT*, November 17, 1993:C17.

8. Schneider K. Stores bar milk produced by drug: five big chains take action—U.S. calls process safe. *NYT*, August 24, 1989:A1,A18. Sun M. Market sours on milk hormone. *Science* 1989;246:876–877.

9. Juskevich DC, Guyer CG. Bovine growth hormone: human food safety evaluation. *Science* 1990;249:875–884. Office of Medical Applications of Research. *Bovine Somatotropin*. In: *National Institutes of Health Technology Assessment Conference Statement*, December 5–7, 1990. Washington, DC, 1991. Miller H. Putting the bST human-health controversy to rest. *Bio/Technology* 1992;10:147.

10. GAO. *Food Safety and Quality: FDA Strategy Needed to Address Animal Drug Residues in Milk* (GAO/RCED-92-209), 1992. *Recombinant Bovine Growth Hormone: FDA Approval Should Be Withheld until the Mastitis Issue Is Resolved* (GAO/PEMD-92-26), 1992.

11. Kimura T, Murakawa Y, Ohno M, et al. Gastrointestinal absorption of recombinant human insulin-like growth factor 1 in rats. *J Pharmacological and Experimental Therapeutics* 1997;283:611–618. Chan JM, Stampfer MJ, Giovannucci E, et al. Plasma insulin-like growth factor-1 and prostate cancer risk: a prospective study. *Science* 1998;279:563–566. Hankinson SE, Willett WC, Golditz GA, et al. Circulating concentrations of insulin-like growth factor 1 and risk of breast cancer. *Lancet* 1998;351:1393–1396. Verdecchia P, Reboldi G, Schillaci G, et al. Circulating insulin and insulin growth factor-1 are independent determinants of left ventricular mass and geometry in essential hypertension. *Circulation* 1999;100:1802–1807. Also see: rbST Internal Review Team, Health Protection Branch. *rbST (Nutrilac) "Gaps Analysis" Report*. Ottawa: Health Canada, April 21, 1998.

12. Cohen R. *Milk: The Deadly Poison*. Englewood Cliffs, NJ: Argus, 1998. Cohen R. Notmilk! Online: www.hungerstrike.com.

13. Blaney DP, Miller JJ, Stillman RP. *Dairy: Background for 1995 Farm Legislation* (USDA Agricultural Economics Report No. 705), 1995. Schneider K. Grocers challenge use of new drug for milk output. *NYT*, February 4, 1994:A1,A14. Over 800 farmers report problems related to rBGH. *Nutrition Week*, June 2, 1995:6.

14. Cohen B. Ben & Jerry's Testifies Before FDA in Favor of BGH Labeling (press release). Waterbury, VT: Ben & Jerry's, May 6, 1993.

15. Kolata G. When the geneticists' fingers get in the food. *NYT*, February 20, 1994:E13. Also see: DuPuis EM. *Nature's Perfect Food*. New York University Press, 2002.

16. OTA. *U.S. Dairy Industry at a Crossroad: Biotechnology and Policy*

Choices—Special Report (OTA-F-470), 1991. BGH moratorium. *Nutrition Week*, August 6, 1993:5.

17. Schneider K. U.S. approves use of drug to raise milk production: gain for biotechnology. *NYT*, November 6, 1993:A1,A9. FDA. Animal drugs, feeds, and related products; sterile sometribove zinc suspension. *FR* 58:59946–59947, November 12, 1993.

18. Benson S, Arax M, Burstein R. A growing concern: as biotech crops come to market, neither scientists—who take industry money—nor federal regulators are adequately protecting consumers and farmers. *Mother Jones*, January/February 1997:36–43,66–71. Feder BJ. Monsanto has its wonder hormone: can it sell it? *NYT*, March 12, 1995:A8. Stauber JC, Rampton S. *Toxic Sludge Is Good for You: Lies, Damn Lies, and the Public Relations Industry.* Monroe, ME: Common Courage Press, 1995:55–59.

19. Engelberg S. Democrats' new overseer is everybody's Mr. Inside. *NYT*, August 19, 1994:A1,A16.

20. Coghlan A. Milk hormone data bottled up for years. *New Scientist* October 22, 1994:4. Millstone E, Brunner E, White I. Plagiarism or protecting public health? *Nature* 1994;371:647–648.

21. Wilson S. Fox in the cow barn. *Nation*, June 8, 1998:20. Montague P. How Monsanto "listens" to other opinions. *Ecologist* 1998;28(5):299–300. Reporters win lawsuit to thwart Fox-TV cover-up. *BGH Bulletin,* undated, accessed December 15, 2001. Online: www.foxbghsuit.com.

22. Schneider K. Lines drawn in a war over a milk hormone. *NYT*, March 9, 1994:A12.

23. Weldon VV. Testimony to the Joint Meeting of the FDA Food and Veterinary Medicine Advisory Committee Meetings, Washington DC, May 6–7, 1993 (written statement distributed at the meeting). Dr. Weldon was then vice president for public policy, Monsanto.

24. After committees meet, BGH decision left to FDA. *Nutrition Week*, May 14, 1993:2–3.

25. FDA. Interim guidance on the voluntary labeling of milk and milk products from cows that have not been treated with recombinant bovine somatotropin. *FR* 59:6279–6280, February 10, 1994.

26. Schneider K. Maine and Vermont restrict dairies' use of a growth hormone. *NYT*, April 15, 1994:A16.

27. Kilman S. Dairy-food concerns launch products from cows not treated with hormone. *WSJ*, May 2, 1994:B7.

28. Burros M. More milk, more confusion: what should the label say? *NYT*, May 18, 1994:C1,C4.

29. King & Spalding. Mandatory labeling of milk and other foods derived from dairy cows supplemented with bovine somatotropin would be unlawful and unwise (memorandum). Washington, DC, April 28, 1993. A cover letter discloses the author as Mr. Richard A. Merrill, the former FDA counsel. These materials were included as part of the briefing materials for the FDA Food Advisory Committee hearings of May 6, 1993.

30. Schneider K. Question is raised on hormone maker's ties to F.D.A. aides. *NYT*, April 18, 1994:A9.

31. GAO. Letter from Acting General Counsel Robert P. Murphy to the Honorables George E. Brown, Jr., David Obey, and Bernard Sanders (B257122), October 19, 1994. Quotations: 15,23.

32. Sanders B. GAO uncovers appearances of impropriety in FDA's approval of rBGH (press release). U.S. House of Representatives, October 30, 1994. The release included detailed summaries of the involvement of the three FDA employees.

33. Bellow D. Vermont, the pure-food state. *Nation*, March 8, 1999:18–21. Brownlee S. Dollars for DNA: biotech seems near to living up to its hype. *US News & World Report*, May 25, 1998:48,50.

34. Aldrich L, Blisard N. Consumer acceptance of biotechnology: lessons from the rbST experience. *Current Issues in Economics of Food Markets* (USDA Agriculture Information Bulletin No. 747-01), December 1998.

35. Hoban TJ. *Consumer Awareness and Acceptance of Bovine Somatotropin (BST)*. Washington, DC: Grocery Manufacturers of America, 1994. Grobe D, Douthitt R, Zepeda L. A model of consumers' risk perceptions toward recombinant bovine growth hormone (rBGH): the impact of risk characteristics. *Risk Analysis* 1999;19:661–673.

36. Gilbert S. Fears over milk, long dismissed, still simmer. *NYT*, January 19, 1999:F7.

37. Kessler DA, Taylor MR, Maryanski JH, et al. The safety of foods developed by biotechnology. *Science* 1992;256:1747–1749, 1832.

38. FDA. Statement of policy: foods derived from new plant varieties: notice. *FR* 57:22984–23005, May 29, 1992. Quotation: 22985.

39. FDA. Premarket notice concerning bioengineered foods: proposed rule. *FR* 66:4706–4738, January 18, 2001.

40. Ingersoll B. New policy eases market path for bioengineered foods. *WSJ*, May 26, 1992: B1,B6.

41. Kim J. Genetic agriculture gets go-ahead. *USA Today*, May 27, 1992:3B.

42. Burros M. Documents show officials disagreed on altered food. *NYT*, December 1, 1999:A18. Druker SM. *Why Food and Drug Administration Policy on Genetically Engineered Food Violates Sound Science and U.S. Law* (presentation to FDA hearing, Washington, DC, November 30, 1999), at www.biotech-info.net/druker.pdf.

43. Millstone E, Brunner E, Mayer S. Beyond "substantial equivalence." *Nature* 1999;401:525–526.

44. Brozan N. Genetically engineered foods? Not in *their* kitchens! *NYT*, July 30, 1992:B6. Chefs urge boycotting new foods. *NYT*, June 3, 1992:C6.

45. FDA. *Foods Derived from New Plant Varieties Derived through Recombinant DNA Technology: Final Consultations under FDA's 1992 Policy*, July 2001, at www.foodsafety.gov/~lrd/biocon.html.

46. Putnam JJ, Allshouse JE. *Food Consumption, Prices, and Expenditures, 1970–97* (Statistical Bulletin No. 965), USDA, 1999. Fisher LM. Developer of the new tomato expects a financial bonanza. *NYT*, May 19, 1994:B7. Hilts PJ. Genetically altered tomato moves toward U.S. approval. *NYT*, April 9, 1994:A7.

47. Martineau B. Food fight. *The Sciences* 2001;spring:24–29. Martineau B. *First Fruit: The Creation of the Flavr Savr Tomato and the Birth of Biotech Food*. New York: McGraw-Hill, 2001. Also see: Charles D. *Lords of the Harvest:*

Biotech, Big Money, and the Future of Food. Cambridge, MA: Perseus, 2001:126–148.

48. Redenbaugh K, Hiatt W, Martineau B, et al. *Safety Assessment of Genetically Engineered Fruits and Vegetables: A Case Study of the Flavr Savr Tomato*. Boca Raton, FL: CRC Press, 1992. Stix G. A recombinant feast: new bioengineered crops move toward market. *Scientific American* 1995;273:38–39.

49. Seabrook J. Tremors in the hothouse. *New Yorker*, July 19, 1993:32–41. O'Neill M. Tomato review: no substitute for summer. *NYT*, May 19, 1994:B7.

50. McMurray S. New Calgene tomato might have tasted just as good without genetic alteration. *WSJ*, January 12, 1993:B1. Fisher LM. Monsanto to acquire 49.9% of biotechnology company. *NYT*, June 29, 1995:D3.

51. Safeway. *A Guide to Safeway Double Concentrated Tomato Puree Produced from Genetically Modified Tomatoes: Help and Advice*. Kent, UK: Safeway, [undated, c. 1998].

52. Rogers D. Stores dodge GM food row. *Marketing* (London), June 18, 1998:14.

53. Whitney CR. Europe loses its appetite for high-tech food. *NYT*, June 27, 1999:D3. Michael A. "GM-free" food labels are value-free. *Nature Biotechnology* 1999;17:420.

54. EPA. Proposed policy: plant-pesticides subject to the Federal Insecticide, Fungicide, and Rodenticide Act; and the Federal Food, Drug, and Cosmetic Act. *FR* 59:60496—60518, November 23, 1994. EPA. Plant-pesticides subject to the Federal Insecticide, Fungicide, and Rodenticide Act: proposed rule. *FR* 59:60519–60535, November 23, 1994.

55. Rissler J, Mellon M. *The Ecological Risks of Engineered Crops*. Cambridge, MA: MIT Press, 1996. National Research Council. *Genetically Modified Pest-Protected Plants: Science and Regulation*. Washington, DC: National Academy Press, 2000.

56. Miller H. A need to reinvent biotechnology regulation at the EPA. *Science* 1994;266:1815–1818. Wadman M. GM advisory panel is slanted, say critics. *Nature* 1999;399:7. Environmental Defense Fund (EDF). EDF Cautiously Praises EPA's Proposed Genetic Engineering Rule (press release). New York, November 16, 1994. Plan to regulate gene-modified plants draws fire. *Illinois Agrinews*, August 1, 1997:A4.

57. Hagmann M. EPA, critics soften stance on pesticidal plants. *Science* 1999;284:249.

58. EPA. Regulations under the Federal Insecticide, Fungicide, and Rodenticide Act for plant-incorporated protectants (formerly plant-pesticides): final rule. *FR* 66:37771–37817, July 19, 2001. Quotation: 37781.

59. EPA. *Biopesticides Registration Action Document*: Bacillus thuringiensis Plant-Incorporated Protectants, October 16, 2001, at www.epa.gov/oppooo01/biopesticides/pips/bt_brad.htm.

60. EPA. Pesticide labeling and other regulatory issues: final rule. *FR* 66:64759–64768, December 14, 2001.

CHAPTER 8. THE POLITICS OF CONSUMER CONCERN: DISTRUST, DREAD, AND OUTRAGE

1. Zepeda L. Don't ask, don't tell: U.S. policy on labeling of genetically engineered foods. In: Buttel FH, Goodman RM. *Of Frankenfoods and Golden Rice: Risks, Rewards, and Realities of Genetically Modified Foods.* Madison: Wisconsin Academy of Sciences, Arts and Letters, 2001:121–130.

2. Poll Shows Broad but Limited Support for Labeling of Bioengineered Foods (press release). CSPI, May 16, 2001, at www.cspinet.org/new/labeling_gefoods .html.

3. International Food Information Council. Most Americans can articulate expected benefits of biotechnology, November 2001, at www.biotech-info.net/ IFIC_research.html.

4. Fox JL. U.S. food labeling policy softens. *Nature Biotechnology* 1999;17:847. Silva C, Leonard R. U.S. prepares to OK labels on GE foods. *Nutrition Week,* October 29, 1999:4–5.

5. *Genetically Engineered Food Right to Know Act.* H.R. 3377, 106th Congress, 1st Session, November 16, 1999.

6. Biotech foods bill would mandate labeling, impose civil penalties. *Food Regulation Weekly,* November 15, 1999:11–12.

7. FDA. Biotechnology in the year 2000 and beyond; public meetings: notice. *FR* 64:57470–57472, October 25, 1999.

8. FDA. *Report on Consumer Focus Groups on Biotechnology,* February 2001, at www.foodsafety.gov/~comm/biorpt.html. The FDA conducted 12 focus groups from May 10 to 24, 2000.

9. FDA. FDA to Strengthen Pre-market Review of Bioengineered Foods (press release). May 3, 2000. White House Briefing Room. Clinton Administration Agencies Announce Food and Agricultural Biotechnology Initiatives (press release). May 3, 2000.

10. Pollack A. F.D.A. plans new scrutiny in areas of biotechnology. *NYT,* January 18, 2001:A12. FDA. Premarket notice concerning bioengineered foods: proposed rule. *FR* 66:4706–4738, January 18, 2001.

11. Kilman S. FDA warns of misleading label on genetically modified foods. *WSJ,* December 20, 2001:B9. Weise E. FDA tries to remove genetic label before it sticks. *USA Today,* October 9, 2002:7D.

12. Nestle M. Food biotechnology: truth in advertising. *Bio/Technology* 1992;10:1056.

13. OTA. *New Developments in Biotechnology: Patenting Life* (OTA-BA-370). U.S. Congress, 1989.

14. Stone R. Sweeping patents put biotech companies on the warpath. *Science* 1995;268:656–658. Rural Advancement Foundation International. Monsanto's "Submarine Patent" Torpedoes Ag Biotech (press release), April 27, 2001, at www.etcgroup.org/en/materials/publications.html?pub_id=262.

15. Moon SE. Seed piracy: biotech industry faces a growing concern. *Illinois Agrinews,* April 17, 1998:A9.

16. Kilman S. Biotech industry shivers at threat to seed patents. *WSJ,* March 3, 1999:B1. *Pioneer Hi-Bred International* v. *J.E.M. Ag Supply (Farm Advan-*

tage). 99-1035 (U.S. Court of Appeals for the Federal Circuit), January 19, 2000. The U.S. Supreme Court confirmed the ruling, December 10, 2001 (534 U.S. 124).

17. Fulmer M. Patent ruling aids seed biotech firms; Courts: analysts say the Supreme Court is taking a tough stance to strengthen intellectual property rights. *Los Angeles Times,* December 11, 2001:C3.

18. Shiva V. *Biopiracy: The Plunder of Nature and Knowledge.* Boston: South End Press, 1997.

19. Basmati patent shrinks. *Science* 2001;293:1761. Kurtenbach E. Patent application raises worries. Yahoo News, December 12, 2001. Online: dailynews .yahoo.com (no longer available).

20. Svatos M. Patents and licensing, ethics, ownership of animal and plant genes. In: Murray TH, Mehlman MJ, eds. *Encyclopedia of Ethical, Legal, and Policy Issues in Biotechnology.* Vol. 2. New York: John Wiley & Sons, 2000:844–854. Also: Ho CM. International intellectual property issues for biotechnology (2000:761–787).

21. Andrews EL. U.S. resumes granting patents on genetically altered animals. *NYT,* February 3, 1993:A1,D5. Also see: Rifkin J. *The Biotech Century: Harnessing the Gene and Remaking the World.* New York: Jeremy P. Tarcher/Putnam, 1998.

22. Thompson PB. *Food Biotechnology in Ethical Perspective.* London: Blackie Academic, 1997. Bruce D, Bruce A. *Engineering Genesis: The Ethics of Genetic Engineering in Non-Human Species.* London: Earthscan, 1998. Shiva V. *Protect or Plunder: Understanding Intellectual Property Rights.* London: Zed Books, 2001.

23. Service RF. Seed-sterilizing "terminator technology" sows discord. *Science* 1998;282:850–851. Steinbrecher RA, Mooney PR. Terminator technology: the threat to world food security. *Ecologist* 1998;28(5):276–279. National Campaign for Sustainable Agriculture. U.S. Department of Agriculture is at it again!! Agency continues to fund terminator technology (leaflet). Pine Bush, NY, August 23, 1999.

24. Food gains for the world's poor are being threatened by furor over genetically modified (GM) foods (press release). New York: Rockefeller Foundation, June 24, 1999, at http://findarticles.com/p/articles/mi_hb5243/is_199906/ai_n20192882.

25. Vidal J. How Monsanto's mind was changed. *Guardian* (London), October 9, 1999, at www.biotech-info.net/mind_change.html.

26. Feder BJ. Monsanto says it won't market infertile seeds. *NYT,* October 5, 1999:A1,C2.

27. Feder BJ. Plant sterility research inflames debate on biotechnology's role in farming, *NYT,* April 19, 1999:A18.

28. Barboza D. After deal of 2 giants, shares plunge. *NYT,* December 21, 1999:C1,C9. Kaiser J. USDA to commercialize "terminator" technology. *Science* 2000;289:709–710.

29. USDA/Agricultural Marketing Service. National organic program: proposed rule. *FR* 62:65849–65967, December 16, 1997. The rules for organic foods went into effect October 21, 2002.

30. Burros M. U.S. proposal on organic food gets a grass-roots review. *NYT,*

March 15, 1998:F10. Fox JL. USDA appeases organic lobby. *Nature Biotechnology* 1999;17:217. Revised organic proposed rule drops GMOs, antibiotics, sewage, irradiation. *Food Regulation Weekly*, March 13, 2000:8–9.

31. Pear R. Tougher labeling for organic food: products of gene engineering cannot carry designation. *NYT*, May 9, 1998:A1,A6.

32. Pollack A. Unapproved canola seed may be on farms, makers say. *NYT, April 16, 2002:* C4. Rieger MA, Lamond M, Preston C, et al. Pollen-mediated movement of herbicide resistance between commercial canola fields. *Science* 2002:296:2386–2388. Carroll J. Gene-altered canola can spread to nearby fields, risking lawsuits. *WSJ*, June 28, 2002:B6.

33. Villar JL. *GMO Contamination around the World*. Amsterdam: Friends of the Earth International, October 2001, 2nd ed, August 2002. Quote: p. 9, at http://stopogm.net/files/GMOContaminationaroundtheworld.pdf. Also see: Barboza D. As biotech crops multiply, consumers get little choice. *NYT*, June 10, 2001:A1,A28.

34. Nigh R, Benbrook C, Brush S, et al. Transgenic crops: a cautionary tale (letters). *Science* 2000;287:1927–1928. Ross J. Tinkering with the tortilla: genetic engineering threatens Mexico's corn culture. *Sierra*, September/October 2001:20–21.

35. Quist D, Chapela IH. Transgenic DNA introgressed into traditional maize landraces in Oaxaca, Mexico. *Nature* 2001;414:541–543. Manning A. Gene-altered DNA may be "polluting" corn: cross-pollination is found in native varieties in Mexico. *USA Today*, November 29, 2001:15D.

36. Suspect evidence of transgenic contamination (letters), and editorial note. *Nature* 2002;416:600–601.

37. Yoon CK. Journal raises doubts on biotech study. *NYT*, April 5, 2002:A21. Chapela's tenure was approved by his department, then denied, appealed, and eventually granted. See *Nature* doi:10.1038/435390b, May 25, 2005. Monbiot G. The fake persuaders. *Guardian* (London), May 14, 2002, at www.guardian.co.uk/politics/2002/may/14/greenpolitics.digitalmedia. Worthy K, Strohman RC, Billings PR. Conflicts around a study of Mexican crops (letter). *Nature* 2002;417:897.

38. Mann CC. Has GM corn "invaded" Mexico? *Science* 2002;295:1617–1619.

39. Christensen E. Food fight: how GATT undermines food-safety regulations. *Multinational Monitor*, November 1990:12–14. Ritchie M. Trading away the family farm: GATT and agriculture (November 1990:26–28). Aaronson SA. *Taking Trade to the Streets: The Lost History of Public Efforts to Shape Globalization*. Ann Arbor: University of Michigan, 2001:142–173. Also see: The World Trade Organization. Online: www.wto.org.

40. Brunner J. What's on WTO's plate regarding agriculture. *Seattle Times*, November 30, 1999:A23. The quotation is attributed to U.S. Secretary of State Madeleine Albright. McKibben B. Don't be fooled. *Seattle Weekly*, November 25, 1999:9.

41. The global food fight. *Time*, July 31, 2000:44–45.

42. Pollack A. Setting rules for biotechnology trade. *NYT*, February 15, 1999:A8. U.S. sidetracks pact to control gene splicing (February 25, 1999:C1,C4). Genetically modified food: food for thought. *Economist*, June 19, 1999:19–21.

43. Pollack A. 130 nations agree on safety rules for biotech food. *NYT*, Jan-

uary 30, 2000:A1,A8. Micklethwait J. Europe's profound fear of food. *NYT*, June 7, 1999:A22.

44. International Organisation of Consumers Unions (I.O.C.U.). *Comments: Implications of Biotechnology for Food Labelling.* Testimony to the Joint FAO/WHO Food Standards Programme Codex Committee on Food Labelling, Ottawa, Canada, October 24–28, 1994. Food fights. *Economist*, June 13–19, 1998:113–114.

45. USDA/FSIS. Codex Committee on Food Labeling: U.S.A., at www.fsis .usda.gov/Codex_alimentarius/Codex_Committee_Food_Labelling/index.asp.

46. Dorey E. EuropaBio unit created to boost agbio defense. *Nature Biotechnology* 1999;17:631. Hencke D, Evans R. How US put pressure on Blair over GM food: special report. *Guardian* (London), February 28, 2000, at www .guardian.co.uk/environment/2000/feb/28/food.freedomofinformation.

47. Citizens' groups: the non-governmental order. *Economist*, December 11, 1999:20–21. Lagnado L. Raising the anti: for those fighting biotech crops, Santa came early this year. *WSJ*, December 14, 1999:A1,A8. Hodgson J. GM roundup. *Nature Biotechnology* 1999;17:939.

48. Environment-consumer coalition launches campaign for labeling, testing of biotech foods. *FCN*, July 24, 2000:10–11. Branch S. Kraft is criticized for genetically modified foods. *WSJ*, February 6, 2002:B18.

49. See, for example, information posted by Ag BioTech InfoNet, online at: www.biotech info.net, and by the Turning Point Project, at http://web.archive.org/ web/*/http://www.turnpoint.org.

50. Books not otherwise mentioned in these chapters are: Charles D. *Lords of the Harvest: Biotech, Big Money, and the Future of Food.* Cambridge, MA: Perseus, 2001. Hart K. *Eating in the Dark: America's Experiment with Genetically Engineered Food.* New York: Pantheon, 2002. Lambrecht B. *Dinner at the New Gene Café: How Genetic Engineering is Changing What We Eat, How We Live, and the Global Politics of Food.* New York: St. Martin's, 2001. Lappé M, Bailey B. *Against the Grain: Biotechnology and the Corporate Takeover of Your Food.* Monroe, ME: Common Courage, 1998. Teitel M, Wilson KA. *Genetically Engineered Food: Changing the Nature of Nature.* Rochester, VT: Park Street, 1999. Ticciati L, Ticciati R. *Genetically Engineered Foods: Are They Safe? You Decide.* New Canaan, CT: Keats, 1998.

51. Lewontin R. Genes in the food! *New York Review of Books*, June 21:2001:81–84.

52. McHughen A. *Pandora's Picnic Basket: The Potential Hazards of Genetically Modified Foods.* Oxford: Oxford University Press, 2000.

53. Nestle M. *Food Politics: How the Food Industry Influences Nutrition and Health.* Berkeley: University of California Press, 2002:120–122.

54. Brand W. FDA holds Oakland hearing to discuss genetic labeling. Media-NewsGroup, December 14, 1999. Pollack A. At U.S. hearing scientists back altered crops. *NYT*, December 14, 1999:A25.

55. Pew Initiative on Food and Biotechnology. State legislative activity in 2001 related to agricultural biotechnology. Pew agricultural biotechnology is at www .pewtrusts.org/our_work_detail.aspx?id=442. Grimm C. Current (February–

March 2001) state GMO legislation in the United States. Ag BioTech InfoNet, March 2001, cached at www.biotech-info.net/current_state_legislation.html.

56. Greenberger RS. Motley group pushes for FDA labels on biofoods to help religious people observe dietary laws. *WSJ*, August 18, 1999:A20. Barboza D. Monsanto faces growing skepticism on two fronts. *NYT*, August 5, 1999:C1,C2. Nixon L. Consumers petition for GM food labels. *Agweek*, July 19, 1999:25. Economics could be key in biotech suit against Monsanto. *Food Regulation Weekly*, December 20, 1999:11.

57. Hoge W. Britons skirmish over genetically modified crops. *NYT*, August 23, 1999:A3. Service RF. Arson strikes research labs and tree farm in Pacific Northwest. *Science* 2001;292:1622–1623. Verhovek SH. S.U.V.'s, golf, and even peas join growing hit list of eco-vandals. *NYT*, July 1, 2001:A1,A15.

58. Peterson M. New trade threat for U.S. farmers. *NYT*, August 29, 1999:A1,A28.

59. Ramey TS, Wimmer MJ, Rocker RM. GMOs are dead. In: Mitsch FJ, Mitchell JS. *Ag Biotech: Thanks, but No Thanks?* Deutsche Bank, July 12, 1999, at www.rag.org.au/baa/gmbank.htm. Also see: GAO. *International Trade: Concerns over Biotechnology Challenge U.S. Agricultural Exports* (GAO-01-727), June 2001.

60. American Corn Growers Association. *Third Annual Survey*, December 21, 2001, and *Corn Growers Concerned Trade Legislation Will Backfire*, January 18, 2002.

61. Wainio J, Gibson P. U.S. exports face high tariffs in some key markets. *FoodReview* 2001;24(3):29–38.

62. Nettleton JA. Food industry retreats from science. *Food Technology* 1999;53(10):24.

CONCLUSION. THE FUTURE OF FOOD SAFETY:
PUBLIC HEALTH VERSUS BIOTERRORISM

1. GAO. *Bioterrorism: Federal Research and Preparedness Activities* (GAO-01-915), September 2001. *Bioterrorism: Review of Public Health Preparedness Programs* (GAO-02-149T), October 10, 2001. *Food Safety and Security: Fundamental Changes Needed to Ensure Safe Food* (GAO-02-47T), October 10, 2001.

2. Green E. Britain details the start of its "mad cow" outbreak. *NYT*, January 26, 1999:F2. Brown P, Will RG, Bradley R, et al. Bovine spongiform encephalopathy and variant Creutzfeldt-Jakob disease: background, evolution, and current concerns. *Emerging Infectious Diseases* 2001;7:6–16. Balter M. Uncertainties plague projections of vCJD toll. *Science* 2001;294:770–771. Projections are imprecise because people ate meat from affected cows from 1980 to 1996, and the disease develops slowly.

3. Brown P. On the origins of BSE. *Lancet* 1998;352:252–253.

4. Other examples are kuru, a human disease specifically associated with ritualistic cannibalism among the Fore people of Papua New Guinea, and prion diseases specific to mink, deer, cats, and a great variety of exotic animals. Two Nobel Prizes honor this work: to Carleton Gajdusek for studies of kuru and

Creutzfeldt-Jakob disease (1976), and to Stanley Prusiner for discovering and naming prions (1997).

5. Prusiner SB. Prion diseases and the BSE crisis. *Science* 1997;278:245–251. But see: Chesebro B. BSE and prions: uncertainties about the agent. *Science* 1998;279:42–43. Prions are believed to cause proteins in the brain and nervous system to fold improperly. Like other proteins, prions should be inactivated by acid in the stomach, and digested (disassembled) to amino acids by intestinal enzymes. They are not. Instead, they survive stomach acid and digestive enzymes, pass through the intestinal wall, get carried intact through the blood stream, and penetrate the "blood-brain barrier" that protects the brain from harmful substances. Prion proteins appear to be so tightly folded that they resist inactivation by acid, enzymes, and cooking temperatures. Their improbable behavior is the basis of skepticism and alternative hypotheses (such as a slow-acting virus), but most evidence now favors the existence of prions.

6. Urry M. Major called for fewer rules on meat hygiene. *Financial Times* (London), June 27–June 28, 1998:7.

7. Collee JG, Bradley R. BSE: a decade on—part 1. *Lancet* 1997;349:636–641 (part 2 is *Lancet* 1997;349:715–721). Nathanson N, Wilesmith J, Griot C. Bovine spongiform encephalopathy (BSE): causes and consequences of a common source epidemic. *Am J Epidemiology* 1997;14;959–969.

8. Will RG, Ironside JW, Zeidler M, et al. A new variant of Creutzfeldt-Jakob disease in the UK. *Lancet* 1996;347:921–925. Anderson RM, Donnelly CA, Ferguson NM, et al. Transmission dynamics and epidemiology of BSE in British cattle. *Nature* 1996;382:779–788. Scott MR, Will R, Ironside J, et al. Compelling transgenetic evidence for transmission of bovine spongiform encephalopathy prions to humans. *Proceedings of the National Academy of Sciences* 1999;96:15137–15142.

9. Less beef, more brain (editorial). *Lancet* 1996;347:915. Darnton J. Britain ties deadly brain disease to cow ailment. *NYT,* March 21, 1996:A1,A7. Lanska DJ. The mad cow problem in the UK: risk perceptions, risk management, and health policy development. *J Public Health Policy* 1998;19:160–183.

10. France will continue beef ban; British pledge to fight in court. *NYT,* December 9, 1999:A6.

11. FDA. Substances prohibited from use in animal food or feed; animal proteins prohibited in ruminant feed. *FR* 62:30935–30978, June 5, 1997. The rules exempted blood, gelatin, cooked meats, and milk, but FDA eliminated the exemption for gelatin later that year (*FR* 62:52345–52346, Oct 7, 1997). Stecklow S. Porous borders: despite assurances, U.S. could be at risk for mad-cow disease. *WSJ,* November 28, 2001:A1,A6.

12. Harvard Center for Risk Analysis. *Evaluation of the Potential for Bovine Spongiform Encephalopathy in the United States: Executive Summary.* USDA/APHIS, November 26, 2001, at www.aphis.usda.gov/newsroom/hot_issues/bse/background/documents/mainreporttext.pdf.

13. Becker E. U.S. mad cow risk is low, a study by Harvard finds. *NYT,* December 1, 2001:A12.

14. GAO. *Mad Cow Disease: Improvements in the Animal Feed Ban and*

Other Regulatory Areas Would Strengthen U.S. Prevention Efforts (GAO-02-183), January 2002:3.

15. Stokes T. Cattlemen continue to beef up efforts to ensure that the U.S. meat supply is safe for consumers. *Nation's Restaurant News,* May 20, 2002: 40,44.

16. USDA/FSIS. Current Thinking on Measures That Could Be Implemented to Minimize Human Exposure to Materials That Could Potentially Contain the Bovine Spongiform Encephalopathy (news release), January 15, 2002, at www.fsis .usda.gov/oa/topics/BSE_thinking.htm. Kilman S, Carroll J. New precautions discussed to bar mad-cow disease. *WSJ,* January 18, 2002:NB2.

17. Ono Y. U.S. beef group raises stakes in Japan. *WSJ,* April 22, 2002:A15. CDC. CDC and Florida Department of Health Investigate a Likely Case of New Variant Creutzfeldt Jakob Disease in a U.K. Citizen Residing in the U.S. (press release), April 18, 2002.

18. Ferguson NM, Donnelly CA, Anderson RM. The foot-and-mouth epidemic in Great Britain: pattern of spread and impact of interventions. *Science* 2001;292:1155–1160. Keeling MJ, Woolhouse MEJ, Shaw DJ, et al. Dynamics of the 2001 UK foot and mouth epidemic: stochastic dispersal in a heterogeneous landscape. *Science* 2001;294:813–817. Lyall S. A tenacious disease finds new victims in British herds. *NYT,* August 5, 2001:A3.

19. Enserink M. Barricading U.S. borders against a devastating disease. *Science* 2001;291:2298–2300.

20. Cowell A. Cattle disaster still felt in Britain. *NYT,* September 10, 2002: W1,W7.

21. Andrews EL. Dutch farmers facing mass foot-and-mouth slaughter. *NYT,* April 6, 2001:A4.

22. Becker E. Prohibited meat entered U.S., a report finds. *NYT,* August 14, 2001:A12. Stone R. Report urges U.K. to vaccinate herds. *Science* 2002;297:319–321.

23. Robert Koch postulated that (1) anthrax bacteria always are present in the blood of animals sick with the disease but not in healthy animals, (2) inoculation of blood from an animal with anthrax into another animal also causes anthrax, (3) inoculation of anthrax bacteria isolated from the blood of a sick animal and grown in culture will transmit anthrax to the new animal, and (4) anthrax bacteria can be isolated from the new animal. "These conclusions are so certain, that no one will dispute them, and the anthrax bacillus will be looked upon by the scientific world as the causal agent of ordinary, typical anthrax infection in both our domestic animals and in man himself." See: Koch R. The etiology of tuberculosis (Koch's postulates), 1884. In: Brock TD. *Milestones in Microbiology: 1556 to 1940.* Washington, DC: American Society of Microbiology, 1998:116–118.

24. Riemann H, Bryan FL. *Food-Borne Infections and Intoxications,* 2nd ed. New York: Academic Press, 1979:235–238.

25. CDC. Human ingestion of Bacillus anthracis-contaminated meat—Minnesota, August 2000. *MMWR* 2000;49:813–816.

26. CDC. Human anthrax associated with an epizootic among livestock—North Dakota, 2000. *MMWR* 2001;50:677–680.

27. Guillemin J. *Anthrax: The Investigation of a Deadly Outbreak*. Berkeley: University of California Press, 1999. Meselson M, Guillemin J, Hugh-Jones M, et al. The Sverdlovsk anthrax outbreak of 1979. *Science* 1994;266:1202–1208. Inglesby TV, O'Toole T, Henderson DA, et al. Anthrax as a biological weapon, 2002: updated recommendations for management. *JAMA* 2002;287:2236–2252.

28. Ala'Aldeen D. Risk of deliberately induced anthrax outbreak. *Lancet* 2001;358:1386–1388.

29. Kristof ND. Profile of a killer. *NYT*, January 4, 2002:A21. Rosenberg BH. Analysis of the anthrax attacks. Federation of American Scientists, February 5, 2002, at www.anthraxinvestigation.com/anthraxreport.htm. Scientist's suicide linked to anthrax inquiry. *NYT*, August 2, 2008. Also see *NYT*, February 20, 2010.

30. Broad WJ, Grady D. Science slow to ponder ills that linger in anthrax victims. *NYT*, September 16, 2002:A1,A13. Greenberg DS. US anthrax scares prompt action on bioterrorism. *Lancet* 2001;358:1435. Lipton E, Johnson K. Tracking bioterror's tangled course. *NYT*, December 26, 2001:A1,B4,B5. Stolberg SG, Miller J. Many worry that nation is still highly vulnerable to germ attack. *NYT*, September 9, 2002:A16.

31. CDC. Investigation of bioterrorism-related anthrax and adverse events from antimicrobial prophylaxis. *MMWR* 2001;50:973–976.

32. Lerner S. Risky chickens. *Village Voice*, December 4, 2001:45. Goldburg R, Florini K. Bayer's Sale of Modified Cipro May Threaten Public Health (press release). New York: Environmental Defense, October 23, 2001. Silbergeld EK, Walker P. What if Cipro stopped working? *NYT*, November 3, 2001:A23. FDA NOOH [Notice of Opportunity for Hearing] for poultry fluoroquinolones (background information), December 7, 2000.

33. Burros M. Poultry industry quietly cuts back on antibiotic use. *NYT*, February 10, 2002:A1,A26.

34. Chiu C-H, Wu T-L, Su L-H, et al. The emergence in Taiwan of fluoroquinolone resistance in *Salmonella enterica* serotype choleraesuis. *NEJM* 2002;346:413–419. McDermott PF, Bodeis SM, English LL, et al. Ciprofloxacin resistance in *Campylobacter jejuni* evolves rapidly in chickens treated with fluoroquinolones. *J Infectious Diseases* 2002;185:837–840.

35. Bayer Signs Financing Agreement for Aventis CropScience Acquisition (press release). Bayer, December 12, 2001.

36. Andrews MS, Prell MA, eds. *Second Food Security Measurement and Research Conference, Volume II: Papers*. USDA/ERS, July 2001.

37. United Nations. Universal Declaration of Human Rights (Adopted by the U.N. General Assembly, December 10, 1948). Reprinted in *JAMA* 1998;280:469–470.

38. Oshaug A, Eide WB, Eide A. Human rights: a normative basis for food and nutrition-relevant policies. *Food Policy 1994;19:491–516*. Drèze J, Sen A. *Hunger and Public Action*. Oxford: Clarendon Press, 1989.

39. *The World Factbook—United States*, 2001. Central Intelligence Agency, at www.cia.gov/library/publications/the-world-factbook.

40. Assefa F, Jabarkhil MZ, Salama P, et al. Malnutrition and mortality in Kohistan district, Afghanistan, April 2001. *JAMA* 2001;286:2723–2728. Ahmad

K. Scurvy outbreak in Afghanistan prompts food aid concerns. *Lancet* 2002;359: 1044.

41. Perlez J. Individual meals from the sky. *NYT,* October 8, 2001:B3.

42. Monbiot G. Folly of aid and bombs. *Guardian* (London), October 9, 2001, at www.guardian.co.uk/politics/2001/oct/09/afghanistan.britainand911.

43. Hungry for peace: with winter near, starving Afghans need more than air-dropped relief. *San Francisco Chronicle,* October 26, 2001:A1,A18. Shanker T, Schmitt E. U.S. warns Afghans that Taliban may poison relief food. *NYT,* October 25, 2001:B2

44. Dao J. Sergeant designs a better box for dropping food to Afghans. *NYT,* October 10, 2001:B3. Waldman A. Food drops go awry, damaging several homes. *NYT,* November 21, 2001:B2. Becker E. Even with roads still open, security fears are choking the flow of food aid. *NYT,* November 30, 2001:B4. Chivers CJ, Becker E. Aid groups say warlords steal as needy wait. *NYT,* January 4, 2002:A1,A15.

45. Nestle M, Dalton S. Food aid and international hunger crises: the United States in Somalia. *Agriculture and Human Values* 1994;11(4):19–27. Lewis P. Downside of doing good: disaster relief can harm. *NYT,* February 27, 1999:B9. McKinlay D. Refugees left in the cold at "slaughterhouse" camp. *Guardian* (London), January 3, 2002. Gall C. Pleas for food, help and a way out. *NYT,* January 20, 2002:A15.

46. Truelsen S. Food aid and the war on terrorism. *The Voice of Agriculture.* American Farm Bureau Federation, November 5, 2001. See www.fb.com.

47. Burros M. A vulnerable food supply, a call for more safety. *NYT,* October 31, 2001: F1,F8. Mitchell A. Bush gives secrecy power to public health secretary. *NYT,* December 12 2001:B6. Mitchell A. Disputes erupt on Ridge's needs for his job. *NYT,* November 4, 2001:B7.

48. Fee E, Brown TM. Preemptive biopreparedness: Can we learn anything from history? *Am J Public Health* 2001;91:721–726 (and letter, 1918–1919). The 2nd National Symposium on Medical and Public Health Response to Bio-Terrorism: Public Health Emergency & National Security Threat. *Public Health Reports* 2001;116 (suppl 2):1–118. Sobel J, Khan AS, Swerdlow DL. Threat of a biological terrorist attack on the US food supply: the CDC perspective. *Lancet* 2002;359:874–880.

49. Henderson DA. The looming threat of bioterrorism. *Science* 1999;283: 1279–1282. National Research Council. *Countering Agricultural Bioterrorism.* Washington DC: National Academy Press, 2002.

50. Henderson DA. Biopreparedness and public health (letter). *Am J Public Health* 2001;91:1917–1918. Also see: Piller C, Yamamoto KR. *Gene Wars: Military Control over the New Genetic Technologies.* New York: William Morrow, 1988. DaSilva EJ. Biological warfare, bioterrorism, biodefence and the biological and toxin weapons convention. *Electronic J Biotechnology,* December 15, 1999:2(3), at www.ejbiotechnology.info/content/vol2/issue3/full/2/index.html. Pollack A. Scientists ponder limits on access to germ research. *NYT,* November 27, 2001:F1,F6.

51. Thompson CJS. *Poisons and Poisoners.* New York: Macmillan, 1931. Jensen LB. *Poisoning Misadventures.* Springfield, IL: Charles C. Thomas, 1970.

Klaassen CD, ed. *Casarett and Doull's Toxicology: The Basic Science of Poisons,* 5th ed. New York: McGraw-Hill, 1996:3–6.

52. Kolavic SA, Kimura A, Simons SL, et al. An outbreak of *Shigella dysenteriae* type 2 among laboratory workers due to intentional food contamination. *JAMA* 1997;278:396–398. Employee sabotage leads to large-scale meat recall. *Nutrition Week,* January 7, 2002:2.

53. Khan AS, Swerdlow DL, Juranek DD. Precautions against biological and chemical terrorism directed at food and water supplies. *Public Health Reports* 2001;116:3–14.

54. Török TJ, Tauxe RV, Wise RP, et al. A large community outbreak of Salmonellosis caused by intentional contamination of restaurant salad bars. *JAMA* 1997;278:389–395. Also see: Miller J, Engelberg S, Broad W. *Germs: Biological Weapons and America's Secret War.* New York: Simon & Schuster, 2001:15–33.

55. Levy T. Health: bioterrorism treatment options besides vaccinations and antibiotics. *Vitality* (supermarket advertiser, Cape Cod, MA), December 2001.

56. The National Library of Medicine provides a list of Web sites dealing with biological and chemical weapons, including one for the National Center for Complementary and Alternative Medicine at www.nim.nih.gov/medlineplus. FTC Cracks Down on Marketers of Bogus Bioterrorism Defense Products (press release), November 19, 2001. The FTC is at www.ftc.gov.

57. Cohen H, Eolis SL, Gould RM, et al. Hyping bioterrorism obscures real concerns: preparedness programs divert time and resources from health care, *Am J Nursing* 2001;101(11):58,60.

58. Douglas M, Wildavsky A. *Risk and Culture: An Essay on the Selection of Technical and Environmental Dangers.* Berkeley: University of California Press, 1982:195.

59. Barnes JE, Bradsher K. Concerns that U.S. food supply is vulnerable to terrorist attack. *NYT,* October 24, 2001:B9.

60. FDA. Frequently asked consumer questions about food safety and terrorism, November 15, 2001, at http://aggie-horticulture.tamu.edu/extension/news letters/foodproc/deco1/art2dec.html. McGinley L. FDA asks the food industry to review safety procedures in the wake of attacks. *WSJ,* October 3, 2001:A3.

61. Mermelstein NH. Terrorism spurs renewed call for single food safety agency. *Food Technology* 2001;55(11):32–36.

62. Cady J. *Federal Food Safety and Security: Can Our Fractured Food Safety System Rise to the Challenge?* Hearing before the Senate Governmental Affairs Oversight Subcommittee. 107th Congress, 1st Session. Alliance for Food Security, October 10, 2001.

63. Pianin E. Food industry resists anti-terror proposals: lobbyist says protections adequate. *Washington Post,* December 6, 2001:A49.

64. Carroll J. FDA issues guidelines to protect food. *WSJ,* January 8, 2002:A2. FDA. *Food Security Preventive Measures Guidance: Importers and Filers,* and *Food Security Preventive Measures Guidance: Food Producers, Processors, Transporters, and Retailers,* January 9, 2002, at www.foodsafety.gov/~lrd/fro 20109.html. USDA/FSIS. *FSIS Security Guidelines for Food Processors,* April 2002, at www.fsis.usda.gov/OA/topics/SecurityGuide.pdf.

65. Pear R. Food industry's resistance stalls bill to protect food. *NYT,* April 16, 2002:A22.

66. Acord D. "Improved" bioterrorism bill sails through Congress. *FCN,* May 27, 2002:1,13–15.

67. Horton R. Public health: a neglected counterterrorist measure. *Lancet* 2001;358:1112–1113.

68. Yach D, Bettcher D. The globalization of public health. I. Threats and opportunities. II. The convergence of self-interest and altruism. *Am J Public Health* 1998;88:735–738, 738–741. McMichael AJ, Beaglehole R. The changing global context of public health. *Lancet* 2000;356:495–499.

69. American Public Health Association. *Guiding Principles for a Public Health Response to Bioterrorism,* October 2001. Online: www.apha.org.

70. Garrett L. *Betrayal of Trust: The Collapse of Global Public Health.* New York: Hyperion, 2000. Quotation: 558.

EPILOGUE

1. Nestle M. Writing the food studies movement. *Food, Culture, and Society* 2010;13(2):162–70. Martin A. Is a food revolution now in season? *NYT,* March 21, 2009:BU1.

2. Monsanto is at www.monsanto.com. Paarlberg R. *Starved for Science: How Biotechnology Is Being Kept Out of Africa.* Cambridge, MA: Harvard University Press, 2009. Lotter D. The genetic engineering of food and the failure of science— Part 1: The development of a flawed enterprise. *International J Sociology of Agriculture and Food* 2009;16:31–49. Gurian-Sherman D, Robinson E. *Failure to Yield: Evaluating the Performance of Genetically Engineered Crops.* Union of Concerned Scientists, April 2009. Online: www.ucsusa.org. Many controversial issues related to GM foods are addressed in National Research Council. *Impact of Biotechnology on Farm Economics and Sustainability.* Washington, DC: National Academies Press, 2010.

3. FDA. Completed consultations on engineered foods, updated December 31, 2009. Online: www.accessdata.fda.gov/scripts/fcn/fcnNavigation.cfm?rpt=bio Listing. USDA/ERS. Adoption of genetically engineered crops in the U.S., July 1, 2009. Online: www.ers.usda.gov/Data/BiotechCrops. USDA/ERS. Briefing room: Sugar and sweeteners: background, updated August 6, 2009. Online: www.ers .usda.gov/Briefing/sugar/background.htm.

4. Developing countries boost spread of GM crops. *Nature* 2009;457:949. Germany joins in with maize moratorium. *Nature* 2009;458:958. Cameron D. Monsanto revives plans to develop wheat seeds. *WSJ,* July 14, 2009.

5. Dyer GA, et al. Dispersal of transgenes through maize seed systems in Mexico. *PLoS One* 2009;4(5):e5734. Online: www.plosone.org. Dalton R. Modified genes spread to local maize. *Nature* 2008;456:149. Stokstad E. Embattled Berkeley ecologist wins tenure. *Science* 2005;308:1239. Waltz E. Battlefield: papers suggesting that biotech crops might harm the environment attract a hail of abuse from other scientists. *Nature* 2009;461:273–2.

6. Caulcutt C. "Superweed" explosion threatens Monsanto heartlands.

France 24, April 19, 2009. Online: www.france24.com. Clapp S. Herbicide diversity called critical to keep Roundup effective. *FCN*, July 20, 2009:7. Gammon C. Weed-whacking herbicide proves deadly to human cells. *Scientific Am*, June 23, 2009. Online: www.scientificamerican.com. The "inert" ingredient is polyethoxylated tallowamine, or POEA.

7. Tang G, et al. Golden Rice is an effective source of vitamin A. *Am J Clinical Nutrition* 2009;89:1776–1783. Enserink M. Tough lessons from Golden Rice. *Science* 2008;320:468–471.

8. Martin A. Fighting a battlefield the size of a milk label. *NYT*, March 9, 2008:BU7. Horovitz B. Companies cut synthetic hormone from dairy products. *USA Today*, March 15, 2009. Online: www.usatoday.com. OTA appeals federal court decision on "rBST-free" labeling. *FCN*, June 3, 2009.

9. The Non-GMO Project is online at www.nongmoproject.org. Neuman W. Biotech-free, mostly. *NYT*, August 29, 2009:B1.

10. CDC. Norovirus activity—United States, 2006–2007. *MMWR* 2007; 56(33):842–846. Widdowson M-A, Monroe SS, Glass RI. Are noroviruses emerging? *Emerging Infectious Diseases* 2005;11:735–737. Hoffmann S. Knowing which foods are making us sick. *Choices* 2009;24(2):6–10. Online: www.choicesmagazine.org.

11. CDC. Surveillance for foodborne disease outbreaks—United States, 2006. *MMWR* 2009;58(22):609–615.

12. Weston Price Foundation. A campaign for real milk. Online. www.real milk.com. Dewell GA, et al. Prevalence of and risk factors for *Escherichia coli* O157 in market-ready beef cattle from 12 U.S. feedlots. *Foodborne Pathogens and Disease* 2005;2:70–76. Reinstein S, et al. Prevalence of *Escherichia coli* O157:H7 in organically and naturally raised beef cattle. *Applied and Environmental Microbiology* 2009;75: 5421–5423 (doi:10.1128/AEM.00459-09). FDA. Questions and answers: Raw milk, March 1, 2007. Online: www.fda.gov/Food.

13. Drape J. Should this milk be legal? *NYT*, August 8, 2007:F1. CDC. *Escherichia coli* O157:H7 infections in children associated with raw milk and raw colostrum from cows—California, 2006. *MMWR* 2008;57(23);625–628.

14. FDA. Backgrounder on measures to eliminate risk caused by *Vibrio vulnificus* infection from consumption of raw molluscan shellfish, October 17, 2009. Online: www.fda.gov/NewsEvents/Speeches/ucm187014.htm.

15. Taylor MR. Remarks, ISSC biennial meeting, October 17, 2009. Online: www.fda.gov/NewsEvents/Speeches/ucm187012.htm.

16. FDA. FDA Statement on Vibrio Vulnificus in raw oysters, November 13, 2009. Online: www.fda.gov/NewsEvents/Newsroom/PressAnnouncements/ucm 190513.htm.

17. FDA recalls are listed online at www.fda.gov/safety/recalls/default.htm. USDA recalls are listed online at www.fsis.usda.gov/FSIS_Recalls/index.asp. The CDC Outbreaks and Incidents page is at http://emergency.cdc.gov/recent incidents.asp.

18. The FDA spinach recall page is at www.fda.gov/NewsEvents/PublicHealth Focus/ucm179124.htm. California Department of Health Services and FDA. Investigation of an *Escherichia coli* O157:H7 outbreak associated with Dole prepackaged spinach, March 21, 2007. Archived online: www.marlerclark.com/2006

_Spinach_Report_Final_01.pdf and www.cdc.gov/ nceh/ ehs/Docs/Investigation _of_an_E_Coli_Outbreak_Associated_with_Dole_Pre-Packaged_Spinach.pdf. One year and millions of dollars later. ThePacker.com, September 7, 2007. USDA disappearance data are at www.ers.usda.gov/Data/FoodConsumption. Per capita availability of spinach was 2.2 pounds in 2005 and 1.8 pounds in 2008.

19. Jay MT, et al. *Escherichia coli* O157:H7 in feral swine near spinach fields and cattle, Central California coast. *Emerging Infectious Diseases* 2007;13(12):1908–1911. California Department of Fish and Game. Preliminary research results find less than one half of one percent occurrences of *E. coli* O157:H7 in wildlife in California Central Coast counties, April 7, 2009. Online: www.dfg.ca.gov/news/news09/2009040702.asp.

20. Solomon EB, Yaron S, Matthews KR. Transmission of *Escherichia coli* O157:H7 from contaminated manure and irrigation water to lettuce plant tissue and its subsequent internalization. *Applied and Environmental Microbiology* 2002;68:397–400. Uhlich GA, et al. Characterization of Shiga toxin-producing *Escherichia coli* isolates associated with two multistate food-borne outbreaks that occurred in 2006. *Applied and Environmental Microbiology* 2008;74:1268–1272.

21. Nestle M. The spinach fallout: Restoring trust in California produce [perspective]. *San Jose Mercury News*, October 22, 2006.

22. Chadwell J. Natural Selection Foods learns from experience. ThePacker.com, September 7, 2007. California Department of Food and Agriculture. Proposed California leafy green products handler marketing agreement, January 24, 2007. Online: www.caff.org/policy/documents/lgph_agreement .pdf. FDA. Guide to minimize microbial food safety hazards for fresh fruits and vegetables, October 26, 1998. FDA. Produce safety: 2004 action plan to minimize foodborne illness associated with fresh produce consumption, October 2004. FDA. Letter to California firms that grow, pack, process, or ship fresh and fresh-cut lettuce, November 4, 2005. FDA. Lettuce safety initiative, August 23, 2006. Online: www.fda.gov/Food. FDA. FDA statement on foodborne *E. coli* O157:H7 outbreak in spinach, September 19, 2006. Online: www.fda.gov.

23. Marler B. Wisconsin woman severely sickened by *E. coli* in spinach forced to sue, September 3, 2009. Online: www.marlerblog.com.

24. FDA. Guidance to industry: Guide to minimize microbial food safety hazards of leafy greens; draft guidance, July 2009. Online: www.fda.gov/Food.

25. Associated Press. *E. coli* outbreak sickens 11 in N.J., December 3, 2007. Online: www.sfgate.com. FDA. FDA investigating *E. coli* O157:H7 infections associated with Taco Bell restaurants in Northeast, December 6, 2006. Online: www.fda.gov. Belson K, Smothers R. Reports of illness spread as search for *E. coli* source narrows. *NYT*, December 8, 2006:B1.

26. Adamy J, Vranica S. Taco Bell faces new questions about *E. coli*. *WSJ*, December 13, 2006:B1. Creed G. Taco Bell food is safe. *NYT*, December 12, 2006:A23. A second advertisement appeared on December 18 announcing the end of the CDC's investigation. The quotation is from DePalma A, Martin A. New Jersey distribution site is scrutinized as more *E. coli* cases are reported. *NYT*, December 8, 2006:B1.

27. CDC. Multistate outbreak of E. coli O157 infections linked to Taco Bell, November–December 2006. Online: www.cdc.gov/ecoli/2006/december/.

28. Schlosser E. Has politics contaminated the food supply? NYT, December 11, 2006. Sickened by fresh produce. NYT, December 9, 2006 (editorial). Burros M. E. coli fears inspire a call for oversight. NYT, December 9, 2006:B1.

29. FDA. Melamine pet food recall of 2007. Online: www.fda.gov/AnimalVeterinary/SafetyHealth/RecallsWithdrawals/ucm129575.htm.

30. Xin H, Stone R. Chinese probe unmasks high-tech adulteration with melamine. Science 2008;322:1310–1311. Ingelfinger JR. Melamine and the global implications of food contamination. NEJM 2008;359:2745–2748. Melamine and food safety in China. Lancet 2009;373:353. Kuehn BM. Melamine scandals highlight hazards of increasingly globalized food chain. JAMA 2009;301:473–475. China executes 2 for role in tainted milk scandal. NYT, November 24, 2009. Online: www.nytimes.com/aponline/2009/11/24/world/AP-AS-China-TaintedMilk.html. The FDA's melamine-in-China page is at www.fda.gov/ohrms/dockets/ac/08/briefing/2008-4386b3.pdf. Melamine scandals continued into 2010.

31. Inspector General. Review of the Food and Drug Administration's monitoring of pet food recalls, August 12, 2009. Online: http://oig.hhs.gov/oas/reports/region1/10701503.pdf.

32. The quotations are from Moss M. E. coli path shows flaws in beef inspection. NYT, October 4, 2009. Stephanie Smith's medical problems and lawsuit are documented online at www.marlerblog.com. USDA recalls are archived online at http://origin-www.fsis.usda.gov/Fsis_Recalls/Recall_Case_Archive/index.asp.

33. USDA/FSIS. Handling the largest meat recall in U.S. history, February 22, 2008. Online: www.fsis.usda.gov. Humane Society of the United States. HSUS investigates slaughterhouse. Online: http://video.hsus.org/.

34. USDA/FSIS. California firm recalls beef products derived from nonambulatory cattle without the benefit of proper inspection, February 17, 2008. Online: www.fsis.usda.gov/PDF/Recall_005-2008_Release.pdf. USDA/FSIS. Statement by Secretary of Agriculture Ed Schafer regarding Hallmark/Westland Meat Packing Company two-year product recall, February 17, 2008. Online: www.usda.gov.

35. Zhang J. Meat inspectors can't keep up, official says. WSJ, April 18, 2008. The quotation is from Healey JR, Schmidt J. USDA orders largest beef recall: 143.4 million pounds. USA Today, February 18, 2008. Online: www.usatoday.com.

36. CDC. Investigation of outbreak of infections caused by Salmonella Saintpaul, update for August 28, 2008. Online: www.cdc.gov/salmonella/saintpaul/jalapeno. The FDA page on this outbreak is at www.fda.gov/NewsEvents/PublicHealthFocus/ucm179116.htm. Maki DG. Coming to grips with foodborne infection—peanut butter, peppers, and nationwide Salmonella outbreaks. NEJM 2009;360:949–953. Weise E. How modern science and old-fashioned detective work cracked the salmonella case. USA Today, June 18, 2008. Online: www.usatoday.com. Jargon J. Grocers and restaurants toss out tomatoes. WSJ, June 10, 2008:B1.

37. CDC. Outbreak of Salmonella serotype Saintpaul infections associated with multiple raw produce items—United States, 2008. MMWR 2008;57(34): 929–934.

38. Acheson D. *Salmonella* Saintpaul outbreak investigation, statement before Committee on Energy and Commerce, House of Representatives, July 31, 2008. Online: www.fda.gov.

39. Goldman LR, Pendergast MK. Breakdown: Lessons to be learned from the 2008 *Salmonella* Saintpaul Outbreak. Pew Charitable Trusts, Produce Safety Project, November 17, 2008. Online: www.producesafetyproject.org/reports?id = 0001 (note the helpful timeline).

40. The FDA page on the peanut butter recalls is www.fda.gov/Safety/Recalls/MajorProductRecalls/Peanut/default.htm. CDC. Multistate outbreak of *Salmonella* infections associated with peanut butter and peanut butter–containing products—United States, 2008–2009. *MMWR* 2009;58(04):85–90. CDC. Investigation update: Outbreak of *Salmonella* Typhimurium infections, 2008–2009, April 29, 2009. Online: www.cdc.gov/salmonella/typhimurium/update.html.

41. Hazardous peanut butters. *NYT*, January 29, 2009. Moss M. Peanut case shows holes in safety net. *NYT*, February 9, 2009.

42. Keefe B. Peanut's firm's chief an advisor. *Atlanta Journal-Constitution,* February 1, 2009. Consumers Union. Consumers Union statement in response to PCA bankruptcy, February 13, 2009. Online: www.consumersunion.org. Severson K, Martin A. It's organic but does that mean it's safer? *NYT,* March 3, 2009. FDA. Guidance for industry: Measures to address the risk for contamination by *Salmonella* species in food containing a peanut-derived product as an ingredient, March 2009. Online: www.fda.gov/Food.

43. *Today.* Obama: "We're suffering from a massive hangover" (transcript), February 2, 2009. Online: www.msnbc.msn.com/id/28975726.

44. Hamburg MA, Sharfstein JM. The FDA as a public health agency. *NEJM* 2009;360:2493–2495.

45. The FDA's pistachios page is at www.fda.gov/Safety/Recalls/MajorProductRecalls/Pistachio/default.htm. CDC. *Salmonella* in pistachio nuts, 2009, April 14, 2009. Online: www.cdc.gov/salmonella/pistachios/update.html. Weise E. FDA: Recall of tainted pistachio nuts far from over. *USA Today,* April 7, 2009.

46. Scott-Thomas C. Setton pistachio knew of salmonella, says FDA. *Food Production Daily,* May 26, 2009. Online: www.foodproductiondaily.com/content/view/print/247755. CAL-PURE and Western Pistachio Association. Important information on FDA pistachio recall, updated August 6, 2009. Online: www.pistachiorecall.org. FDA. FDA warns consumers not to eat California Prime Produce and Orange County Orchards brands of pistachios: Products linked to the previous recall by Setton Pistachio of Terra Bella Inc., June 22, 2009. Online: www.fda.gov.

47. FDA. Letter to processors about current GMPs, April 3, 2009. Online: www.fda.gov/Safety/Recalls.

48. Big surprises in recall of cookie dough. *Consumer Reports,* September 2009. Online: www.consumerreports.org.

49. CDC. Multistate outbreak of *E. coli* O157:H7 infections linked to eating raw refrigerated, prepackaged cookie dough. Updated August 7, 2009. Online: www.cdc.gov/ecoli/2009/0807.html. FDA. *E. coli* in Nestlé Toll House cookie dough: Background, July 13, 2009. Online: www.fda.gov. Layton L. This woman might die from eating cookie dough. *Washington Post,* September 1, 2009. Online: www.washingtonpost.com. Flour (or chocolate bits) were considered likely sources.

50. Marler B. More bad raw milk stories, August 29, 2009. Online: www.marler blog.com.

51. USDA/FSIS. California firm recalls ground beef products due to possible *Salmonella* contamination, August 6, 2009. Online: www.fsis.usda.gov/News _&_Events. The USDA/FSIS recall page is at www.fsis.usda.gov/FSIS_RECALLS.

52. Burke G. Calif. meat plant cited for cow handling problems. *Pawtucket Times,* August 12, 2009.

53. Morrison B, Eisler P, DeBarros A. Why a recall of tainted beef didn't include school lunches. *USA Today,* December 2, 2009.

54. Gabbett RJ. USDA still considering calling E. *coli*–positive primals adulterated. Meatingplace, August 20, 2009. Online: www.meatingplace.com.

55. Pew Commission on Industrial Farm Animal Production. *Putting Meat on the Table: Industrial Farm Animal Production in America,* 2008. Online: www .ncifap.org/_images/PCIFAPFin.pdf.

56. Salvage B. A.M.I. opposes bill curbing antibiotic use, July 20, 2009. Online: www.meatpoultry.com. Johnston T. Animal antibiotics improve food safety, coalition tells White House, August 17, 2009. Online: www.meatingplace .com. American Veterinary Medical Association. *Response to the Final Report of the Pew Commission on Industrial Farm Animal Production,* August 2009. Online: www.avma.org/advocacy/PEWresponse.

57. Branigin W, Allen M, Mintz J. Tommy Thompson resigns from HHS. *Washington Post,* December 3, 2004. FDA food defense information is at www .fda.gov/Food/FoodDefense/default.htm.

58. Taylor MR. The recent *Salmonella* outbreak: Lessons learned and consequences to industry and public health. Testimony before the House Subcommittee on Oversight and Investigations, Committee on Energy and Commerce, July 31, 2008. Online: http://energycommerce.house.gov.

59. FDA Science Board. *Science and Mission at Risk: Report of the Subcommittee on Science and Technology,* November 2007; and *Food Protection Plan: An Integrated Strategy for Protecting the Nation's Food Supply,* November 2007. Online: www.fda.gov. Taylor MR. Testimony. Committee on Health, Education, Labor and Pensions, U.S. Senate, December 4, 2007. Online: http:// help.senate.gov/Hearings/2007_12_04/Taylor.pdf.

60. FDA. Egg safety final rule, July 7, 2009; and FDA issues draft guidances for tomatoes, leafy greens, and melons, July 31, 2009. Both online: www.fda.gov/ Food. Scott-Thomas C. FDA publishes details of warning letter overhaul, August 11, 2009. Online: www.foodproductiondaily.com/content/view/ print/256120. USDA. Proposed marketing agreement for leafy greens, September 3, 2009. Online: www.ams.usda.gov. Cornucopia Institute. Proposed federal rules could competitively injure small, local, and organic fresh market produce growers, September 3, 2009. Online: www.cornucopia.org.

61. Congress introduced bills to modernize the FDA in 2009. In July, the House passed H.R. 2749, the Food Safety Enhancement Act. Early in 2010, the Senate was still considering a similar bill, S. 510. Online: www.govtrack.us. National Sustainable Agriculture Coalition (and 70 other organizations). Letter to Senators Tom Harkin and Michael Enzi, Senate Committee on Health, Education, Labor, and Pensions, November 16, 2009. Online: http://sustainableagriculture.net.

APPENDIX. THE SCIENCE OF PLANT BIOTECHNOLOGY

1. I cannot resist an example. Here are the crucial steps in construction of the vector used to insert the genes for beta-carotene synthesis into rice, as given in the paper cited as note 3: "Finally, *crtI* and *psy* expression cassettes were isolated with Kpn I/Not I digestion and inserted into Kpn I/Not I-digested pUC18M and designated as pBaal3. pBin19hpc was made by insertion of a Kpn I fragment originally from pCIB90 containing aphIV selectable marker gene into pBaal3 followed by digestion of the I-Sce fragment of the resulting plasmid and insertion into I-Sce I-digested pBin19M." This description is fully intelligible to any scientist who works with plasmids; table 17 gives a rough explanation of what it means.

2. A particularly lucid account of these concepts is given in Alberts B, Bray D, Johnson A, et al, eds. *Essential Cell Biology: An Introduction to the Molecular Biology of the Cell.* New York and London: Garland Publishing, 1998.

3. Ye X, Al-Babili S, Klöti A, et al. Engineering the provitamin A (β-carotene) biosynthetic pathway into (carotenoid-free) rice endosperm. *Science* 2000;287: 303–305.

4. Beyer P, Al-Babili S, Ye S, et al. Golden Rice: introducing the β-carotene biosynthesis pathway into rice endosperm by genetic engineering to defeat vitamin A deficiency. *J Nutrition* 2002;132:506s–510s.

5. Chawla HS. *Introduction to Plant Biotechnology.* Enfield, NH: Science Publishers, 2000.

LIST OF TABLES

LIST OF FIGURES

INDEX

Note: Page numbers in *italics* refer to figures; page numbers in **boldface** refer to tables.

CALIFORNIA STUDIES IN FOOD AND CULTURE

Darra Goldstein, Editor

Compositor: BookMatters, Berkeley
Indexer: Andrew Joron
Text: Sabon
Display: Futura
Printer and binder: Maple-Vail Book Manufacturing Group